Disentangling Dyslexia

Linguistic Insights

Studies in Language and Communication

Edited by Maurizio Gotti,
University of Bergamo

Volume 212

PETER LANG
Bern · Bruxelles · Frankfurt am Main · New York · Oxford · Warszawa · Wien

Maria Vender

Disentangling Dyslexia

Phonological and Processing Deficit in Developmental Dyslexia

PETER LANG
Bern · Bruxelles · Frankfurt am Main · New York · Oxford · Warszawa · Wien

Bibliographic information published by die Deutsche Nationalbibliothek
Die Deutsche Nationalbibliothek lists this publication in the Deutsche Nationalbibliografie; detailed bibliographic data is available on the Internet at ‹http://dnb.d-nb.de›.

British Library Cataloguing-in-Publication Data: A catalogue record for this book is available from The British Library, Great Britain.

Library of Congress Control Number: 2017947148

Published with a grant of the Department of Cultures and Civilizations, University of Verona.

ISSN 1424-8689 pb.
ISSN 2235-6371 eBook
ISBN 978-3-0343-2064-1 pb.
ISBN 978-3-0343-2963-7 eBook
ISBN 978-3-0343-2965-1 MOBI
ISBN 978-3-0343-2964-4 EPUB

This publication has been peer reviewed.

Wabernstrasse 40, CH-3007 Bern, Switzerland
info@peterlang.com, www.peterlang.com

Contents

Acknowledgments

This book is an extended version of my PhD Dissertation at the University of Verona, which was submitted and defended in the spring of 2011. Although the general structure of the dissertation is preserved, several modifications have been added, thanks to the many constructive comments and suggestions that I have received in these years.

I am very grateful to Denis Delfitto, my thesis advisor, who always supported my work, encouraging me to follow my intuitions, and who suggested me to transform my dissertation in this book: significant parts of it are based on joint work with him.

Writing this book has proven to be a big challenge and a valuable experience, to which I devoted most of my time, energies and passion. As every small and great challenge, this work would not have been possible without the precious help of many people. I am very obliged to Chiara Melloni, who supported me in the idea to publish this book, offering constant help and mindful suggestions. A special thank you also to my colleagues, Federica Mantione and Maria Scappini, and to all the people who have assisted me in this adventure and during the PhD, discussing and supporting my projects and ideas with interesting comments and suggestions: Birgit Alber, Adriana Belletti, Pier Marco Bertinetto, Camilla Bettoni, Sibilla Cantarini, Roberto Cubelli, Elise de Bree, Maria Teresa Guasti, Gaetano Fiorin, Francesca Forza, Giorgio Graffi, Shenai Hu, Karin Martin, Elena Menegazzo, Jacques Moeschler, Paola Paradisi, Stefan Rabanus Anne Reboul, Danilo Reggiani, Christian Retoré, Silvia Savazzi, Alessandra Tomaselli, Jacopo Torregrossa, Francesco Vespignani, Mirta Vernice, Frank Wijnen.

I am very indebted to all the people and institutions that helped in the organization of the experiments presented in this work: first of all, I wish to thank all the children who participated in the experimental sessions with great enthusiasm and all their families. I am also grateful to the directors and the speech-therapists of the "Centro Audiofonetico" in Trento, of the "Dipartimento di Neuropsichiatria Infantile" ULLS 20 in Verona, and of the "U.O. di Neuropsichiatria Infantile" in Rovereto (Trento), who helped in the recruitment of the dyslexic children. Thanks to all the directors and the teachers of the schools who collaborated with us and helped in the recruitment of the children: "Istituto Comprensivo di Fondo" in Romeno (Trento), "Istituto Comprensivo di Revò" in Revò and Banco (Trento), "Istituto Comprensivo di Cles" in Livo (Trento), "Scuola Elementare Aleardi" in Quinto di Valpantena (Verona), "Scuola Materna Paolo Crosara" in S. Bonifacio (Verona) and "Scuola Equiparata dell'Infanzia" in Cles (Trento).

Thanks to Gaetano Fiorin, Karin Martin, Luisa Piccoli and Danilo Reggiani, who helped administering the experiments.

A final and special thanks goes to my whole family and to my friends, to my husband Nicola, who has always supported me, and to my children, Gabriele, Angelica and Aurora, my real source of inspiration.

Preface

In this book, I will review some of the most peculiar aspects concerning developmental dyslexia, focusing on its distribution and, especially, on its manifestations and possible causes.

Observing that dyslexic individuals appear to manifest severe deficits in those cognitive tasks which require a fine phonological analysis and which are particularly demanding in terms of processing resources, I will propose an original hypothesis to account for the cognitive impairment underlying this disorder, the Phonological and Executive Working Memory Deficit Hypothesis, reported below.

> The Phonological and Executive Working Memory Deficit Hypothesis
>
> Dyslexic individuals suffer from a limitation affecting their Working Memory and hampering in particular their phonological memory and their executive functions. As a consequence, this impairment disrupts their phonological competence, as well as their performance in complex tasks that are particularly demanding in terms of Working Memory resources. On the contrary, dyslexics can rely on a spared visuo-spatial memory, to which they can resort for the accomplishment of compensatory strategies.

As I will discuss in this book, Working Memory is the brain system engaged in the temporary storage and manipulation of the information that is necessary for cognitive tasks such as reasoning, learning, problem solving, language comprehension. Specifically, I will adopt as a starting point for my analysis Baddeley and Hitch's (1974) influential Working Memory Model, according to which Working Memory is constituted by two short-term stores, the Phonological Loop and the Visuo-Spatial Sketchpad, and a limited capacity attentional controller supervising all the activities, the Central Executive. The two short-term stores, which are independent from each other, are concerned respectively with the temporary storage of phonological information and of visuo-spatial information. The Central Executive, instead, is involved in executive functions, that is in the control of attention, detecting the relevant stimuli and filtering out those that are irrelevant, in the supervision of the activities carried out by the two slave-subsystems and in the manipulation and execution of the operations. In a subsequent version of the model, these functions are partially accomplished by a fourth component, the Episodic Buffer, which is a subsystem supporting a multimodal code and concerned with the manipulation and integration of the information provided by the two short-term stores.

Adopting this framework, I will review recent experimental results demonstrating that Working Memory, and in particular the Central Executive, plays a fundamental role in human cognition. Individual differences in cognitive tasks are determined by the general capacity of the individual's Working Memory: people whose Working Memory is limited or less efficient are more likely to show lower speed and accuracy in the execution of complex tasks that are demanding in terms of processing resources.

In the Phonological and Executive Working Memory Deficit Hypothesis, I propose that developmental dyslexia is characterized by the presence of two main impairments affecting dyslexics' Working Memory. On the one side, in fact, dyslexic individuals suffer from a phonological memory deficit, preventing them from correctly analyzing the internal structure of words and nonwords. On the other side, instead, they show an impairment affecting their executive functions and hampering their performance in complex and demanding tasks. The severity of these impairments determines the severity of the disorder itself.

A clear consequence of this hypothesis is that dyslexic individuals are expected to exhibit difficulties whenever they are asked to perform complex operations or to execute more than one task simultaneously. Nevertheless, some compensation is allowed by the general plasticity of the system: an individual with a high IQ score, for instance, can learn to use alternative strategies to perform a task in order to circumvent her difficulties.

Throughout this discussion, I will show that the Phonological and Executive Working Memory Deficit Hypothesis is able to account for all the core manifestations of developmental dyslexia, explaining not only the well-known reading and spelling difficulties that characterize the disorder, but also the frequently reported phonological deficits, vocabulary and naming disorders, grammatical impairments and attention problems.

The book is organized as follows. In Chapter 1, I will present a detailed introduction to developmental dyslexia, discussing the manifestations of the disorder, and focusing on recent studies developed to identify the precursors of dyslexia.

Chapter 2, instead, will be dedicated to the illustration of the main theories proposed to explain the causes of dyslexia, ranging from the Visual and Auditory Deficit Hypotheses and moving to the more recent approaches, such as the Magnocellular Deficit Hypothesis, the Phonological Deficit Hypothesis, the Double Deficit Hypothesis and the Working Memory Deficit Hypothesis. Discussing both strengths and weaknesses of each proposal, I will argue that none of them is able to capture all the difficulties associated with dyslexia, except for the Working Memory Deficit Hypothesis. However, I will suggest that this proposal should be reformulated more precisely and that it is actually in need of some further experimental corroboration, by means of experimental protocols designed to accurately test dyslexic children's and age-matched typically developing children's Working Memory.

The results of this experimental protocol will be presented in Chapter 3. As I will observe, findings provide uncontroversial evidence in favor of an impairment affecting dyslexics' Phonological Loop and Central Executive, but leaving their Visuo-Spatial Sketchpad spared and normally functioning.

Considering these results as a starting point, I will propose my hypothesis, the Phonological and Executive Working Memory Deficit Hypothesis outlined above, in Chapter 4. Specifically, I will argue that dyslexics' poorly functioning phonological memory and executive functions hamper their performance in tasks requiring a good phonological competence and demanding a high amount of cognitive resources. I will note, therefore, that dyslexics' deficits are more likely to arise in complex tasks.

In order to further test the Phonological and Executive Working Memory Deficit Hypothesis I decided to assess dyslexic children's performance in linguistically complex tasks, developing three experimental protocols whose results will be presented in the subsequent chapters.

In Chapter 5, I will discuss the result of a first protocol testing dyslexic children's ability to compute scalar implicatures, an operation remarkably expensive in terms of processing resources, comparing their performance to that shown by age-matched typically developing children, a group of younger children and a group composed by adults.

In Chapter 6, I will present a second experiment testing the interpretation of negation in dyslexic children and age-matched typically developing children, considering their ability to comprehend negative active and passive sentences.

Finally, in Chapter 7, I will expose the results of a last protocol assessing dyslexic children's competence in the interpretation of pronouns, comparing their performance to that shown by age-matched control children, control adults and two groups of younger children.

As I will argue throughout the discussion, all three experiments provided results that are consistent with the Phonological and Executive Working Memory Deficit Hypothesis, demonstrating that dyslexics are indeed remarkably more impaired than their peers in the comprehension of complex sentences. Moreover, their performance is strikingly similar to that shown by children who are 2 or 4 years younger.

Finally, Chapter 8 will be dedicated to the concluding remarks: I will summarize the considerations put forward throughout the book and I will propose a new definition of developmental dyslexia, which focuses on the phonological and executive Working Memory impairment exhibited by dyslexic individuals. I will also briefly introduce and discuss the Cerebellar Deficit Hypothesis developed by Nicolson and colleagues (1995, 2001, 2008) to explain dyslexia.

I will argue that the Cerebellar Deficit Hypothesis and the Phonological and Executive Working Memory Deficit Hypothesis present both commonalities and differences and that further research is needed to analyze more thoroughly the distinct predictions made by the two proposals.

Chapter 1

An Introduction To Developmental Dyslexia

1. Introduction

Developmental Dyslexia is a learning based disability that interferes in particular with the acquisition of language. This disorder, which has a clear neurologic and genetic origin, affects around 5–15% of the population and it is highly inheritable. It is namely widely acknowledged that dyslexia runs in families: it is estimated that a child with a dyslexic parent or sibling has 50% probability of being dyslexic (Gayan and Olson 1999).

A difference between the sexes has also been found, with a sex ratio of approximately three or four males to one female (Wolff and Melngailis 1994). This discrepancy appears to increase in parallel to the severity of the disorder and to the IQ of the subject: as the reading deficit becomes more severe, the IQ tends to be lower and the male ratio tends to be higher (Olson 2002). However, the imbalance between the sexes may sometimes be overestimated, due to the tendency reported by teachers to identify boys as being more problematic than girls in class.

One of the most easily detectable symptoms of dyslexia, to which this disorder actually owes its name, is the failure to acquire properly reading and spelling skills. This impairment appears to be particularly surprising in those children, as dyslexics, who are otherwise intelligent and adequately exposed to literacy. Specifically, as we will observe throughout this book, dyslexics perform very poorly when asked to read irregular words or non-words. Obviously, these difficulties are even more evident in languages with an 'opaque' orthography, as English, where there is more than one possible mapping between a letter and its sound (consider the pronunciation of the phoneme /əʊ/ in the words "so", "road", "bowl", "though"). In these languages phoneme-grapheme correspondence rules are less reliable than in transparent languages, such as Italian, where mappings between phonemes and graphemes are more regular and children have more chances to read properly both regular and irregular words.

This cross-linguistic discrepancy can be held responsible for the different percentages concerning the distribution of dyslexia that can be found across countries: in Italy, in fact, it is argued that dyslexia affects 3–4% of the population[1], whereas the percentage raises to reach 15–20% in the USA[2]. Of course, this discrepancy does not imply that dyslexia is more widespread in one country than in another one; it simply reflects the fact that it is easier to detect reading difficulties in children whose mother-tongue has an opaque orthography. On the contrary, the difficulties experienced by those children whose mother-tongue has a transparent orthography may go unnoticed.

However, although it appears that reading difficulties are the most significant and important problem exhibited by dyslexics, we will observe throughout the discussion that reading failure is just one of the symptoms of dyslexia, which is definitely a more complex and multifaceted disorder. Other frequently reported manifestations of dyslexia are impairments in those speech processes which require both accuracy of phonological processing and speed, such as picture naming tasks (Swan and Goswami 1997a), tasks tapping phonological awareness (Swan and Goswami 1997b), testing the repetition of words and nonwords (Miles, 1993) and verbal working memory performance (Nelson and Warrington 1980, Gathercole et al. 2006).

We will also notice that dyslexic children exhibit a poor performance in comparison to their peers in linguistic tasks assessing for instance the comprehension of complex structures and the sensitivity to morphological errors.

Furthermore, I will review some of the most influential studies conducted on very young children at familial risk of dyslexia, i.e. children who have at least one parent or sibling suffering from dyslexia and who are therefore genetically more likely to manifest dyslexia as well. A number of interesting experiments designed to assess the linguistic competence in these children have revealed that at-risk children, who had been indeed diagnosed as dyslexics some years later, were actually more impaired than their peers in tasks tapping phonological

1 www.aiditalia.org

2 www.dyslexia-usa.com

awareness, syntactic competence, sensitivity to grammatical violations and rapid naming. Importantly, these findings suggest that it is possible to recognize some precursors of dyslexia that will permit to identify the disorder during the late preschool period and therefore prior to literacy instruction, contrary to what is generally believed.

For what concerns the etiology of dyslexia, instead, different theories have been developed to explain the disorder throughout the last two centuries; in the second chapter of this book I will discuss the most well-known and influential ones, as the Visual Theory, the Auditory Theory, the Magnocellular Theory, the Phonological-Deficit Hypothesis and the Double-Deficit Hypothesis.

Taking into consideration both strengths and weaknesses of each proposal, I will argue that none of them is able to capture adequately and completely the intricate range of impairments shown by dyslexics and that all symptoms manifested by impaired children seem to be due to a working memory inefficiency.

The experiments that I performed on dyslexic and normally achieving subjects and that I will present in the following chapters aimed precisely to provide insights into the question whether dyslexia is associated with a verbal working memory deficit. As we will observe, the results of my experimental protocols point precisely in this direction.

In the remaining part of this chapter, I would like to briefly introduce the topic: I will first discuss the difficulty to find a comprehensive definition of developmental dyslexia; then I will illustrate the major manifestation of the disorder, devoting a special attention to the linguistic competence of dyslexic children. Finally, I will present the studies conducted on children at familial risk of dyslexia, which show that it is possible to identify some precursors of reading failure in very young boys and girls.

2. On the difficulty to find a comprehensive definition of Developmental Dyslexia

One of the major concerns of researchers studying developmental dyslexia is the need to find a generally valid, accepted and all-embracing definition. Despite decades of in-depth studies, there is, in fact, no universally agreed definition of dyslexia, presumably because the population of poor-readers in not homogeneous.

Consider the following attempts, elaborated through the years, to define dyslexia:

> Developmental dyslexia is a disorder in children who, despite conventional classroom experience, fail to attain the language skills of reading, writing and spelling commensurate with their intellectual abilities (World Federation of Neurology, 1968).

> Developmental dyslexia is a specific impairment affecting the acquisition of reading and spelling skills, despite adequate intelligence, opportunity and social background, which occurs in absence of physical, neurological, emotional and socio-economical problems (Vellutino 1979).

> Developmental dyslexia, or specific reading disability, is defined as an unexpected, specific and persistent failure to acquire efficient reading skills, despite conventional instruction, adequate intelligence and socio-cultural opportunity (American Psychiatric Association, 1994).

> Dyslexia is evident when accurate and fluent word reading and/or spelling develops very incompletely or with great difficulty, despite appropriate learning opportunities – that is, learning opportunities which are effective for the great majority of children. (British Psychological Society, 1999).

Evidently, these much-quoted definitions of developmental dyslexia are far from being sufficiently specific to capture the broad range of deficits experienced by dyslexic people. At least two problems can be recognized in these definition: first, they seem to regard reading (and spelling) failure as the only characterizing feature of dyslexia, and secondly they are designed by exclusion, that is, excluding from the dyslexic sample those individuals who display additional problems or conditions.

As we will observe throughout this chapter, in fact, reading disabilities can be considered neither the necessary nor the sufficient symptoms of dyslexia. On the one side, in fact, there can be individuals who fail to be diagnosed as dyslexic although they display poor reading, whereas, on the other side, it is not rare to meet people who should be diagnosed as dyslexic because they manifest the wide range of impairments typical of dyslexia, but who aren't considered dyslexics since their reading and spelling abilities are relatively spared. This is the case, for instance, of children whose mother-tongue has a transparent orthography and whose reading difficulties may thus go unnoticed.

As mentioned above, moreover, these definitions attempt to identify dyslexia by exclusion, that is excluding from the population of dyslexics all those individuals whose reading problems can be caused independently by physical or neurological problems, or by a subnormal intelligence, or again by a lack of socio-cultural opportunities and conventional instruction.

The exclusionary criterion adopted in these definitions has been object of debate. On the one hand, it is justified since it has the purpose to identify a more valid and pure research sample: reading difficulties, in fact, can also result from poor instruction or physical impairments other than dyslexia, and therefore a diagnosis of dyslexia would be more reliable, if reading disabilities occur in the absence of other negative factors. On the other hand, however, the use of this criterion can be tricky: since, as nowadays generally accepted, dyslexia is a genetically inherited disorder, it is in fact evident that it can occur at any level of intelligence, exposure to instruction and socio-economical conditions. As a consequence, it would not be correct to exclude from the dyslexic sample individuals who manifest the same difficulties as dyslexics but have a lower intelligence or, above all, have received a worse instruction or live in poor socio-economical conditions. This consideration led some researchers to admit that dyslexia is simply *easier* to be diagnosed in those subjects who are "intellectually, socially and educationally advantaged than in those who are not" (Seymour 1986).

These unresolved controversies provide us with some initial evidence that research on dyslexia is still undergoing a phase of rapid growth, especially since the exact locus of the impairment causing the difficulties that characterize this disorder has not been identified yet.

As I will discuss in the second chapter, different theories have been developed to explain the etiology and the manifestations of dyslexia, even though none of these is generally accepted. However, it is necessary to emphasize that important and interesting steps have been made: it has been demonstrated that dyslexia is genetically inheritable, that it has a neurological basis and that the phonological competence is compromised in the totality of the population affected by dyslexia.

Bearing all these aspects in mind, I will propose an alternative definition of dyslexia, which will be outlined and discussed in Chapter 8.

In this work, I will report the results of studies showing that dyslexia is mainly a language-learning disability, which interferes with linguistic competence at different levels. Moreover, I will present these considerations in a wider perspective, arguing that dyslexia is definitely related to an impairment of the verbal and processing component of working memory.

Before presenting this hypothesis, I will introduce and discuss the major manifestations of developmental dyslexia.

3. Manifestations of Developmental Dyslexia

Developmental Dyslexia is a complex and multifaceted disorder. Although they are the most evident and well-known symptoms of dyslexia, reading and spelling difficulties constitute only the tip of the iceberg of the more widespread impairments exhibited by dyslexic individuals. It has been ascertained, in fact, that their phonological and, more generally, linguistic competence is remarkably poor, and that they show marked deficits in vocabulary and naming tasks. Moreover, dyslexic subjects appear to be impaired in those tasks that require the automation of a skill and they frequently present motor and attention deficits.

In the following paragraphs, I will discuss thoroughly these impairments.

3.1. Reading difficulties

As argued in the previous section, the poor development of reading skills is one of the most studied impairments shown by dyslexic individuals. Specifically, dyslexics' difficulties seem to be due to a basic impairment in learning to decode print, causing problems in word identification (Vellutino et al. 2004). As evidenced by a great number of studies, dyslexic children exhibit a very slow, inaccurate and effortful reading. Reading errors typically concern a poor capacity to discriminate: (i) similar graphemes which are differently oriented (e.g. "b" and "d"), (ii) similar graphemes which differ only for small details (e.g. "m" and "n") and (iii) graphemes that correspond to similar phonemes (e.g. "b" and "p"; "v" and "f").

Moreover, dyslexics tend to substitute similar-looking, even if unrelated, words in place of the right ones (e.g. "play" for "pay", "what" for "that", but also "republic" for "publicity"). Remarkable difficulties, moreover, arise when they are asked to read nonwords, whereas their reading is more accurate with frequent words.

As mentioned above, reading errors are more frequent in those languages that have an opaque orthographic system, like English. A number of studies (Wimmer 1993, Wimmer and Goswami 1994, Seymour et al. 2003) have in fact tested word and nonword reading in dyslexic children across different languages: significantly, results demonstrated that the accuracy rate was only 40% for English children at the end of Grade 1, whereas it was close to ceiling for children speaking languages with a more consistent orthography, such as German, Spanish and Italian.

Moreover, it has been found that the most sensitive variable when comparing reading performance across languages is not reading accuracy, but rather reading speed, especially in those languages with a transparent orthography (see Wimmer and Schurz 2010 for a detailed review).

In a study by Ziegler and colleagues (2003), both German and English speaking dyslexics have exhibited a marked speed deficit in comparison not only to chronological age-matched children but also to reading age-matched children, suggesting that dyslexia is characterized by a fundamental deficit that cannot be simply ascribed to a general developmental delay. Not surprisingly, moreover, dyslexics have manifested a striking word-length effect, indicating that difficulties increase proportionally to the stimulus length. Analyzing the stimulus length in both words and nonwords, the authors were able to estimate the processing costs required by each additional letter, showing that it increases dramatically in a linear fashion. The processing times needed to read long words, in fact, were up to 11 times greater for German dyslexics and up to 7 times for English dyslexics than for age-matched controls. Ziegler and colleagues conclude arguing that reading is extremely serial and letter-by-letter based in dyslexics, whereas it is much more parallel for control children.

Summarizing, the main deficit exhibited by dyslexic children across countries appears to be poor reading fluency, characterized by a slow and effortful decoding process. Moreover, dyslexics generally manifest great difficulties when asked to read nonwords and unfamiliar words, their problems increasing proportionally to the stimulus length. Finally, poor readers' errors seem to reveal that they do not obey the orthographic-phonologic conversion rules and that they tend to replace similar-looking but unrelated words instead of the meant one.

To better understand the difficulties manifested by dyslexic individuals, it can be useful to analyze the cognitive mechanisms underlying reading. In the next paragraph, I will present one of the most well-known theoretical approaches to reading, the Dual-Route Model, and the influential model of learning to read developed by Frith (1989).

3.1.1. A theoretical approach to reading: the Dual-Route Model

To be a competent reader, one must be able to extract and construct meaning starting from printed words; therefore, in order to understand what she reads, she should be able to identify the words arranged in the text with the accuracy and fluency necessary to allow the computation of the text's meaning.

During the last century, a number of hypotheses and models have been elaborated with the aim to represent how the brain processes reading. Currently, one of the most well-known approaches to reading is the Dual-Route Model (Coltheart, 1985, Humphreys and Evett 1985), subsequently implemented in Coltheart's Dual-Route Cascade (DRC) Model (Coltheart et. al. 2001).

According to this model, there are essentially two distinct mechanisms underlying the decoding and pronunciation of letter strings[3]: a *lexical route* and a *sublexical route*. Despite the label *dual-route model*, a third route has been subsequently added, referred to as the *lexical nonsemantic route*.

3 I prefer to employ the expression "letter strings" instead of "words", since the latter entails the notion of access to meaning. The model, in fact, is mainly concerned with the ability to decode sequences of letters, such as non-words, independently from their meaning.

The model is represented in Figure 1.1.

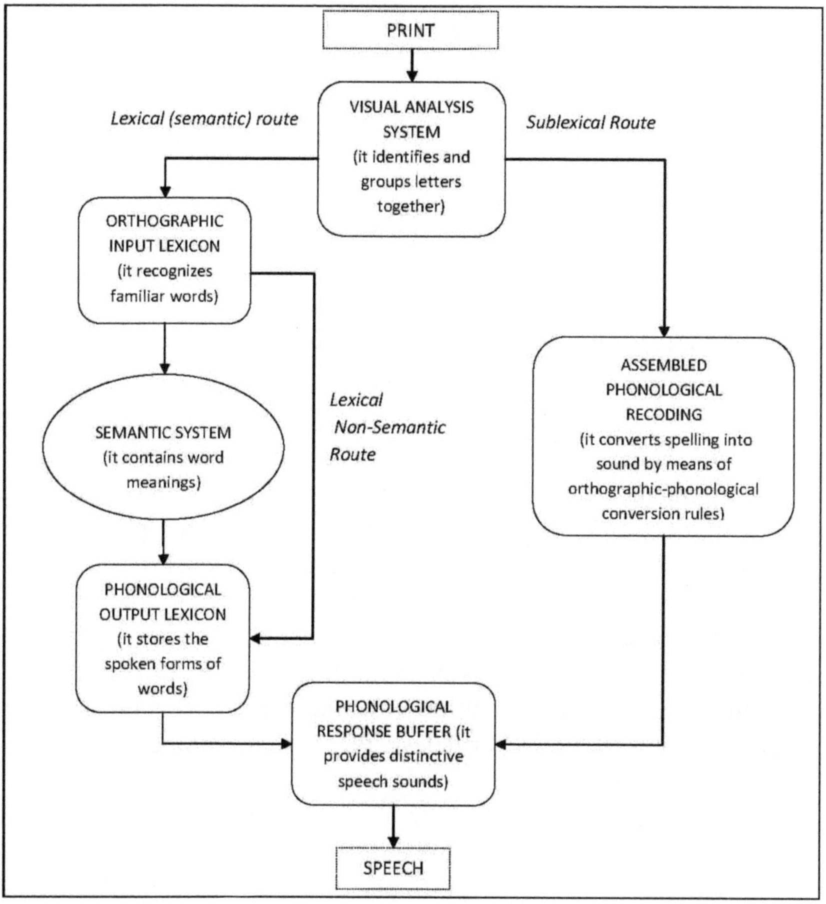

Figure 1.1. The Dual-Route Model.

According to dual-route theorists, letter strings are first analyzed by the visual analysis system, which identifies and groups letters together. Afterwards, words can be read through a lexical or a sublexical route; generally, familiar words whose phonological form has already been stored in the lexicon are read thorough the lexical route, whereas unfamiliar strings are read by the sublexical route.

The lexical route treats each string as a whole, i.e. as an indivisible unit. Words are recognized by accessing an entry in the orthographic input lexicon, a sort of memory storage for all known words. The orthographic input lexicon, then, feeds into the semantic system, which contains word meanings and which in turn activates the phonological form of the word stored in the phonological output lexicon. Since the string is perceived as a whole, each letter being processed at the same time, it is possible to say that this kind of mechanism processes words in parallel rather than sequentially. The lexical route is generally used to read already familiar words and it is indispensable to decode idiosyncratic exception words, such as *enough* or *caveat*, that cannot be pronounced properly relying simply on the orthographic-phonological conversion rules.

Differently from the lexical route, the sublexical process breaks down the string in its minimal components, resorting to a set of conversion rules to retrieve the pronunciation of each unit. Basically, the string gets first decomposed in smaller units (i.e. single graphemes, subsyllabic components or syllables); then, every unit is pronounced according to a set of context-dependent rules, dubbed orthographic-phonological conversion rules[4]. Evidently, this mechanism processes strings serially, considering each letter at a time, and it operates in a left-to-right sequential manner. The sublexical route is assumed to be required for the pronunciation of nonwords or pseudowords, which are clearly not stored in the orthographic input lexicon and do not have a lexical entry in the semantic system. Nevertheless, this process can be used as well to read regular words.

The existence of a third route, the lexical nonsemantic route, has been added to account for the results of behavioral studies conducted on patients suffering from dementia. In particular, the patient W.L.P. could read correctly 95% of the words, comprising both high and low frequency words as well as regular and irregular words, although she could not understand the meaning of those words (Schwartz, Saffran and Marin 1980). This and other similar cases point to the existence of a third nonsemantic lexical route that connects directly the orthographic input lexicon to the phonological output lexicon, bypassing the semantic system.

4 I use the expression "orthographic-phonological conversion rules" instead of "grapheme-phoneme conversion rules", since it is not always the case that single graphemes are translated into sound units.

Even though there are general tendencies, the choice of which route to use is not necessarily determined by the nature of the stimulus to be read, but it may be, to some extent, under the control of the reader. If irregular and exception words must necessarily be read by the lexical route and nonwords by the sublexical route, in fact, regular words can be read equally well using one route or the other.

Evidence for this analysis is provided by neuropsychological studies showing that the routes may be selectively impaired. Cases of double dissociations have namely been reported: there can be patients who can read properly both regular words and nonwords but are not able to read exception and irregular words, suggesting that they suffer from an impairment to the lexical route that leads them to resort consistently to the sublexical route.

Conversely, other patients can exhibit problems when asked to read nonwords, but are able to pronounce properly familiar regular and irregular words, indicating that they can rely only on the lexical route.

The range of reading problems exhibited by dyslexics and reviewed above seems to suggest that both routes are impaired, at least to some extent, in dyslexic children. The tendency to read better familiar and short words may indicate that they resort mainly to the lexical route, perhaps relying on some visual features, as the initial letters of the stimuli, to identify the word. This procedure, of course, is not completely reliable and it constitutes a source of errors, as reflected by the frequent tendency to confuse similar-looking words shown by dyslexics. In other words, dyslexics exhibit a particularly poor performance when asked to read nonword stimuli, but they can read highly familiar words definitely better (Bruck and Treiman 1990, De Gelder and Vrooman 1991). This discrepancy seems to indicate that dyslexics suffer from an impairment affecting the sublexical route of reading: as we have observed above, in fact, the Dual-Route model predicts that nonwords cannot be read through the lexical route, since they do not have a phonological representation stored in the orthographic input lexicon. Nonwords, in fact, can be read only through the sublexical route, by applying the orthographic-phonological conversion rules. Dyslexics' inability to read nonwords seems thus to suggest that some aspects of their sublexical route are damaged, preventing them from relying on conversion rules.

However, dyslexics cannot always resort to the lexical route: the evidence for a slow, serial and effortful reading procedure reported by Ziegler and colleagues suggests that in some cases they are forced to use the sublexical route, which is not working properly. This is arguably due to the fact that the knowledge of conversion rules is not completely acquired or automatized, or to the fact that the processing resources needed to complete the decoding and pronunciation of the word surpasses the child's abilities.

The intuition that dyslexics' difficulties are linked to processing deficits is also supported by the finding that longer words, which require higher processing resources, are read much slower and worse by dyslexics than by normally developing children. A strong length effect has been reported by another recent study conducted by Araùjo et al. (2014) who found that Portuguese-speaking dyslexics' performance is significantly slower than controls' in reading long stimuli. According to the authors, both the lexical and the sublexical routes are disrupted in dyslexia; moreover, they propose that dyslexics seem to be less flexible than controls in switching from one route to the other according to the demand of the stimuli.

To summarize, results seem to indicate that dyslexics' sublexical route is impaired and, specifically, that they are not able to apply quickly and automatically the orthographic-phonological conversion rules as the other children do. As a consequence, their reading is slow and effortful and they commit phonological errors. Alternatively, they can resort more frequently to the lexical route to read words that they recognize as familiar: however, as we have seen, simply relying on gross visual cues is often a source of confusion and mistakes.

3.1.2. The development of reading: Frith's model of learning to read

The acquisition of reading depends upon a number of distinct skills and may take several years to be completely mastered. Before a child starts to read, she generally already has some of the necessary skills in place and some basic concepts about print that she can exploit in learning to read. For instance, she may already know that words have a written version – perhaps she is able to write her name or some familiar and simple words – and she can also move her eyes to fixate the words printed on the page.

Starting from these considerations, Frith (1986) proposed one of the most influential models to account for the acquisition of reading proficiency, according to which the development of reading has to go through three main stages: the logographic stage, the alphabetic stage and the orthographic stage.

In the logographic stage the child learns to read words as a whole, treating them as single units. As a consequence, in this first phase words are perceived as logos, or icons, and they are recognized on the basis of some salient visual features. A typical example of a salient feature is the first letter of the word, even though other letters can act as salient visual cues as well. Significantly, a word can be recognized irrespective of the precise order of the letters composing it: a typical example is reported by Coltheart (1986), who argues that in this stage a child may recognize the logo "Harrods" both when the word is properly written and when its letters are scrambled as in "Hrorads".

In the alphabetic stage the child learns to decode a word into single graphemes, acquiring and applying the regular correspondences between graphemes and phonemes. Consequently, she learns the mechanisms required to blend sounds to evoke the target word through the orthographic-phonological conversion rules. Therefore, mastering this level, the child is able to establish direct mappings between letters and sounds. Crucially, this ability rests upon her underlying level of phonological skills.

In the orthographic stage the child learns to break down the word into syllables or morphemes, rather than decoding it letter by letter. In this stage, the child is able to analyze words into orthographic units without the need to resort to a letter-by-letter phonological conversion. Moreover, the orthographic strategy enables instant word recognition, as the logographic strategy, even though not merely relying on salient visual cues but rather on morphemes.

Note that according to Frith's model the development of reading is not simply the result of a gradual and constant enhancement of the child's skills, since qualitative changes occur while moving from one stage to the other.

According to Frith, the reading difficulties shown by dyslexic children are caused by the failure to successfully master the conversion rules that are normally acquired in the alphabetic stage. Therefore, she argues that the mastering of the alphabetic stage is critically impaired in dyslexic children, proposing that they are not able to attend the "subtle phonological analysis" indispensable for this process. This impairment gives rise to problems in applying conversion rules, thus causing the poor reading of non-words often detected in dyslexia. Consequently, impairments at the alphabetic stage affect spelling abilities as well, resulting in difficulties to properly represent sounds and to reproduce the correct sequence of letters making up words.

It is possible to draw some interesting parallelisms between Frith's model of the development of reading and the Dual-Route proposal for the cognitive mechanisms underlying reading discussed above. Even though the two models have been elaborated in different periods and for different purposes, some correspondences between them can be found. Specifically, the competence acquired in Frith's alphabetic stage rests on the same assumption underlying the mechanism of the sublexical route in the Dual-Route Model. In both models, in fact, it is necessary to acquire a set of orthographic-phonological conversion rules in order to read irregular words or nonwords. Crucially, both hypotheses postulate that this ability is impaired in dyslexic individuals, accounting for the difficulties that they typically exhibit. Frith, in particular, argues that the alphabetic strategy is a necessary precondition for attaining reading skills and she suggests that its complete mastery is not attained by dyslexic children, who may never reach a sufficient competence to move on to the orthographic strategy. Dyslexics, in fact, do not develop the ability to make quick and automatic links between the letters and their sounds.

However, it is important to bear in mind that dyslexic individuals may well reach, throughout the years, a satisfactory level of reading and spelling skills that grants them the possibility to cope with ordinary life. Actually, in both models a compensatory strategy is allowed: even though their sublexical route is impaired, dyslexics can read familiar words relying on the lexical route in the Dual-Route Model. Similar predictions are made by Frith, who argues that compensatory strategies are allowed and expected: an earlier, mastered stage could namely be capable of a further development. Specifically, if a dyslexic is unable to master the alphabetic stage, compensation may "take the form of over-development of the earlier strategy", that is the logographic stage.

Another important parallelism that can be found between the two models concerns the involvement of phonological skills, which are considered essential requisites for the successful acquisition of reading and spelling competence. In both theories, phonological skills are crucial for the acquisition of conversion rules and the ability to read unfamiliar words or nonwords. In particular, Frith argues that the unsuccessful attempt to master the alphabetic stage noticed in dyslexics is due to the inability to carry out the necessary phonological analysis, which is also responsible for the non-word reading deficit.

According to Frith, there is indeed strong evidence suggesting that the problems manifested in the acquisition of reading skills are related to the ability to segment words in speech sounds and therefore to the domain of phonology.

> The main task that a child has to master, when learning to read in an alphabetic system, is to understand how to represent speech sound by letters and how to translate precisely between written and spoken language. Syntax, semantics and pragmatics, the other – hugely important – components of language processing, do not come into this task. Only phonology does.
> (Frith 1999: 202)

The centrality of phonological abilities as a founding deficit of dyslexia has been postulated by a huge number of researchers and it has become the main issue of one of the most accredited theories of dyslexia, the phonological deficit hypothesis, which will be presented and discussed in the following chapter.

To summarize so far, dyslexic children manifest great difficulties in the acquisition of reading skills, which appear to depend on a phonological impairment preventing them to learn and apply the phonologic-orthographic conversion rules.

3.2. Spelling difficulties

The inability to acquire properly spelling skills is the other major symptom generally associated with developmental dyslexia. In comparison to reading, spelling is further complicated by the fact that there is often more than one possibility to write a word in a phonologically acceptable way, especially in languages characterized by phoneme-grapheme inconsistencies, as English (e.g. “main” and “mane”).

As evidenced by Caravolas and colleagues (2001), spelling is affected by a variety of skills, as the familiarity with grapheme-phoneme correspondences, the ability to recognize the letters of the alphabet and the knowledge about orthography derived through reading. Moreover, they argue that proficient spelling demands, beyond phonological skills, also attention, motor skills (in case of written spelling) and visual memory. Given that dyslexics exhibit poor phonological decoding and poor phonological awareness, poor spelling is also expected, indicating that spelling is inextricably linked to reading development, as underlined by Ehri (1991, 1997).

Bourassa and Treiman (2003) tested both oral and written spelling performance of 30 dyslexic children (mean age 11 years and 1 month) and 30 spelling level matched younger children (mean age 7 years and 5 months). They found that dyslexic children performed at the same level of younger children, producing the same kind of spelling errors. The misspellings produced by both groups of children were generally reasonable and linguistically motivated. Similar findings have been reported by Friend and Olson (2008) who tested 77 pairs of children, each including one older child with spelling disability and one spelling-level-matched younger child with normal spelling ability. As Bourassa and Treiman, they found that impaired children’s error were very similar to that of younger controls. Typical misspellings included the omission of the second consonant in a complex cluster (“trip” spelled as “tip”), the omission of double consonants (e.g. “dinner” as “diner”), the confusion of graphemes corresponding to similar phonemes (e.g. “tomato” spelled as “tomado”) and irregular spellings (e.g. “packed” as “packt”). Significantly, although dyslexic children were on average more than 3 years older than control children, they produced the same kind of errors, making it impossible to distinguish between the two groups. Interestingly, then, Bourassa and Treiman found that both groups of children tended to represent words better than nonwords, suggesting that they were making use of orthographic strategies to retrieve the visual shape of the intended word. Obviously, in fact, it is not possible to resort to visual aspects to recover the spelling of an invented stimulus, whence the greatest difficulty found with nonwords.

Finally, Plisson et al. (2013) analyzed the spelling abilities shown by a group of 26 French-Canadian dyslexics, reporting that they scored more poorly than two groups of controls composed respectively of chronological-age and reading-age matched children. The authors argue that the difficulties manifested by dyslexics prevent them from developing stable spelling representations, resulting in a poorer performance.

These finding can be interpreted within the framework of the Dual-Route Model, introducing interesting parallelisms with reading. As observed in the previous section, dyslexic children appear to rely more heavily on the lexical route for reading, retrieving the phonological form of the word from the orthographic input lexicon, which stores the spoken forms of familiar words. Given that dyslexics are more impaired with the spelling of nonwords, it seems plausible to assume that they adopt a similar strategy, recovering the visual form of the words from a phonological input lexicon, corresponding to the orthographic input lexicon, which is linked to an orthographic output lexicon, storing the written forms of words. Postulating the existence of a lexical route for spelling, similar to the lexical route of the Dual-Route Model, contributes to explain why dyslexic children, as well as younger children who have just started acquiring literacy, are better at spelling familiar and frequent words, whereas they are particularly poor at spelling nonwords.

As discussed for reading, than, it seems that the sublexical route, which relies heavily on orthographic-phonological conversion rules, is particularly weak in dyslexic children.

3.3. Phonological deficits

It is well known that phonological deficits are very widespread in dyslexia; illuminating in this respect is the study performed by Ramus et al (2003) revealing that 100% of dyslexics suffer from phonological impairments.

The most distinctive phonological feature exhibited by dyslexics is the very poor phonological awareness. Phonological awareness can be defined as a metalinguistic skill concerning the individual's conscious knowledge of the phonological structure of words, that is, of the precise sequence of sounds making up words. As discussed above, phonological awareness skills are necessary to accomplish reading: the decoding of words, in fact, demands the knowledge of their internal structure, since it involves linking graphemes to phonemes. Typical tasks testing phonological awareness require the subject to identify the initial, final or middle sound of words, to detect and produce words that rhyme, to segment words into syllables and sounds, to blend syllables and sounds into words, and to delete or substitute syllables or sounds in words.

A compelling body of evidence, indeed, confirms that dyslexics perform very poorly in phonological tasks and that their phonological awareness is significantly low, suggesting that their difficulties in analyzing the sound structure of words are responsible for their incapacity to acquire the systematic correspondences between orthography and phonology. Consistently, studies have demonstrated that children with poor phonological awareness are generally poor at reading, whereas children with a higher phonological awareness are more proficient readers; conversely, poor readers are significantly impaired in phonological awareness tasks (Snowling 1995; Blachman, B. A. 1994, 1997, 2000; Rispens 2004).

A recent study conducted by Ramus and colleagues (2013) confirms that phonological deficits are very widespread in dyslexia and particularly evident in tasks assessing phonological awareness, such as spoonerisms and rhymes detection.

Interesting insights come also from studies conducted on preschool children at familiar risk for dyslexia: in a longitudinal research Rispens (2004) reported that at-risk children performed more poorly than their peers on tasks tapping phonological awareness and letter knowledge. After one year of reading instruction the results were re-examined and it appeared that the children who did not manifest normal reading progress were the ones who had shown the worst performance.

A strong correlation between phonological awareness and letter knowledge has been reported also by other researchers (Bowey 1994; Johnston et al. 1996; De Jong and Van der Leij 1999). Moreover, remediation studies have shown that facilitating phonological awareness and orthographic-phonological conversion through direct instruction enhances performance in reading and spelling (Torgesen et al. 1999, 2001). In particular, Bus and Van Ijzendoorn (1999) conducted a meta-analysis of experimental training studies and reported that improvement was higher when phonological awareness was trained in parallel with letter-sound correspondences.

Such findings have led researchers to argue that the impaired phonological competence showed by dyslexic children is the most influential cause of their reading and spelling deficits (Rack et al. 1992).

Notice that poor phonological awareness can also account for the non-word reading deficit typically detected in dyslexic individuals: the ability to read nonsense pronounceable words, in fact, depends strongly on phonological processes and consequently on phonological awareness. This is supported by findings showing that nonword reading is highly predictive of reading proficiency. In particular, dyslexic children perform more poorly than younger children matched for reading-age: Rack et al. (1992) reviewed 10 different studies involving a total of 428 dyslexics ranging from 8;5 years old to 13;2 years old and testing nonwords reading accuracy. Significantly, results show that dyslexics performed remarkably worse than reading-level matched normal readers, who ranged from 1;3 years to 5 years younger than them.

Furthermore, a number of researchers investigated the phonological coding in dyslexic children, administering speech perception and production tasks. Results showed that dyslexics perceived phonetic boundaries less sharply than normal readers did (Manis et al. 1988; Adlard and Hazan 1997) and that they were worse than controls in the verbal repetition of both high and low frequency words and, especially, nonwords (Brady et al. 1983, Elbro 1997).

As the reader may have observed, in the experiments reviewed here phonological deficits have been typically assessed using metalinguistic tasks, relying basically on phonological awareness skills. A different perspective has been adopted by Desroches and colleagues (2006), which pursued a novel approach, measuring phonological competence using eyetracking. In their experiment, subjects were instructed to look at named items that were presented in a visual display, which contained the target item (e.g. *candle*), a cohort competitor that shared the initial syllable of the target items (e.g. *candy*) and/or a rhyme competitor (e.g. *sandal*). Results demonstrated that both dyslexics and age-matched control children showed lower recognition rates when a cohort competitor was present, suggesting that they were sensitive to this phonological overlap. Significantly, however, only control children showed slower fixation rates in presence of the rhyme distractor, whereas dyslexics did not, performing as fast as in the baseline condition, where no distractors were introduced, and thus demonstrating that they were not sensitive to the presence of rhyme competitors. This finding indicates that dyslexics are less sensitive than controls in detecting rhyming relationships among words and, consequently, that they are less sensitive to phonological suprasegmental information.

Moreover, Paulesu et al. (2001) performed an interesting study to test both reading and phonological competence in English, French and Italian adult dyslexics. As expected, they found that Italian subjects were less impaired than French and English subjects on reading tests, due to the greater transparency of their orthographic system. However, Italians performed worse than controls and as poorly as English and French dyslexics in all phonological measures (i.e. word and nonword reading speed, digit naming, short-term memory and spoonerisms), lending further support to the idea that dyslexia is associated with a phonological deficit, which appears to persist across languages and orthographic systems. Moreover, differences between the three groups of dyslexics and the respective groups of controls have been confirmed with the PET technique, showing a significantly greater activation for controls in the left hemisphere, with the maximum peak in the middle temporal gyrus. No areas of significantly greater activation, instead, have been found in dyslexics in comparison to controls.

To summarize, dyslexic children manifest great and widespread difficulties in the domain of phonology, affecting their phonological awareness, which are persistent across ages and languages, as reflected by different neural circuits activation.

3.4. Vocabulary development and lexical retrieval

Vocabulary deficits and word-finding problems are often reported in the literature on dyslexia and they are frequently referred to as early predictors of later reading achievements. In particular, dyslexic children's vocabulary has been found underdeveloped in comparison to that of age-matched typically developing children. Moreover, poor readers displayed a significant word-length effect (i.e. the longer the word, the poorer the performance) and a frequency effect (i.e. the lower the frequency of the word, the poorer the performance) (Wolf and Obregon 1992). Interestingly, vocabulary knowledge in preschool children has been also found predictive of early reading achievements (Scarborough 1990, Snowling et al. 2003).

However, the most interesting research on this topic concerns the performance shown by dyslexics and unaffected individuals in rapid naming tasks. The focus on naming speed deficits originally stems from the work implemented by Denkla (1972) and Denkla and Rudel (1976a, 1976b), who created the Rapid Automatized Naming (RAN) tests to measure serial speed naming. In the RAN tests subjects are asked to name as quick as possible visually presented stimuli such as alphanumeric characters, colors, and drawings of simple objects.

Rapid naming tasks have been administered to dyslexic individuals obtaining interesting results. A huge body of evidence, in fact, demonstrates that both children and adults suffering from dyslexia are significantly slower than unaffected subjects on all RAN measures. In particular, Denkla and Rudel found that dyslexic children across ages and languages were slower at picture naming not only in comparison to chronological age-matched controls, but also to reading age-matched controls.

An early poor performance in rapid naming tasks can also predict later reading difficulties, as shown firstly by Wolf, Bally and Morris (1986) and confirmed by more recent studies reporting a high correlation between naming speed and reading performance (Manis et al. 1997). Moreover, naming deficits persist also in adolescence and adulthood, as shown by Wolff and colleagues (1990), who reported digits and letters naming deficits in adult dyslexics.

In an interesting study, Fawcett and Nicolson (1994) analyzed three groups of dyslexic children aged 8, 13 and 17 years old, comparing their performance to the performance shown by three groups of typically developing children matched for age and IQ, and a group of 10-year-old children with mild learning difficulties (full IQ comprised between 70 and 90), matched for reading age with the 8-year-old dyslexics. Subjects were asked to rapidly name objects, colors, digits and letters. Results showed that dyslexic children were significantly slower at naming colors, digits and letters in comparison to age-matched control children, whereas they performed as younger but reading age-matched controls. Remarkably, they showed a significantly poorer performance also in comparison to reading age-matched controls when asked to rapidly name pictures. Specifically, 17-year-old dyslexics performed only at the level of 8-year-old controls in letters and pictures naming, suggesting that naming deficits are persistent and very severe. The 10-year-old slow learners, instead, performed as 8-year-old dyslexics, compatibly with their reading age.

As the authors suggest, the longer latencies shown by dyslexics across age seem to reflect a less automatic or less efficient lexical access or an impaired lexical retrieval or assembly of the sequence of phonemes making up words.

Another interesting aspect to reflect on is the greater difficulty shown by dyslexics when they are asked to rapidly name pictures of simple objects, in comparison to colors and alphanumeric stimuli. Presumably, this can be due to the fact that there is a limited number of colors, digits and letters, whereas in the case of objects the number of possible alternatives increases radically. Dyslexics' slowness, then, seems to increase proportionally to the number of possible responses, suggesting that the deficit affects the amount of processing required, more than the speed of reaction.

3.5. Grammatical deficits

More recent studies have shown that linguistic deficits in dyslexia are not confined just to the domain of phonology, but that they affect grammatical competence as well, influencing dyslexics' performance in tasks tapping morphology, syntax and semantics.

The correlation between syntactic or grammatical ability and reading proficiency was originally suggested by Fry, Johnson and Muehl (1970), who reported that poor readers produced significantly less complex constructions that their peers, as it was further confirmed by Muter and Snowling (1998), who found that grammatical competence in early childhood was predictive of reading achievements. The same consideration was supported also by Bishop (1991), who carried out a series of researches pointing to the existence of a correlation between semantic and syntactic abilities and reading problems.

In this section I will report the results of some of the most interesting experimental studies administered to test dyslexic children's grammatical competence comparing their performance to that shown by chronologically age-matched or reading age-matched typically developing children.

3.5.1. The Interpretation of Tough Sentences

One of the most discussed proposals about the causes underlying development dyslexia focuses on the phonological weaknesses exhibited by poor readers and maintains that they are also responsible for the other impairments characterizing the disorder. To test this hypothesis, Byrne (1981) conducted an interesting experiment assessing good and poor readers' interpretation of the English though constructions, reported in (1), which are characterized by having a very similar phonological structure but a completely different underlying syntactic structure.

(1) a. The snake is glad to bite.
b. The snake is hard to bite.
c. The snake is horrible to bite.

The surface parsing of the three sentences in (1) is identical, but the underlying grammatical relations differ: in (1a) *the snake* is both the surface subject and the logical subject of the action of biting. This type of sentence is classified by Byrne as S-type construction, since the adjective *glad* can only yield a subject interpretation. In (1b), instead, *the snake* is the surface subject but it is not the underlying subject of the infinitive verb *to bite.* In this sentence *the snake* is, in fact, the object of the action of biting. This construction is called O-type since an adjective like *hard* can only yield an object interpretation. Sentence (1c), finally, is labeled A-type, since it is ambiguous: the adjective *horrible*, in fact, can yield both a subject and an object interpretation.

Acquisition studies have demonstrated that O-type constructions are more difficult to interpret than S-type constructions: specifically, young children are not able to process the more complex structure of O-type sentences and they tend to treat the surface subject as if it was the logical subject (Chomsky 1969; Cromer 1970). The higher complexity of

(1b) is due to the presence of two linguistic dependencies to be computed. It is argued, in fact, that the role of the subject is carried out by an arbitrary PRO, which is not phonetically realized and which gets a generic interpretation (Chomsky 1980). While processing (1b), then, the human parser must compute first the linguistic dependency between the silent subject PRO and the verb *to bite* and secondly the one between the object *the snake* and the verb *to bite.* While processing (1a), instead, the parser must simply compute the dependency between the subject *the snake* and the verb *to bite.*

Bearing this in mind, we can now consider the experiment performed by Byrne, who tested S-type, O-type and A-type constructions in good and poor readers. The subjects who took part in the experiment were 24 dyslexic children (mean age 7;11) and 20 typically developing children (mean age 7;7). As for the methodology, an act-out task was used: participants were presented with the target sentences and then they were asked to act it out using hand puppets.

The results revealed that all children showed a perfect competence of S-type constructions, but that dyslexic children made significantly more errors with O-type sentences in comparison to control children. Moreover, poor readers manifested a marked tendency to interpret ambiguous sentences (i.e. A-type constructions) as S-type, whereas on the contrary good readers tended to interpret them as O-type. These results indicate that the difficulties shown by dyslexics in this experiment cannot be attributed to their impaired phonological competence, since the three sentences have a very similar phonological structure, but they must be related to the different degrees of syntactic complexity of the sentences at issue.

Summarizing, dyslexic children performed differently from their peers, interpreting more frequently the surface subjects as logical subjects. Interestingly, they displayed the same behavior observed in young children, suggesting that their linguistic competence is less mature, or that their processing resources are more limited.

3.5.2. The Interpretation of Pronouns

The interpretation of pronouns by dyslexic children has been investigated in an interesting study, presented by Waltzman and Cairns (2000) and revealing that poor readers are remarkably more impaired than good readers in the interpretation of pronouns.

Before we consider the experimental protocol and its results, it can be useful to remind the linguistic principles underlying the computation of the sentences tested by the authors. According to the Binding Theory formulated by Chomsky (1981), three different principles determine the possibility or impossibility for anaphors, pronouns and referential expression[5] to be bound in their minimal domain, as reported below.

(2) Binding Theory
Principle A: An anaphor is bound[6] in its governing category[7].
Principle B: A (non-reflexive) pronoun is free (i.e. it cannot be bound) in its governing category.
Principle C: A referential expression must be free everywhere.

5 According to the Principle B of the Binding Theory formulated by Chomsky (1981), Nominal Phrases are divided in three categories:
Anaphors, which include reflexive pronouns (such as *myself, herself, itself*...), reciprocal pronouns (such as *each other*) and DP-traces.
Pronouns, which comprise personal (*he, she*...) and possessive (*his, her*...) pronouns.
Referential expressions (R-expressions), which are all other nominal expressions that can choose a referent and that have an independent semantic content (*Lisa, the queen of England, a baby*...).
The main difference between the first two classes and the third one is precisely that R-expressions have an independent semantic content, while anaphors and pronouns depend for their interpretation on the denotation of other elements in the sentence or in the discourse context. In other words, in order to be able to interpret them, it is necessary to retrieve their semantic content from the context.

6 The traditional definition of binding is reported below:
Binding
α binds β if and only if
(i) α and β are coindexed,
(ii) α c-commands β.
The notion of c-command, instead, is defined as follows:
C-command
α c-commands a node β if and only if
(i) α does not dominate β,
(ii) β does not dominate α,
(iii) the first node dominating α also dominate β

7 The governing category of α is the minimal clause containing a governor of α and an accessible subject, where α qualifies as an accessible subject if the co-indexation of α and the subject does not violate any grammatical principle.

Principle A states that anaphors (i.e. reflexives and reciprocals) must be coindexed with a c-commanding antecedent within their local domain. For instance, the sentence in (3a) is grammatical, since the reflexive *herself* is coindexed with the DP *Lisa*, and thus it is interpreted as a bound variable. (3b), instead, is ruled out by principle B, being the pronoun *her* coindexed, and hence bound, by the R-expression *Lisa* in its governing category.

(3) a. $Lisa_i$ admires $herself_i$.
b. *$Lisa_i$ admires her_i.

Principle B states that a pronominal expression must be free in its governing category; hence, it cannot be bound nor coindexed with a c-commanding antecedent.

The sentence reported in (4a) is acceptable according to Principle B, because the pronoun is not bound in its local domain; on the contrary, (4b) is ruled out because the pronoun *her* is bound and coindexed with the R-expression *Anna*.

(4) a. $Anna_j$ admires her_i.
b. *$Anna_j$ admires her_j.

Finally, Principle C asserts that a referential expression can never be bound. In (5a) and (5b), Principle C is violated since the DPs are bound by their antecedents. Sentence (5c) instead is correct, being the R-expression *Lisa* free.

(5) a. *She_i admires $Anna_i$.
b. *She_i thinks that Anna admires $Lisa_i$.
c. Anna admires Lisa.

Language acquisition studies have shown that children obey Principle A and C from around age 4, but that, quite surprisingly, they violate Principle B even after age 5 and 6, accepting as grammatical sentences like (4b) around 50% of the times. This phenomenon is known as the "Delay of Principle B Effect" and it is reported in a variety of languages, such as English (Chien and Wexler, 1990), Russian (Avrutin and Wexler, 1992) and Dutch (Philip and Coopmans, 1996).

Interestingly, the experiment performed by Waltzman and Cairns on dyslexic children yielded the same results obtained in previous acquisition studies. Poor readers, aged 8 years and 7 months, were remarkably more impaired than age-matched good readers in the condition testing Principle B, accepting a sentence like (4b) in a context in which Anna admires herself.

As younger children, instead, they performed adultlike in the conditions testing Principle A and C. This parallelism between acquisition findings and Waltzman and Cairns' experiment indicates again that dyslexic children behave as preschool children in tasks testing their interpretation of pronouns and that their grammatical competence is impaired or, more likely, that it is yet immature.

To explain children's violations of Principle B, Grodzinsky and Reinhart (1993) argue, in fact, that their difficulties arise from the immaturity of their pragmatic and/or general processing system. Grodzinsky and Reinhart state that this behaviour cannot be explained from a syntactic point of view, but rather they claim that children's failure is determined by the complexity of the processing required by Rule I (Intransentential Coreference).

Very briefly, Rule I has been proposed to account for those cases in which a pronoun receives an interpretation that should be excluded by the Binding Principles. In (6), for instance, Principle C is violated, since the R-expression *Oscar*, which should be free, is instead coindexed with the pronoun *he*.

(6) Everyone has finally realized that Oscar is incompetent. Even *he* has finally realized that *Oscar* is incompetent.

According to Reinhart and Grodzinsky, this coreferential reading is obtained by means of Rule I, reported below.

(7) Rule I
α and β cannot be covalued in a derivation D, iff
a. α c-commands β
b. α cannot bind β in D, and
c. The covaluation interpretation is undistinguishable from what would be obtained if α binds β.

[To check c, construct a comparison-representation by replacing β, with a variable bound by α].

Rule I entails that if just one of these three clauses is violated, coreference is possible. Specifically, in (6) the first and the second conditions are satisfied, since *he* c-commands *Oscar* and *he* cannot bind *Oscar* (given that *Oscar* is not a free variable). To check clause (c) a comparison-representation should be constructed by replacing β (i.e. Oscar) with a variable bound by α, as shown below:

(8) Even *he* has finally realized that *Oscar* is incompetent.
Covaluation: Even he (λx (x thinks that **Oscar** is incompetent) & he = Oscar
Binding-comparison: Even he (λx (x thinks that **x** is incompetent) & he = Oscar

In other words, the coreferential interpretation of (6) is obtained because clause (c) is violated: the property of believing Oscar incompetent, corresponding to the covaluation construal, is what is pragmatically relevant in the context (6), and this property is certainly not equivalent to the property of believing oneself incompetent.

Let us now consider the procedure required to establish whether (4b) is grammatical or not. The first and the second conditions of Rule I are respected, since *her* is c-commanded by *Anna* but it cannot be bound by the DP (since the pronoun must be free in her governing category). Therefore, it is necessary to construct a comparison representation, reported below.

(9) Anna admires her.
Covaluation: Anna (λx (x admires **her**) & her = Anna
Binding-comparison: Anna (λx (x admires **x**)

Since the two readings obtained respectively by covaluation and binding are equivalent and thus undistinguishable, clause (c) is satisfied and the coreference derivation is filtered out.

Following this procedure through the three steps involved, you may have noted that the computation required to process Rule I is quite complex and thus very expensive in terms of working memory resources.

In particular, it has been argued that the most demanding step is the third one, requiring the construction of the comparison representation. This stage, in fact, requires to construct, keep in memory and compare two different representations in order to establish which is the correct one, an operation known as Reference-Set Computation, which has proven to be especially challenging for children (see Chapter 5 for more details).

While processing Rule I, for instance, children are asked to hold the sentence in memory and, at the same time, to construct two representations, the one for variable binding and the other for covaluation. Finally, they have to compare them and to decide if they are distinguishable or not.

According to Grodzinsky and Reinhart, Rule I is innate and children do know precisely what they have to do, but the need to hold and compare two distinct representations at the same time exceeds their processing abilities. Hence, they get stuck during the execution of the task, they are forced to give up and thus they try to guess, as demonstrated by the chance-rate performance reported in experiments testing the mastery of Principle B.

To summarize, the work by Waltzman and Cairns demonstrates that dyslexic children show an adult competence in assigning the correct reference to anaphors and referential expressions, correctly applying Principles A and C of the Binding Theory, whereas they are considerably impaired when they have to interpret pronouns whose reference assignment is governed by Principle B. Interestingly, dyslexics seem to replicate the behaviour of young children, who manifest exactly the same tendency. This finding can be explained, following Reinhart and Grodzinsky, arguing that pronoun interpretation is governed by Rule I, whose computation is very demanding in terms of processing resources. Young children and dyslexics' behaviour seems to point to a lack of the processing resources required to accomplish this task.

An inefficient working memory has been held responsible also for the results reported by Fiorin (2010), who tested dyslexic and control children's performance with ambiguous sentences, like the one in (10), where the pronoun "his" can be interpreted as referring both to the DP *Francesco* and to the DP *every friend*. In (10), both variable binding and coreferential readings are indicated.

(10) Every friend of Francesco painted his bike.
Binding: For every x, if x is a friend of Francesco, then x painted **x**'s bike
Coreference: For every x, if x is a friend of Francesco, then x painted **Francesco**'s bike

In Fiorin's experimental protocol the subject was told a short story at the end of which a puppet uttered the target sentence. The participant's task was to decide if the puppet described correctly what happened in the story. There were two experimental conditions. For instance, in Condition A the experimenter told the subject that two of Francesco's friends painted both their own bike and Francesco's bike, whereas the third friend painted only his own bike. In condition B, instead, two out of three boys painted both their own bike and Francesco's one, whereas a third boy decided to paint only Francesco's bike.

At the end of the story, the puppet uttered the target sentence in (10) and the subject had to decide if it described the story correctly or not. Note that both judgments are correct, since (10) is ambiguous. However, the subject's response reveals which strategy she used to interpret the sentence, that is, if she chose the variable binding reading, or rather the coreference reading.

If (10) is judged correct in Condition A, it is possible to infer that the subject interpreted *his* as referring to *every friend of Francesco*, that is, that she adopted a bound-variable reading. If (10) is judged correct in Condition B, instead, this entails that the subject chose the coreference reading, since she interpreted *his* as referring to *Francesco*.

Fiorin administered the experiment both in Italian and in Dutch: the subjects of the Italian group were 18 dyslexic children (mean age 9;4) and 20 age-matched control children (mean age 9;2), whereas the Dutch group was composed by 10 poor readers at familiar risk of dyslexia (mean age 8;4), 22 good readers at familiar risk of dyslexia (mean age 8;4) and 17 good readers non at-risk of dyslexia (mean age 8;4).

Results showed that both Italian dyslexic children and Dutch poor readers displayed a constant tendency to assign the same interpretation to most or all of the experimental items, choosing constantly the variable binding or the coreferential reading. Italian control children and Dutch good readers (both at-risk and non at-risk), instead, did not manifest this tendency and performed at individual chance level.

To explain this difference, Fiorin observes that dyslexics and poor readers were able to access both interpretations, but that they tended to stick to the same interpretation due to their limited processing resources. More specifically, he proposes that dyslexics assigned to the target sentence the same interpretation chosen for the preceding one in order to avoid the process of resolving the ambiguity of the sentence, that is, due to a limitation of the processing resources that are involved in the ability to constantly shift between two interpretations of the very same sentence.

To summarize so far, both the experiment conducted by Waltzman and Cairns and that administered by Fiorin show that dyslexics display a different performance in the interpretation of pronouns in comparison to normally achieving children, presumably due to their limited processing resources. In Waltzman and Cairns' experiment, they displayed an impaired ability to properly interpret pronouns according to Principle B of the Binding Theory, performing as younger children. In Fiorin's experiment, instead, they tended to interpret ambiguous sentences sticking consistently to the same interpretive strategy, avoiding resource-consuming shifting between two different interpretations of the very same sentence.

3.5.3. Comprehension and Production of Relative Clauses

The comprehension of relative clauses has been investigated in a number of studies revealing that poor readers have more difficulties than good readers (Mann et al. 1984, Bar-Shalom et al. 1993) and that their performance resembles that shown by younger children (Sheldon 1974).

Four main types of relative clauses can be distinguished: (i) Subject-modifying-subject clauses (SS), (ii) subject-modifying-object clauses (SO), (iii) object-modifying-subject clauses (OS) and (iv) object-modifying-object clauses (OO). An example for each type of relative clauses, taken from Stein et al. (1984), is reported below.

(11) a. SS: *The lion* that hits the bear__rolls the ball.
b. SO: *The bear* that the lion hits__rolls the ball.
c. OS: The lion hugs *the bear* that__rolls the ball.
d. OO: The bear bites *the lion* that the ball hits__.

It is important to note that one of the syntactic features characterizing relative clauses is the presence of a superficially missing noun phrase, which is not phonetically realized. Consider for instance (11c): to understand correctly this sentence the hearer must first recognize that there is a phonetically empty Determiner Phrase (DP) in the subject position of the relative clause, and then she must interpret it as coreferential with the overt object DP *the bear* in the main clause. This computation is arguably quite difficult for young children, as confirmed by acquisition studies showing that SS clauses are acquired before OO clauses, which are in turn acquired before SO and OS clauses (Sheldon 2004). The same reasoning seems to be valid also for dyslexic children, who appear to have troubles with the interpretation of SO, OS and OO relative clauses, as demonstrated by Mann et al. (1984), who tested poor and good readers' competence by means of an act-out task. To explain dyslexics' poor performance, the authors refer to the concept of working memory, arguing that their limited phonological memory hinders their language comprehension.

In a subsequent study, Smith et al. (1989) performed a slightly different experiment, analyzing the same relative clauses but inserting them in more felicitous contexts. The authors proposed two methodological changes to verify if the decreased load on working memory had an effect on dyslexics' performance. First, they reduced the number of DPs mentioned in the sentence from three to two, and secondly they satisfied the presupposition associated with relative clauses, which states that restrictive relative clauses are felicitous only when more than one object corresponding to the relativized element is present in the context. For instance, sentence (12) is not uttered felicitously when there is only one girl in the context.

(12) The boy kissed the girl that was wearing a red dress.

Stein and colleagues demonstrated that dyslexic children performed as well as control children when the context of utterance was manipulated, suggesting that their difficulties with the experimental settings provided by Mann and colleagues were due to the infelicity of these contexts.

Relative clauses have been further tested by Bar-Shalom et al. (1993). In their experiment, again an act-out task, the authors adopted only one of the two methodological changes introduced in Stein and colleagues' study, reducing the number of animate DPs from three to two, but without satisfying the presupposition of the relative clause contained in the test sentence (i.e. there was only one character corresponding to the relativized DP). This choice was motivated by the need to determine which of the two modifications was responsible for dyslexics' enhanced performance reported in Smith et al.'s paper. In addition, Bar-Shalom and colleagues tested also production, eliciting relative clauses to verify if dyslexics' problems were confined to comprehension or whether they extended to production as well.

Results revealed that dyslexics were significantly worse than controls on SO, OS and OO relative clauses, as found by Mann et al.: this finding indicates that reducing the number of DPs is not sufficient to eliminate poor readers' problems, which appear to be rather due to the pragmatic infelicity of the context of utterance. Moreover, the results of the elicitation task showed that dyslexics were able to produce relative clauses, indicating that their competence was intact, even though they produced less SO relatives in comparison to controls, preferring to passivize. Specifically, they uttered (13a) instead of (13b), arguably due to the higher complexity of the SO clause.

(13) a. The salesman that was met by the doctor departed.
b. The salesman that the doctor met departed.

Discussing these results, Bar-Shalom and colleagues argue that dyslexics' difficulties with relative clauses are mainly due to pragmatic rather than syntactic factors. Poor readers display indeed an intact comprehension of relative clauses, but they manifest problems when the sentences are uttered out of an appropriate context. In particular, the authors propose that the absence of the extra character, which would satisfy the presupposition required by restrictive relative clauses, forces the subject to augment their mental model to accommodate the unsatisfied presupposition. This extra computation necessitates of additional working memory resources and it is therefore responsible for dyslexics' and young children's errors.

Keeping in mind this consideration, it remains unexplained why both poor readers and preschool children perform better with SS clauses and manifest the greatest difficulties with object-extracted relative clauses, i.e. OS and OO clauses.

This problem is successfully handled by Gibson (1991, 1998), who provides one of the most successful approaches to sentence comprehension, arguing that the online computation of an utterance involves the temporary storage of the partial information obtained during the comprehension process, in order to allow the human parser to compute the necessary linguistic dependencies between the elements in the sentence.

Let us see how the human parser computes each kind of relative clause we have examined.

(14) a. SS: *The lion* that___hits the bear rolls the ball.

In (14a) the presence of the complementizer *that* informs the parser that the relativized DP *the lion* is the argument of an embedded verb and that therefore it must be temporarily stored. When the parser finds the embedded verb *hits* the DP *the lion* is retrieved from memory and analyzed as the subject of *hits*.

b. SO: *The bear* that *the lion* hits___rolls the ball.

In (14b) the complementizer signals again that *the bear* must be stored, and that we must wait for the embedded verb. However, the parser encounters first the DP *the lion*, which must also be stored, since it is expected to be the subject of the embedded verb. Finally, when the parser finds *hits*, both DPs must be retrieved and analyzed respectively as the object and the subject of the embedded verb.

c. OS: The lion hugs *the bear* that___rolls the ball.

In (14c) *the bear* is stored until the verb *rolls* is encountered by the parser.

d. OO: The bear bites *the lion* that the ball hits___.

In (14d) both DPs *the lion* and *the ball* are stored until the parser finds the embedded verb *hits*. They must then be retrieved and analyzed respectively as the object and the subject of the embedded verb.

On these grounds, given the computations performed by the parser, it can be argued that relative clauses involving object extraction (e.g. SO and OO) are more difficult than those involving subject extraction (e.g. SS and OS), since in object extraction structures the parser has to temporarily store and analyze two DPs instead of only one. This approach immediately explains why SS are generally interpreted with fewer difficulties in comparison to the other types of clauses.

A more recent study reported in Cardinaletti and Volpato (2015) focused both on comprehension and production of relative clauses, comparing the performance shown by a group of dyslexic adults (aged between 22 and 25 years old) to that of two control groups composed by adolescents (mean age 15;5) and adults (mean age 24;11). For what concerns the interpretation of relative sentences, all three groups of subjects showed a similar performance, with more difficulties in the case of object relatives in comparison to subject relatives. Problems appeared more clearly in production, where dyslexics underperformed in comparison to age-matched controls, performing similarly to adolescents. The authors suggest that their difficulties may be due to processing deficits, related to the need to compute long-distance dependencies, which are arguably expensive in terms of cognitive costs.

A difficulty in the production of relative clauses has also been reported in another study conducted on Italian by Guasti et al. (2015), evidencing that children with dyslexia overall produced a lower number of correct relative clauses in comparison to controls, showing more marked deficits with object relatives than with subject relatives. A similar result was reported by Pivi and Del Puppo (2014), who analyzed the production of restrictive relative clauses in dyslexic and control children, suggesting that deficits appeared only in the production of object relatives, whereas the production of subject relatives was spared.

To summarize, dyslexics, both children and adults, have been found impaired with relative clauses, both in comprehension, especially in those contexts in which the sentence was uttered infelicitously, and in production. In both cases, difficulties are more marked with object relatives than with subject relatives. The impairments displayed by dyslexics, as stated by Gibson (1991, 1998), are arguably due to processing deficits.

3.5.4. *The Interpretation of Passive Sentences*

The interpretation of passive sentences in dyslexic children was originally investigated by Stein et al. (1984), who reported that poor readers performed as well as good readers with both reversible and non-reversible passive sentences.[8]

However, the results of this study have been recently challenged by Reggiani (2010), who found that dyslexics are remarkably impaired in the interpretation of reversible non-actional passive sentences, performing at the same level of preschool children, four years younger than them. Reggiani observes that Stein and colleagues tested only long[9] actional passives, which are interpreted without difficulties even by 3 years old children. Based on this consideration, Reggiani included in his experimental protocol a picture selection task, with more complex passive sentences, divided in four conditions, as reported below with an example for each condition:

(15) a. Non-reversible passive sentences with actional verbs:
"Winnie the Pooh is eaten by honey".
b. Non-reversible passive sentences with non-actional verbs:
"Donald Duck is heard by the alarm clock".
c. Reversible passive sentences with actional verbs:
"The girlfriend is kissed by Donald Duck".
d. Reversible passive sentences with non-actional verbs:
"Winnie the Pooh is seen by the bees".

The protocol was administered to a group of dyslexic children (mean age 9;7), a group of age-matched controls (mean age 9;7), a group of young controls (mean age 5;8) and a group of adults (mean age 35;8).

8 Reversible passive sentences are those constructions in which the agent and the patient can be switched while maintaining a semantically plausible meaning. Conversely, this exchange cannot take place with non-reversible sentences, as shown by the examples below.
(a) The girl is kissed by the boy.
(b) The apple is eaten by the boy.
The sentence in (a) is said to be *reversible*, since if the patient *the girl* is exchanged with the agent *the boy*, the sentence remains semantically plausible. The utterance in (b), instead, is classified as non-reversible, since if the subject *the apple* is switched with the agent *the boy*, the sentence does not make sense anymore.

9 Passive constructions are considered to be *long* if they include a by-phrase.

The method used was a Truth Value Judgment Task: the subject was shown a picture portraying two characters performing some actions and then she was asked to evaluate a target sentence pronounced by a clumsy puppet to determine what happened in the story. Results showed that age-matched controls performed adultlike in all conditions, whereas dyslexic children were significantly impaired in those tasks involving reversible non-actional passives as the one reported in (15d). Specifically, dyslexics subjects, as well as younger children, accepted a sentence like (15d) as a correct description of a picture portraying Winnie the Pooh that sees, without being seen, some bees. This finding, discarding the hypothesis that dyslexics do not manifest problems with the interpretation of passives proposed by Stein et al., suggests that dyslexic children suffer instead from the so-called Maratsos Effect.

Very briefly, the Maratsos Effect accounts for the greatest difficulty met by young children with passives involving psychological non-actional verbs in comparison to actional verbs. Different theories have been developed to account for this phenomenon. The most plausible explanation, supported also by Reggiani (2010), argues that the Maratsos Effect is due to a processing deficit: due to their limited processing resources, children are not able to handle both psychological verbs and the non-canonical word order typical of passive sentences. The interaction of these two factors imposes too high processing costs and it is thus responsible for the failure found in the interpretation of reversible non-actional passives.

To summarize, Reggiani (2010) demonstrated that dyslexic children are impaired in the comprehension of passive sentences and that they display the Maratsos Effect at an age at which they should have exhibited an adultlike comprehension of passive sentences, as shown by age-matched controls, suggesting that their difficulties are determined by a processing deficit.

3.5.5. The Interpretation of Grammatical Aspect

A recent experiment conducted by Fiorin (2010) has demonstrated that dyslexic children show a significantly poor performance when asked to interpret grammatical aspect. Specifically, Fiorin tested the comprehension of the Italian past tenses *Imperfetto* (IMPF), which is used to encode past tense and imperfective aspect as reported in (16a), and *Passato Prossimo* (PP), which encodes past tense and perfective aspect, as shown in (16b).

(16) a. IMPF: Marco mangiava il gelato.
'Marco ate-IMPF the ice-cream'.
b. PP: Marco ha mangiato il gelato.
'Marco ate-PP the ice-cream'.

In his experimental protocol, Fiorin used the methodology of the picture selection tasks: a puppet uttered a target sentence and the subject had to choose the most appropriate one between two different pictures. For instance, with the target sentence in (16a), the subject could choose between a picture portraying an ongoing situation with Marco eating the ice-cream (the correct one) and a picture depicting a complete situation, in which Marco has eaten up the ice-cream. Two groups of subjects took part in the experiment: a group of dyslexic children (mean age 9;8) and a group of age-matched control children (mean age 9;3). As shown by the results, control children displayed an adultlike performance with both past tenses, whereas dyslexic children performed as good as their peers with PP sentences, but significantly more poorly with IMPF sentences. Specifically, they associated consistently the picture depicting a complete situation to IMPF sentences as (16a).

This finding echoes back the results reported in the acquisition studies conducted by Hollebrandse and van Hout (2001), who showed that IMPF is acquired later than PP and that 5-year-old children correctly associated PP sentences with complete situations but still judged IMPF as appropriate with complete events. This data can be explained by resorting to the hypothesis proposed by Delfitto (2002, 2004), who argues that PP is used to encode past and complete event, whereas IMPF conveys the neutral information that the sentence can be used both for complete and ongoing events. However, the reference to complete events with IMPF is filtered out by the Gricean Principle of Cooperation. According to the Maxim of Quantity, the speaker is assumed to be as informative as possible: therefore, while computing a sentence with IMPF, the hearer reasons out that if the speaker had wanted to refer to a complete situation, she would have used a PP, which is more informative, instead of the IMPF. The fact that she chose to use the IMPF means that the PP wouldn't have been appropriate and thus that the reference to a complete event has to be discarded in favor of the ongoing event. Within this line of explanation, then, the association of IMPF sentences with ongoing situations involves a quite complex computation, which appears to be too costly to compute for both young children and dyslexic children. This hypothesis is further supported by the results that I will present more thoroughly in Chapter 5 and that confirm that dyslexic children meet significant difficulties when they are asked to interpret scalar implicatures.

To summarize, the results of the experiment performed by Fiorin indicate that dyslexic children are more impaired than their peers in the interpretation of IMPF sentences, given their difficulty to compute scalar implicatures. Again, dyslexic children appear to display a behavior that is more typical of younger children.

3.5.6. Morphosyntactic Agreement

Morphosyntactic impairments have been detected in dyslexic subjects by a number of studies that I will briefly review.

The first research, conducted by Joanisse and colleagues (2000), was administered on a large sample of 61 dyslexics (mean age 8;7), a group of chronological age-matched normal readers (mean age 8;5) and a group of reading age-matched controls (mean age 6;11). Subjects were administered a test on inflectional morphology, in order to evaluate their abilities to apply past tense agreement rules and plural rules to both familiar words and nonwords. Specifically, subjects were shown a picture portraying two or more of the same objects, and they were prompted to provide the plural of the noun. Both regular (e.g. fish>fishes) and irregular plurals (e.g. foot>feet) were tested; in the case of nonwords, subjects were presented with an invented noun corresponding to a fictitious creature. Similarly, they were asked to provide the past tense of regular verbs (e.g. bake>baked), irregular verbs (e.g. drive>drove) and nonsense verbs (filp>filped). Results showed that dyslexics performed remarkably worse than age-matched controls on both tasks, whereas their performance was slightly but not significantly worse than the performance of reading age-matched younger children.

The same findings is reported by Jiménez et al. (2004), who tested gender and number agreement in a group of reading disabled children (mean age 9;8), chronological age-matched controls (mean age 9;7) and younger reading age-matched controls (mean age 7;6). Participants were asked to complete truncated sentences with two alternatives differing in gender or in number. The authors tested also the ability to assign syntactic roles, presenting subjects with a picture and a series of sentences varying in that subject and object roles were reversed. Finally, they focused on function words proposing two kinds of tests: in the first task, subjects were shown two pictures and a sentence and they were asked to decide which picture corresponded to the sentence. In order to accomplish this kind of task, they had to be able to understand the meaning of the function word used in the sentence. In the second task, they had to complete a sentence with one out of two function words. The authors found that children with reading disabilities had a very poor performance, committing more errors than chronological age-matched controls and even than reading age-matched control in all tasks.

A morphosyntactic impairment has been detected also by Rispens (2004), who tested morphosyntactic agreement in Dutch children by means of a grammaticality judgment task. Her experiment was performed on a group of dyslexic children (mean age 8;09), a group of chronological age-matched control (8;11) and a group of reading age-matched controls (mean age 7;01). Participants were presented with grammatical and ungrammatical sentences and were instructed to press a button with a smiling face for correct sentences and a button with a frowning face for incorrect sentences. Moreover, the author evaluated the children's spontaneous speech, elicited by a fixed set of questions about holidays, family, hobbies and so on. Results revealed that dyslexic children always underperformed in comparison to both groups of control children in the grammaticality judgment task, failing to recognize agreement errors. Dyslexics displayed a poor behavior also in production, uttering an incorrect inflection in 17% of the instances, compared to the 99% correct performance of control children. Their errors comprised principally the omission of agreement markers and the substitution of the plural inflection with a singular inflection.

To summarize, the experiment performed by Joanisse et al. (2000), Jiménez et al. (2004) and Rispens (2004) reveal that dyslexic children's morphosyntactic competence is highly impaired in comparison to both chronological age-matched and reading age-matched control children. Moreover, the significant difference found between dyslexics and reading age-matched controls shows that impaired children underperform also in comparison to younger children (around two years younger in the experiments discussed above). Moreover, the poorer performance shown by dyslexics in comparison to younger controls confirms that their difficulties cannot be ascribed to their reading deficits.

3.6. *Attention deficits*

Attention can be defined as the ability to direct resources to the required tasks, retaining the relevant information and filtering out the irrelevant and distracting stimuli.

Inattentive behavior has been often reported as a typical symptom exhibited by children affected by dyslexia. Specifically, dyslexics appear to show lacks of concentration, high levels of distractibility and shorter attention spans in comparison to normally achieving children. These attention disorders bring about a stronger tendency to forget the content of the instructions, to lose the focus on the tasks in hand and to abandon an activity before completing it, which are behaviors typically reported by parents and teachers. In addition, difficulties have been reported in shifting the attention from one task to another, in organizing and monitoring the activity and in inhibiting irrelevant stimuli.

Heiervang and colleagues (2001), for instance, report highly significant attention problems in dyslexic children, as revealed by three questionnaires on behavior completed respectively by parents, teachers and by the children themselves. Beyond attention disorders, both internalizing and externalizing problems have also come to light, consistently with other studies showing that dyslexics manifest an antisocial and depressive behavior more frequently than normally achieving children (Maughan et al. 1996).

For the purposes of the present discussion, however, I will concentrate solely on the attention problems, given that aggressive or anxious behaviors could be interpreted as psychological consequences of academic and reading failure, causing poor self-esteem and frustration. On the contrary, attention deficits appear to have a distinct and independent etiology, affecting also the performance in multisensory tasks.

In an interesting study, Everatt and colleagues (1997) examined the incidence of the so-called Stroop Effect in dyslexic and control children.

The Stroop Phenomenon is named after the psychologist John Ridley Stroop, who tested the effect of interference examining subjects' performance under different conditions: in a first control condition, they were asked to read color words printed in black ink, while in the second experimental condition they were required to name the ink color of words which were printed in a tint different from the one denoted by the word itself (see Figure 1.2). That is, if the word "blue" was printed in a red ink, the subject should say "red" instead of "blue".

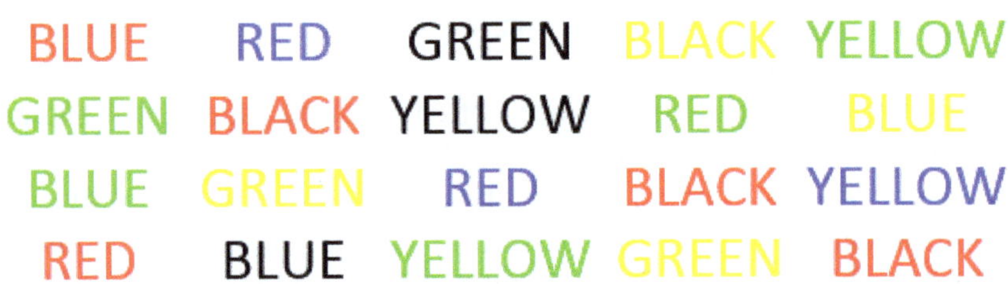

Figure 1.2. A classical example of the material used to analyze the Stroop Effect.

Stroop found that response times were dramatically longer in the experimental condition than in the control condition. To explain it, he proposed that the increase in response times was caused by the interference of the tendency to read the word with the recognition of the color. Specifically, he argues that this interference is determined by the automatic association of the read word with its semantic content: basically, the subject reads "blue" and thinks automatically of the color "blue". However, she has to inhibit the semantic content of the word he reads, since her task is to name the color ink in which the word is printed. This inhibition process, therefore, is necessary in order to accomplish the task, as it permits to filter out those information that are irrelevant for the purposes of the experiment, and to retain only the relevant ones. As argued above, this mechanism is governed by attention.

Everatt and colleagues administered the Stroop Test on a group of 20 dyslexic children (mean age 10 years and 6 months), on a group of 20 typically developing age-matched children and on a third group composed by younger control children matched for reading age (mean age 8 years and 1 month). Interestingly, they found that dyslexic children were significantly slower even in comparison to younger controls matched for reading age in naming the color ink of words. In other words, they exhibited larger effects of interference, leading the authors to suggest that they are less able to control and inhibit the processing of the word meaning and hence that the control process is "detrimentally affected" in dyslexia (228). It follows that attention processes are impaired in dyslexic individuals.

The same conclusion is reported by Hari and colleagues (1999), who tested a group of 18 dyslexic adults and a group of 22 control adults in an attentional blink task. In this typology of task, the subject is asked to identify a first target and a second one in a close temporal succession. Psychological studies demonstrated that response times typically increase when the subject has to switch the attention from one target to another: it has been demonstrated, in fact, that when the attentional resources are focused on a target, they are unavailable for the second target for 400–600 milliseconds.

In Hari et al.'s experiment subjects were asked to identify a first target, which could be any letter of the English alphabet except for "X" or "K", and simultaneously also a second target, which was an "X" present amongst the other letters. They found that dyslexics performed significantly worse than controls when the different target stimuli were presented at intervals shorter than 1 second, suggesting that their attentional dwell time was radically longer, so that they were remarkably slower in disengaging the attention from previous items and switching from one target to another.

Disorders in attention shifting have been found not only in visual tasks, but also in spatial and auditory tasks (Facoetti et al. 2000, Asbiornsen and Bryden 1998). Attentional disorders have been reported also by Moores and colleagues (2003), who confirmed that dyslexics are impaired in shifting attention tasks, but not in focus attention tasks. They found that dyslexics did not perform differently from controls in terms of either accuracy or speed in focus attention tasks, requiring them to attend selectively to one single stimulus (e.g. a specific shape or color). Problems, instead, arose in shifting attention tasks, in which subjects were asked to identify two different stimuli alternately (e.g. white ovals and blue squares in a sequence of ovals, squares and other shapes painted in different colors). However, the authors propose that the attention shifting deficits were not determined by the rapid processing required to switch from one target to another, as proposed by other scholars, but rather they claimed that the problems shown by dyslexics seem to involve a more "central" component of attention. Specifically, they observed that the shifting attention task is more complex than the focus attention tasks, requiring the subject to maintain two targets in memory, instead of only one, while performing the detection task. Therefore, the shifting attention condition involves more attentional resources, which are evidently less readily available for dyslexic individuals.

To summarize, a number of studies have corroborated the teachers' reports of inattentive behavior in dyslexic children, confirming that dyslexics appear to have less attentional resources in comparison to their peers. Arguably, this deficiency can affect dramatically their performance in demanding tasks, leading to the high levels of distractibility and lack of concentration so typically reported.

3.7. Motor deficits

The range of deficits detected in dyslexic individuals is not only confined to the verbal and attentional domain; these deficits often extend to motor impairments as well.

Motor deficits, together with evidence of clumsiness, are frequently reported in the literature, even though their relationship to developmental dyslexia is still controversial, especially because many dyslexics can perform successfully in sports and in tasks requiring high degrees of manual dexterity.

Slight motor deficits associated with dyslexia include speed of tapping, rapid thumb-finger opposition, heel-toe placement and handwriting, as reviewed by Denckla (1985) and Rudel (1985), who argue that dyslexic children, even those who show athletic ability, suffer from a "non-specific developmental awkwardness" and are poorly coordinated. However, these deficits appear to be more marked during the acquisition of new skills, when performance is generally more effortful and requires more conscious attention. Once the skill is acquired, instead, the awkwardness gradually disappears and the child exhibits a normal performance. A fine-motricity deficit is also held responsible for the handwriting and copying difficulties so often exhibited by dyslexic children: the graphic performance, in fact, requires a good oculo-manual coordination. The same holds for tying shoelaces, another difficult task for dyslexic children, which involves also bimanual coordination. Early coordination difficulties are reported also in gross motor activities, such as riding a bicycle or swimming.

Haslum (1989) carried out a longitudinal study on a group of 12,905 children and found that performance on two motor coordination tests highly correlated with dyslexia at age 10. In the first test, the child had to catch a ball, throw it in the air and clap a specified number of times before catching it again: results showed that poor readers performed significantly worse in comparison to normally developing children. In the second task, instead, the subject had to walk backwards along a straight line for six steps: again, dyslexic children displayed more difficulties than controls.

Balance has been investigated by Nicolson and Fawcett (1990), who monitored the performance of dyslexics and normally-achieving children in three distinct tasks: standing on both feet with one foot directly in front of the other, standing on one foot and walking on a low beam. Both single task balance and dual task balance were performed: in the former, the child had merely to balance, whereas in the latter she had to balance while performing another secondary tasks, such as counting.

Results showed that dyslexic children performed as well as controls in single task balance, but that they were strikingly impaired under dual task conditions. Even more interestingly, this pattern applied to almost all the participants: 22 out of 23 of the dyslexics displayed a worsening under dual task conditions, whereas most controls actually improved. Similar results have been reported in a later work, with blindfolded balance replacing dual-task balance (Fawcett and Nicolson 1992).

In a further experiment Nicolson and Fawcett (1994) tested a whole range of motor skills in three groups of dyslexics aged 8, 12 and 16 years old and in three groups of age-matched normally achieving children. Specifically, they tested bead-threading, considering how many beads the child was able to thread in one minute, and pegboard peg moving, measuring the time needed by the subject to move a row of 10 pegs to the next row of a pegboard. The motor skill tests included also a variety of static balance tasks, standing on both feet or on one foot, on both feet blindfolded and dual task balance. Comparing dyslexic children's and control children's performance, the authors found an "extraordinarily poor performance" of all three dyslexic groups on all measures, and especially in bead threading, blindfold balance and dual task balance. Moreover, they argue that dyslexics show severe initial deficits but that they make progresses, improving with age in pegboard manipulation and normal balance, suggesting that learning processes are essentially intact. However, deficits persist in blindfold balance, with the oldest group of dyslexics, aged 16 years old, performing worse than the youngest group of controls, aged 8 years old. These results have been replicated in a later study, conducted by Fawcett and Nicolson (1995), who tested 8, 13 and 17 years old dyslexics and control children, in bead threading, pegboard peg moving and articulation rate. In this last task, subjects were asked to say a given word several times, as quickly as possible; stimuli included monosyllabic words (e.g. *bus*), two-syllable words (e.g. *monkey*) and three-syllable words (e.g. *butterfly*). As in the previous experiment, the authors found persistent deficits in all three groups of poor readers; the articulation rate task revealed difficulties even with the monosyllabic word, which affected also the performance of 17-year-old dyslexics. Fawcett and Nicolson take these results as a strong evidence for the presence of severe motor skill deficits in dyslexic children, which persist at least into late adolescence.

However, the relationship of motor impairments to developmental dyslexia is still unclear and debated. Ramus et al. (2003), in particular, tested motor skills in 16 dyslexics and 16 control university students and found that only four of the poor readers exhibited clear deficits. Specifically, they tested balance (both single task and dual task), bead threading, finger-to-thumb opposition (subjects had to touch the index finger of one hand with the thumb of the other hand and vice versa; then they had to rotate one hand clockwise and the other anticlockwise until index and thumb touched again), repetitive finger-tapping (subjects had to press repeatedly and quickly with one finger on a response box) and bimanual finger tapping (subjects had to tap for 30 seconds in synchrony with a metronome and when the metronome stopped they had to continue for 30 seconds at exactly the same speed). The authors reported motor problems just in some of the dyslexics (4 out of 16), taking this result as evidence for the fact that motor deficits are independent from dyslexia and that they affect only a part of dyslexic people.

However, the contrast between the results reported by Fawcett and Nicolson and the data found by Ramus and colleagues can be due to the different ages of the subjects tested in the experiment: the subjects who took part in Ramus et al.'s experiment were namely 21 years old. It should be kept in mind, in fact, that dyslexic children are generally said to display marked motor deficits during their infancy and adolescence, with their difficulties gradually disappearing in adulthood.

In a subsequent experiment White and colleagues (2006) reported a dissociation between sensorimotor impairments and reading abilities. They tested 23 dyslexic children, 22 autistic children (divided in good readers and poor readers) and 22 control children, all aged between 8 and 12 years. The experimental protocol comprised literacy tests (i.e. reading and spelling), phonology tests (i.e. rhyme, spoonerisms, non-word reading and rapid naming), auditory tests (i.e. categorization of phonemes), visual tests (e.g. motion coherence and form coherence: subjects viewed two panels on a screen and they had to judge which one contained the coherent signal) and motor tests, which involved bead threading, finger-to-thumb opposition, one-legged balance and heel-to-toe balance (subjects had to walk along a line with heel and toe touching). Results showed that dyslexics were impaired in literacy and phonology tasks, whereas they did not exhibit deficits in auditory and visual tasks. For what concerns motor tasks, instead, the authors found that 48% of dyslexics, 54% of autistic poor readers and 67% of autistic good readers were impaired in one or more tasks, whereas only 15% of controls showed problems. Moreover, they failed to find a correlation between sensorimotor abilities and reading difficulties, reporting that 6 autistic children displayed normal reading despite having one or more sensorimotor impairments and that 12 dyslexics had reading deficits without sensorimotor impairments.

In conclusion, White and colleagues argue that sensorimotor impairments do not necessarily cause reading abilities, since only a subset of dyslexics had sensory and/or motor impairments. Rather, they propose that sensorimotor impairments can be regarded as "more general nonspecific markers of neurodevelopmental disorders" and that they are secondary and independent from reading and phonological deficits.

However, one could object to the methodology used for this experiment: it is not clear, in fact, why the presence of a correlation has been searched considering also autistic subjects, in addition to dyslexics and controls. Furthermore, White and colleagues did not consider "pure" motor deficits, taking into account also visual and auditory deficits that were completely absent in dyslexic children.

To summarize, the presence of motor deficits in dyslexia is still controversial. Even though a number of studies have reported widespread and severe deficits in dyslexic children and adolescents, other works have failed to find links between dyslexia and motor deficits. However, it is wise to acknowledge the presence of additional motor disorders in certain dyslexic subjects: a complete theory of dyslexia, in fact, should also be able to explain why sensorimotor impairments occur more often in the dyslexics than in the general population, as recognized by Ramus himself in a subsequent work (Ramus 2003).

4. Precursors of Dyslexia

One of the major problems related to developmental dyslexia is that it can be diagnosed only after literacy exposure has started and therefore only in children older than 8 years old. However, a number of studies (Scarborough 1989, 1990, 1991a, 1991b; De Bree 2007; Wilsenach and Wijnen 2003; Rispens 2004) have demonstrated that it should be possible to recognize dyslexia during preschool years: there are, in fact, some signals that can be considered precursors of dyslexia and that would allow to identify the disorder in very young children.

This finding is supported by the longitudinal studies conducted on the so-called "at-risk children", that is those children who have dyslexic parents and/or older siblings with dyslexia. In the studies that I will review in this section, at-risk children's performance on a series of phonological and syntactic tasks is compared to the performance shown by children without family incidence of dyslexia. Interestingly, the experiments conducted comparing at-risk to control children have revealed that significant differences between the two groups are evident and identifiable already by the third year of life.

In a first longitudinal study, Scarborough tested 34 children at risk of dyslexia and 44 children from non-dyslexic families and demonstrated that reading abilities were strongly affected by family type: 65% of the at-risk children were actually diagnosed as dyslexics (23 out of 34), whereas only 5% of the control children manifested reading difficulties (2 out of 44). In order to identify the precursors of dyslexia, Scarborough divided the subjects into three groups: the "Dyslexic" group included those at-risk children who became poor readers, the "Family" group comprised the at-risk children who became instead good readers and the "Control" group was composed by children from non-dyslexic families who became good readers. Analyzing several natural language samples, the author found that at 30 months the "Dyslexic" children showed a syntactically and phonologically poorer proficiency in comparison to the children of the "Control" and the "Family" groups, who manifested a very similar, and more correct, behavior. In particular, dyslexics' utterances were shorter, less complex from a syntactic point of view and with a restricted range of syntactic constructions than those produced by their peers. Moreover, they showed a poorer vocabulary, were more impaired when asked to detect and produce rhymes and less accurate in the pronunciation of words.

At 60 months, in addition, the "Dyslexic children" performed more poorly than both groups of controls in tasks tapping phonemic awareness, knowledge of letter-sound correspondences, letter identification and picture naming accuracy. When 5 years old, in particular, the

"Dyslexic" group was less skilled than the "Control" group in identifying letters and in pairing pictures with the initial phonemes and graphemes of the corresponding words. Phonological difficulties in at-risk children have been also reported by De Bree (2007): in a first experiment she assessed speech production by means of a speech production task and she found that, consistently with the results presented by Scarborough, at-risk children manifest a delayed phonological behavior at 3–4 years old, producing shorter utterances and more phonological errors. In a further study, she reported a delay in word stress acquisition in at-risk children, who had more difficulty than controls at repeating non-words with irregular stress patterns and illegitimate stress. In addition, at-risk children appear to be remarkably poor when asked to repeat non-words, a task that is considered by the author as the most powerful predictor of reading failure.

Syntactic deficits have been reported by Wilsenach and Wijnen (2003), who found that at-risk children aged 18–23 months were not able to correctly discriminate between grammatical and ungrammatical sentences. In addition, sensitivity to subject-verb agreement has been found to be a reliable predictor for reading disabilities: Rispens (2004) reported that at-risk children were less able to recognize sentences containing agreement violations from grammatical sentences and that they performed more poorly than controls also in phonological awareness tasks and in letter knowledge tasks.

To summarize, a number of studies have demonstrated that early syntactic and phonological production abilities are strong predictors of upcoming reading and spelling disabilities and that it is possible to identify children who will be later diagnosed as dyslexics already by the age of two-three years old. These results are of crucial importance mainly for two reasons: first, they indicate that dyslexics' impairments are not confined to reading and that linguistic competence is generally affected. Secondly, they show that it is possible to identify dyslexia also in preschool years, before the child has begun to acquire reading and spelling skills.

5. Summary and Conclusions

In this chapter we have introduced the main topic of this book, developmental dyslexia, discussing its distribution, manifestations and precursors. We have observed that it is not easy to find a comprehensive definition of dyslexia able to capture all of its peculiarities.

First, we have noticed that reading and spelling difficulties can be more or less severe, depending on the transparency or opaqueness of the orthographic system adopted by each language. An English child, for instance, will have more reading and spelling problems in comparison to an Italian child, since the orthography of its mother-tongue is opaque and characterized by the presence of more than one possible mapping between graphemes and phonemes. Conversely, the difficulties experienced by an Italian child, whose mother-tongue has a transparent orthography, will be less evident and may go unnoticed. We have then argued that this discrepancy is responsible for the different percentages regarding the distribution of dyslexia as reported across different countries (e.g. 3–4% in Italy, 15–20% in USA).

Moreover, we have observed that reading and spelling difficulties are only the tip of the iceberg of the less well-known deficits manifested by dyslexic individuals. Linguistic competence, in particular, is so dramatically impaired that developmental dyslexia can be defined in terms of a learning disability that interferes especially with the acquisition of language skills.

The totality of the dyslexic population has been found to suffer from phonological deficits, which are persistent across ages and languages. Vocabulary disorders are also very widespread and predictive of dyslexia, as well as poor sensitivity to morphosyntactic violations. Moreover, dyslexics manifest remarkable difficulties in those tasks that appear to be particularly demanding in terms of processing resources, such as the interpretation of tough sentences, relative clauses, passive clauses, grammatical aspect and pronouns. In addition, attention deficits have been reported extensively in the dyslexic population.

Other symptoms, finally, affect the motor domain, even though the available evidence is in this respect still controversial. Given that motor deficits are not consistently acknowledged by researchers, I will not consider them as a typical manifestation of dyslexia and I will discuss them separately in Chapter 8.

We have then remarked that an early detection of dyslexia is possible, thanks to the presence of predictors, which signal reading and spelling difficulties even before the child starts to acquire literacy. Amongst these predictors, we have mentioned phonology and syntactic production skills, vocabulary development and letter knowledge.

To summarize, the major symptoms exhibited by dyslexic subjects concern:

(i) Reading deficits;
(ii) Spelling deficits;
(iii) Phonological deficits;
(iv) Vocabulary and naming speed deficits;
(v) Grammatical deficits;
(vi) Attention deficits.

In the following chapter, I will present the most important theories developed to account for developmental dyslexia, discussing how they explain dyslexics' difficulties and verifying to which extent they are capable of providing a justification for all of these symptoms.

Chapter 2

Developmental Dyslexia: Theoretical Perspectives

1. Introduction

The first speculations on developmental dyslexia are relatively recent: they date back to the nineteenth century, when some scholars began to study the cases of patients who lost their reading skills after a brain insult. The term "dyslexia", in fact, was coined in 1872 by the German physician Rudolf Berlin to describe the pathology of an adult affected by a sudden loss of reading ability, due to a brain lesion. The label "dyslexia" was then used to refer to an acquired disorder that was neurological in origin, since it was caused by a cerebral trauma.

The first mention of developmental dyslexia goes back to 1895, when the English optic surgeon James Hinshelwood published an article in the journal "The Lancet" referring to a "strange blindness for words" affecting some children who weren't able to acquire reading skills as efficiently and successfully as their peers. As the term "blindness" suggests, Hinshelwood was convinced that dyslexics' difficulties were caused by a deficit concerning the visual system.

This opinion was shared by another British physician, W. Pringle Morgan, who is generally considered the father of developmental dyslexia, and who reported the case of a fourteen boy named Percy unable to properly acquire reading despite showing a normal intelligence.

Another key figure in dyslexia's history persuaded of its visual origin was Samuel Torrey Orton, who coined the term "strephosymbolia", which literally means "twisted signs", maintaining that individuals with dyslexia had difficulty in associating the visual forms of words with their spoken forms (Orton 1925).

After Orton's studies, dyslexia became an interesting matter of analysis and debate also for psychologists, sociologists and educators, who began to consider environmental and psychological factors, such as the educative method and the family life, as possible causes of the disorder. Moreover, there was a general belief that dyslexia could be cured.

A radical shift in the hypothesis elaborated about dyslexia took place in the 1960s, when the French scientist Alfred Tomatis argued that dyslexia was due to a disorder affecting the auditory system and proposed a method (known as Tomatis' method) to solve dyslexics' problems.

These first hypotheses on dyslexia, which gave input respectively to the Visual and to the Auditory Theories of dyslexia, have been the most influential ones until the 1970s, when they were both discarded in favour of the more modern theories of dyslexia, as the Magnocellular Hypothesis, the Phonological Hypothesis, the Double Deficit Hypothesis and the more recent Working Memory Deficit Hypothesis.

In this chapter I will expose and discuss the most important theories that have been developed through the decades to explain developmental dyslexia. In order to discuss and evaluate both strengths and weaknesses of each proposal developed so far, I will refer to their ability to account for the manifestations of dyslexia examined in Chapter 1 and reported here for convenience:

(1) Manifestations of Dyslexia
(i) Reading deficits;
(ii) Spelling deficits;
(iii) Phonological deficits;
(iv) Vocabulary and naming speed deficits;
(v) Grammatical deficits;
(vi) Attention deficits.

I will first consider the Visual Deficit Hypothesis (paragraph 2.), the Auditory Deficit Hypothesis (paragraph 3.) and then the Magnocellular Deficit Hypothesis (paragraph 4.), which represents a more modern approach to the sensory (i.e. visual and auditory) deficits reported in dyslexic individuals. I will then concentrate more thoroughly on the Phonological Deficit Hypothesis, which focuses on the poor phonological awareness exhibited by dyslexia (paragraph 5.), and on the Double Deficit Hypothesis, which maintains that both phonological and naming disorders are crucial in dyslexia (paragraph 6.).

Finally, I will introduce the Working Memory Deficit Hypothesis, which claims that dyslexia is intimately linked to an inefficiency affecting the working memory system. I will illustrate the concept of working memory, discussing the influential model developed by Alan Baddeley and the peculiarities of its components. I will also focus on the development of working memory skills considering the disorders found in individuals suffering from working memory impairments. Finally, I will present McLoughlin and colleagues' (2002) proposal, according to which dyslexia can be defined as a working memory inefficiency and Fiorin's (2010) Verbal Working Memory Deficit Hypothesis.

I will then argue that these last proposals, which will be further refined and discussed in Chapter 4, constitute the most complete and reliable account of developmental dyslexia and provide the most adequate basis of explanation for all its manifestations.

2. The Visual Deficit Hypothesis

In the framework of the Visual Deficit Hypothesis, visuo-perceptual impairments are held responsible for the difficulties experienced by dyslexics in learning to read. Specifically, dyslexia is considered primarily as a deficit affecting visuo-spatial processing and causing a faulty visual perception, which in turn determines the difficulties in acquiring reading skills.

As anticipated in the Introduction, the Visual Deficit Hypothesis basically constitutes the first approach proposed to explain developmental dyslexia, starting from scholars as Hinshelwood, who noted that dyslexic children seemed to manifest a strange "blindness" for words, and Orton, who suggested that dyslexics perceive letters and words as reversed forms. Other researchers have argued that dyslexics suffer from visual processing deficits affecting visual sequences and visual memory, like erratic eye movement and eye convergence deficits, and that these problems cause their reading difficulties.

The visual theory of dyslexia was widely accepted until the 1960s-1970s, when it was severely criticized by Vellutino's seminal work (1979), in which he proved that visuo-perceptual disorders do not really play a significant role in dyslexia. Replicating some of the experiments conducted by the supporters of the Visual Deficit Hypothesis, Vellutino found that there were few significant differences between dyslexics and controls when the influence of verbal coding was controlled. For instance, he noted that dyslexics underperformed when they were asked to recall orally a sequence of visually presented similar letters (e.g. "b" and "d"), whereas they performed as well as controls when a written response was required. This difference seems to suggest that the difficulties found in dyslexics are due to phonological more than to strictly visual reasons.

Moreover, it has been demonstrated that visual skills are poor predictors of reading abilities, indicating that reading difficulties cannot be determined by visual factors, but are more likely due to a linguistic impairment.

However, low-level visual deficits such as oculomotor deficiencies and visual-tracking problems have been recently found in dyslexic individuals. The presence of these disorders has given input to a modern proposal about the causes of dyslexia, the Magnocellular Deficit Hypothesis, which will be discussed below.

To summarize, the Visual Deficit Hypothesis cannot be considered as a valid account for developmental dyslexia, since it is not able to explain its core manifestations reported in (1).

3. The Auditory Deficit Hypothesis

The father of the Auditory Deficit Hypothesis of dyslexia is Alfred Tomatis. At the end of the 1960s, he proposed that dyslexia was caused by an auditory deficit, interfering with the child's phonological competence. Specifically, Tomatis and the other supporters of the Auditory Deficit Hypothesis proposed that auditory perception deficits were the core disorder characterizing dyslexia: an impaired perception of the distinctive speech sound could, in fact, determine phonological deficits and, as a consequence, reading and spelling problems. Supporters of the Auditory Deficit Hypothesis, therefore, do not deny the existence of phonological deficits in dyslexics, but rather claim that these deficits are secondary to a more general auditory impairment in sound perception.

A number of studies have examined auditory perception in dyslexics, even if only a fraction of them showed poor performance in auditory tasks. Tallal (1980, 1984), for instance, found that dyslexic children display deficits affecting the rate at which they can process incoming auditory information, since dyslexics' auditory processing was mainly impaired on short sounds and fast transitions. For this reason, the disorder exhibited by dyslexics was dubbed as "rapid" or "temporal" auditory processing deficit, giving rise to the Auditory Temporal Processing Deficit Hypothesis or Rapid Auditory Processing Hypothesis of dyslexia (Tallal 1980).

Nevertheless, this theory presents problems as well: only a part of dyslexic children, in fact, have been found impaired in auditory tests in further studies. Moreover, Snowling (2001) and Ramus and colleagues (2003) have shown that there is no reliable relationship between dyslexics' performance on rapid auditory processing tasks and speech categorization and discrimination, indicating that there cannot be a causal connection between the auditory deficit and the phonological impairment. On the contrary, they observed that some dyslexics do preserve auditory abilities despite phonological difficulties. This fact demonstrates unequivocally that phonological deficits can arise in absence of auditory impairments and that therefore the poor phonological competence cannot be secondary to auditory deficits, as the Auditory Deficit Hypothesis claims. However, auditory deficits have been more recently reconsidered in the framework of the Magnocellular Deficit Hypothesis, which will be discussed below.

To summarize, the Auditory Deficit Hypothesis cannot account for the manifestations of dyslexia reviewed in (1) and cannot thus be considered an adequate framework for developmental dyslexia.

4. The Magnocellular Deficit Hypothesis

As anticipated above, low-level visual processing deficits have been recently reported in dyslexic individuals, leading researchers to the formulation of an influential hypothesis, known as the Magnocellular Deficit Hypothesis, which develops and revises some aspects of the Visual Deficit Hypothesis and, partly, of the Auditory Deficit Hypothesis as well. Many of the visual and auditory deficits detected in dyslexic people, in fact, have been interpreted as symptoms of an impairment affecting the magnocellular system (see Nicolson and Fawcett 2008 and Beaton 2004 for a review).

In this paragraph, I will review this hypothesis very briefly, introducing the subdivision between the visual and auditory systems and reporting some data pointing to a magnocellular deficit in dyslexia. Then I will show how the hypothesis tentatively explains reading deficits as a consequence of magnocellular impairments.

4.1. The Magnocellular Systems and its disruption in Dyslexia

In neurological terms, the visual system and the auditory system are served by two distinct pathways, the magnocellular and the parvocellular systems. The magnocellular system is characterized by large neurons (whence their name) with high conduction velocity and great sensitiveness to low spatial frequencies, as rapid changes and movements in the visual field. In other words, they are able to transmit visual information very quickly, but they convey less detailed signals. Conversely, the parvocellular system consists of smaller neurons that respond better to high spatial frequencies and are more sensitive to color and fine spatial details.

Different studies have revealed that dyslexic people seem to suffer from an impairment affecting the magnocellular system, which is responsible for the low-level visual processing deficit mentioned above (see Stein and Walsh 1997; Stein 2001). Dyslexics, in fact, have been found to show reduced sensitivity to low spatial frequencies, especially at slow level of luminance, suggesting that there is an impairment affecting the magnocellular system. Lovegrove and colleagues (1986), and Martin and Lovegrove (1987) reported that dyslexics are less sensitive to the contrast between a series of narrow black and white gratings in comparison to controls and that their sensitivity is further reduced when these gratings flickered. Similarly, Evans and colleagues (1994) found that dyslexics show minor sensitivity to low and medium spatial frequencies; moreover, they are worse than controls at detecting flicker and slower when asked to identify a digit from an array of digits. Since identifying rapidly changing visual stimuli depends on the activity of the magnocells, it has been proposed that the magnocellular system is impaired in dyslexics.

A similar proposal has been developed to account for the deficit affecting the processing of rapid auditory stimuli reported by Tallal and colleagues (1980, 1984), who found that dyslexic children are slower than controls at identifying rapidly changing auditory stimuli. Therefore, they formulated the Rapid Auditory Processing Hypothesis, arguing that the phonological difficulties exhibited by dyslexics may be caused by an inability to distinguish and identify speech sounds, due to their defective rapid auditory processing. However, as mentioned in the preceding section, this proposal has been contradicted by the finding that only a part of dyslexics suffer from auditory disorders.

To capture both visual and auditory aspects, it has been proposed that a "pansensory" magnocellular abnormality is responsible for the difficulties experienced by dyslexics in rapid processing of both types of stimuli (cf. Nicolson and Fawcett 2008). In the following section, we will see how these anomalies are claimed to account for reading deficits.

4.2. Reading deficits as a consequence of magnocellular disorders

The Magnocellular Deficit Hypothesis claims that dyslexic people suffer from an impairment affecting their magnocellular system and causing a reduced sensitivity to rapidly changing stimuli. According to the proponents of the theory, this deficit is also responsible for the reading difficulties experienced by dyslexics. The magnocellular system, in fact, is highly operative during reading, being involved in the saccadic movement of the eyes, whereas the parvocellular system is operative during fixation and generates a visual trace that persists for approximately 250 milliseconds. One of the tasks performed by the magnocells during reading is to inhibit the activity of the parvocells when the eyes are in motion, in order to suppress this trace and to avoid the visual confusion that it could create. Proponents of the Magnocellular Deficit Hypothesis, thus, argued that precisely this mechanism is defective in dyslexia: it has been suggested, in fact, that a specific impairment prevents the magnocellular system from suppressing the visual trace left by the parvocellular system, creating a masking effect that makes reading a much more difficult task (cf. Vellutino 2004). Arguably, this would have a dramatic impact on the acquisition of reading skills.

However, this proposal has been severely criticized, in particular by Hulme (1988), who observed that it would not predict reading difficulties when words are presented one at a time. Since dyslexics commit errors also in single words and nonwords reading, it cannot be argued that their difficulties are due to the masking effect created by a malfunctioning of the magnocellular system. It could rather be, as Vellutino and colleagues argue, that the persistence of the visual trace is a correlate, rather than a cause, of reading disabilities.

Although it is one of the most investigated models of dyslexia, the Magnocellular Deficit Hypothesis has been judged inadequate to explain the disorder for the following reasons. First, it is not the case that all dyslexics suffer from magnocellular deficits and that magnocellular problems affect only people with dyslexia. Secondly, it is implausible that the deficit causing dyslexia is related exclusively to the magnocellular system, as shown by Skottun (2000).

Moreover, referring to the manifestations of dyslexia reported in (1), we can observe that the Magnocellular Deficit Hypothesis could only explain (to some – and not uncontroversial – extent) reading difficulties and phonological difficulties, whereas it could not justify the other main manifestations of dyslexia discussed in Chapter 1, like vocabulary, grammatical and attention deficits.

Therefore, this hypothesis cannot be considered a convincing and exhaustive framework for dyslexia.

5. The Phonological Deficit Hypothesis

The Phonological Deficit Hypothesis has been considered the dominant explanatory framework for dyslexia and it has obtained wide consensus in the last decades, since it provides a reliable account for the difficulties experienced by dyslexic individuals in reading and spelling tasks, as well as for their poor phonological awareness.

In short, this approach claims that the underlying cause of developmental dyslexia is poor phonological coding[1]; as a consequence, dyslexics would suffer from a specific impairment affecting the representation, storage, manipulation and retrieval of speech sounds. In other words, the hypothesis maintains that dyslexics code phonological information less precisely and less efficiently than unimpaired individuals; their weak phonological coding is thus held responsible for reading and spelling difficulties.

As discussed in Chapter 1, phonological deficits are indeed very widespread among dyslexics, affecting the totality of the dyslexic population. The central issue of the Phonological Deficit Hypothesis is the belief that poor reading and spelling arise precisely from a weakness in the phonological domain. Specifically, the incapacity to acquire the regular relationships between spelling and sound, which is typical of dyslexia, has been attributed to a difficulty in analyzing the sound structure of the target language.

This proposal is also consistent with the predictions made by Frith's model discussed in Chapter 1, which claims that phonological segmentation and blending skills are crucial in the acquisition of reading, suggesting that poor phonological awareness may hinder the acquisition of the alphabetic strategy and, as a consequence, the development of reading.

As argued in Chapter 1, phonological awareness is a metalinguistic skill concerning the individual's conscious knowledge of the phonological structure of words and is fundamental for a correct and effective acquisition of reading and spelling. Significantly, preschool children at

1 Phonological coding is the ability to use speech code to analyze and represent the structure of words.

risk of dyslexia, dyslexic children and adults have been found impaired in tasks assessing phonological awareness, suggesting that their poor performance has a dramatic effect on phonological competence, as well as on reading and spelling.

Two different hypotheses have been provided to explain phonological deficits in dyslexic people: a first proposal argues that phonological representations are underspecified, whereas a second approach claims that they are intact but more difficult to be accessed.

Before we analyze these hypotheses, we will try to answer two important questions. First, are dyslexic children really impaired in comparison to control children, or are they simply lagging behind their chronological age-matched peers? And secondly, are reading difficulties caused by phonological problems or, conversely, are phonological deficits caused by reading difficulties?

5.1. Deficit or delay? The Developmental Lag Hypothesis

Observing dyslexic children's performance in phonological tasks, as well as in reading and spelling task, it appears that they perform as children younger than them, suggesting that they are simply lagging behind age-matched normally achieving children. This argument is defended by the proponents of the so-called Developmental Lag Hypothesis, claiming that dyslexic children's deficits are not caused by a persistent phonological disorder, but rather by a developmental delay that is responsible for the differences detected between them and their peers.

However, this hypothesis has been criticized and disconfirmed by the results of longitudinal studies showing that dyslexics' deficits persist over time. The Developmental Lag Hypothesis, in fact, predicts that dyslexics' performance would improve and that they could eventually catch up with normal readers. Contrary to this expectation, longitudinal studies have demonstrated that dyslexic children persistently fall behind both chronological-age and reading-age peers (Manis et al. 1993; Snowling et al. 1996). In this respect, studies on adults are particularly interesting, since they show that phonological deficits are persistent also in adulthood. Specifically, Felton and colleagues (1990) found that adult dyslexics are significantly impaired in phonological awareness, non-word reading and rapid naming tasks, whereas Gross-Glen and colleagues (1990) report that the most sensitive measure of deficits in dyslexic adults is non-sense passage reading. Even those dyslexics who successfully employ compensation strategies to bypass their initial literacy difficulties, showing normal reading and spelling skills, in fact, perform remarkably poorly in phonological awareness tasks (Paulesu et al. 1996).

Similar results were reported by Snowling and colleagues (1997), who administered a set of phonological tests to a group composed by dyslexic university students, showing that they perform worse than age and educationally matched controls on all of the tasks, and in particular on phonological awareness tasks, phonemic and semantic fluency[2] tasks and non-word reading.

These findings are important for two reasons: on the one side they permit to confute the Developmental Lag Hypothesis, and on the other side they confirm that poor phonological sensitivity is one of the most distinctive aspects persisting also in adult dyslexics, even when they have reached a satisfactory reading level.

5.2. Phonological deficits causing or caused by poor reading?

Another question to be answered concerns the causal chain linking phonological competence and reading failure. It may in fact be unclear whether poor phonological skills are the cause or rather the consequence of poor reading.

However, this dilemma can be easily solved by recalling the main studies on the phonological deficits exhibited by dyslexics, which have been discussed in Chapter 1. A first evidence demonstrating that reading difficulties do not cause phonological difficulties is provided by the studies conducted on children at familiar risk of dyslexia, showing that phonological deficits are evident also in preschool children and therefore much before reading instruction.

2 In phonemic fluency tasks subjects are given a phoneme and asked to produce as many words as possible starting with that phoneme in a limited period of time. In semantic fluency tasks participants are asked to provide as many examples of a category as possible in a limited period of time.

Another source of evidence is provided by the studies testing phonological awareness in dyslexic children and control children matched for reading age. The results reported in these studies reveal that impaired children display a very poor performance also in comparison to reading age-matched controls, demonstrating that reading difficulties cannot be considered the cause of phonological deficits. If it were the case, in fact, we would expect that children matched for reading age perform at the same level in phonological tasks.

Finally, the results of cross-linguistic and intervention studies further confirm that phonological deficits are not determined by reading deficits. First of all, it has been found that dyslexic children whose mother-tongue has a transparent orthography are highly impaired in phonological tasks, despite showing a relatively spared reading competence.

Summarizing, there is uncontroversial evidence that reading difficulties are not the cause of phonological deficits. Rather, it appears that prior existing phonological deficits are responsible for reading and spelling difficulties, in full agreement with the proponents of the Phonological Deficit Hypothesis.

5.3. Underspecified phonological representations or difficulties in accessing them?

Once ascertained the presence of remarkable phonological deficits in dyslexic children, another question arises, regarding the exact nature of the impairment causing these difficulties. It has been originally proposed that phonological representations are underspecified or degraded in dyslexic individuals, but a more recent hypothesis claims that their representations are intact and that problems rather concern their ability to correctly access them.

The first hypothesis claims that poor phonological awareness might reflect an underspecification of phonological representations, rather than a lack of phonological analysis skills (Elbro 1996; Snowling and Hulme 1994). Specifically, phonological representations may be fuzzier, or noisier, or underspecified, or degraded due to a sparser or insufficient resolution (i.e. their units of phonological representation may be larger than phonemes). Assuming that phonological representations are underspecified, it should not be surprising that dyslexics have trouble while performing operations on those representations, as in phonological decoding and phonological awareness tasks. Evidence in favour of this hypothesis comes from the experiment conducted by Swan and Goswami (1997a), aiming at verifying whether the phonological awareness skills of dyslexics and both chronologically age matched controls and reading age matched controls were better on fully specified or underspecified words. The central experimental question was to discover whether dyslexics would make errors also when asked to read words whose phonological representations had been already accurately specified. To assess the accuracy of phonological representations, in fact, Swan and Goswami asked each participant to name the pictures of the words that they were going to use in the phonological awareness tasks. Afterwards, they presented subjects with a set of phonological awareness tasks. Results showed that dyslexics' performance is indeed affected by the nature of their phonological representations: in fact, they perform better when they have a precise phonological representation of the word tested in the experiment. This finding, therefore, seems to suggest that dyslexics' errors are caused by underspecified phonological representation.

However, as stated by Fowler (1991), the quality of phonological representations can be enhanced over time, gradually becoming more detailed and organized; consequently, the representations of familiar words may become fully specified, whereas the representations of less familiar items are more likely to remain fuzzier and incomplete. This would explain why dyslexics show greater difficulties when asked to read unfamiliar words and non-words, whereas they exhibit a relatively spared performance with more frequently used items. Nevertheless, the phonological representations deficit persists also in adulthood, as shown by the study conducted by Snowling and colleagues (1997), who argue that dyslexics' phonological difficulties stem from a developmental inability to establish phonological representations, which remain underspecified and therefore difficult to access, disturbing the generalization of orthography to phonology mappings.

An alternative and more recent hypothesis is proposed by Ramus and Szenkovits (2008), who claim that phonological representations are in themselves intact, suggesting that dyslexics' difficulties are rather due to a deficit in the access to phonological representations, related to a lower capacity of their short-term memory[3]. In fact, the results of a whole series of experiments conducted in their lab show that dyslexics' phonological representations are basically intact and that problems arise only under certain conditions, requiring high short-term memory resources, conscious awareness and time constraints. Specifically, they wanted to assess if dyslexics manifested the phonological similarity effect[4] normally shown by unimpaired people. Therefore, they asked a group of adult dyslexics and a group of controls to discriminate two sequences of nonwords differing only for one phonetic feature (e.g. [taz] vs. [taʒ]) and two sequences of maximally different nonwords (e.g. [taz] vs. [gum]).

Results showed that dyslexics were more impaired than controls in discriminating between the two sequences but that they did show a phonological similarity effect as controls; in particular, dyslexics' performance improved by the same magnitude as for controls when the phonological similarity decreased. These data are consistent with the results of other experimental protocols revealing that dyslexics do not behave differently from controls in tasks assessing the phonological similarity effect (Hall et al. 1983, Johnston et al. 1987). Ramus and Szenkovits interpreted these results as evidence for the fact that phonological representations are not degraded in dyslexics: if they were, the confusion and hence the phonological similarity effect should have been higher in dyslexics than in controls. Conversely, they proposed that the deficit does not lie in the phonological representations as such, but rather in the short-term memory processes operating on these representations, indicating that the difficulties typically exhibited by dyslexics arise from an impairment affecting their verbal short-term memory.

Similar results have been reported more recently by Ramus et al. (2013), who tested dyslexic children's performance in tasks assessing their phonological competence, comparing their performance to that

3 Short-term memory refers to the ability to temporarily maintain sequences of items for immediate recall. For more details, see section 7.

4 The Phonological similarity effects predicts that the ordered recall of items is poorer when they are phonologically similar than when they are dissimilar. For a detailed review of this effect, see section 7.

shown by children suffering from Specific Language Impairment (SLI)[5] in order to analyze the presence of differences between the two populations. The authors found that dyslexics' phonological deficits are more evident in tasks assessing their phonological awareness (e.g. rhyme detection, spoonerisms, digit naming and digit span) than in tasks assessing the integrity of their phonological representations. Their phonological representations were tested using tasks specifically designed to decrease the load on verbal short-term memory. Consistently with previous results, data demonstrated that dyslexics' phonological representations do not appear to be degraded, as they are in SLI children.

This consideration provides further support to the hypothesis according to which the phonological problems exhibited by dyslexics are not due to the representations themselves, but more likely to some cognitive skills applying to them, such as verbal short term memory and working memory (Ramus et al. 2013; Ramus and Ahissar 2012, Mundy and Carroll 2012).

This second hypothesis, which I find more convincing, will be discussed more thoroughly in the following sections. For the time being, I would like to conclude this paragraph identifying both strengths and weaknesses of the Phonological Deficit Hypothesis.

5.4. *Strengths and weaknesses of the Phonological Deficit Hypothesis*

Undoubtedly, the Phonological Deficit Hypothesis has the advantage of offering a coherent framework for developmental dyslexia, which is able to account for reading and spelling difficulties and for phonological deficits. The fact that phonological deficits are so common and widespread in the dyslexic population provides further convincing evidence in favor of this hypothesis.

5 SLI is a neurodevelopmental disorder affecting approximately 7% of the population and characterized by language abilities below age expectations, despite normal cognitive abilities and absence of physical and neurological deficits (Leonard, 1998; Rice 2004). Children with SLI present a delay in their language, which does not get resolved over time and display deficits in comparison to their typically developing peers in the phonological, lexical and morphosyntactic domains.

However, although it represents the most influential and investigated theory on dyslexia, the Phonological Deficit Hypothesis cannot provide a complete account for all the problems that dyslexics must face, as summarized in (1) above. Representative in this regard is the comment by Scarborough (1990) who argues that "plausible though this hypothesis might be, it may not provide a complete explanation of reading failure" (1739).

The two most relevant limits of this theory, in fact, are that phonological deficits cannot explain all the symptoms manifested by dyslexics and, moreover, that they are not specific to dyslexia, since they are shared by those non-dyslexic individuals whose phonological competence is impaired. Phonological deficits alone, for instance, cannot explain either the language comprehension difficulties or the vocabulary/naming deficits or the attention disorder reviewed in Chapter 1. Particularly significant in this respect is the experiment conducted by Byrne (1981) to assess the comprehension of the so called "tough sentences", which are characterized by similar phonological structure but different syntactic structure (see Chapter 1, paragraph 3.5.1.). As shown by Byrne, those sentences that are more complex from a syntactic point of view are much more difficult to understand for dyslexics in comparison to less complex, but phonologically similar, sentences. If phonological limitations were the only deficit characterizing dyslexia, one should not expect this difference. Dyslexics, in fact, should rather show the same performance with syntactically more complex and simpler sentences, given that their phonological structures are very similar.

The same reasoning holds also for the other experimental protocol discussed in Chapter 1 and demonstrating that dyslexics' grammatical competence is impaired: the Phonological Deficit Hypothesis alone, in fact, cannot explain the difficulties manifested in the interpretation of pronouns and grammatical aspect and in the comprehension of relative and passive clauses. Furthermore, a phonological disorder can explain neither vocabulary deficits nor difficulties with rapid naming tasks.

Summarizing, the Phonological Deficit Hypothesis can account for a range of symptoms manifested by dyslexics, comprising reading and spelling problems and phonological deficits, including poor phonological awareness, difficulties in analyzing the internal word structure and identifying the sequence of phonemes. Nonetheless, it cannot be considered an adequate theory of dyslexia, since it is not able to explain all the deficits manifested by dyslexic individuals. In this regard, and to conclude, I would like to report a particularly effective metaphor proposed by Nicolson and Fawcett.

> We know there is pollution (phonological difficulties) at the river's estuary, but to establish its cause we seem to have no alternative to tracing the river and tributaries back to the source of pollution.
> (Nicolson and Fawcett 2008: 153)

6. The Double Deficit Hypothesis

The Double Deficit Hypothesis has been developed by Wolf and Bowers (1999) to account for both phonological and naming deficits in dyslexic individuals and it represents a development and an extension of the Phonological Deficit Hypothesis. The proponents of the Double Deficit Hypothesis, indeed, point out that the phonological deficit is not the core disorder in dyslexia, as claimed by the proponents of the Phonological Deficit Hypothesis: there is, actually, a second fundamental disorder, the naming speed deficit, which is independent from the phonological deficit and even more effective and reliable in predicting dyslexia.

As reviewed in Chapter 1, naming speed deficits are detected by means of the Rapid Automatized Naming test, during which subjects are asked to name as quickly as possible visually presented stimuli such as alphanumeric characters, colors and drawings of simple objects. Dyslexic children and adults have been found to be considerably slower than their peers on all RAN measures (see Wolf et al. 2000 for a detailed and comprehensive review of the studies performed between 1972 and 1999).

In the framework of the Phonological Deficit Hypothesis, naming speed deficits are generally subsumed under phonological deficits. However, Wolf and colleagues (1999; 2000) challenged this view, arguing that the internal complexity of naming speed tasks goes beyond phonological processing, requiring attentional, visual, conceptual, memory, lexical and articulatory processes. In their model, attentional processes activate the visual processes necessary to identify the symbol or picture to name and immediately afterwards conceptual processes are accessed to recognize the stimulus and match it with its already stored mental representation. Lexical processes are then activated, involving both the phonological form of the word, its semantic content and retrieval mechanisms. Finally, motor commands allow the articulation of the phonological information in a known word. The demands of rapid and serial processing typical of the RAN tasks contribute to increase the general processing complexity of this task.

According to Wolf and colleagues, the processes required to accomplish these tasks show that rapid naming involves radically different resources in comparison to phonological tasks. Moreover, they argue that the distinct processes required for rapid naming explain why this kind of task is able to predict reading disabilities, given that both rapid naming and reading involve rapid and serial processing, engaging attentional, visual, conceptual, memory, lexical and articulatory processes. The authors propose that naming speed deficits reflect a larger systemic timing deficit, which goes beyond language. They observe, in fact, that differences between dyslexics and controls arise when stimuli are presented serially at fast levels of speed and disappear when they are presented at longer intervals. This finding suggests that the requisites of rapidity and seriation are particularly demanding for dyslexic children. Moreover, they observe that deficits appear also in the other domains in which speed is involved; therefore, they propose that dyslexics' difficulties may indeed be determined by a general timing deficit, even though they admit that more evidence is needed before any conclusion can be drawn.

Beyond the different cognitive requirements entailed by RAN and phonological processes, Wolf and colleagues provide other sources of evidence to demonstrate that naming deficits cannot be subsumed under phonological disorders. First, they observe that the naming deficit occurs across different ages and, most of all, it appears to be specific to dyslexia. In fact, studies conducted on nondiscrepant readers (i.e. poor readers whose reading level is expected on the basis of their general intellectual development) were faster than dyslexics and closer to average readers' latencies. Similarly, other learning disabled children without reading disabilities were unimpaired in RAN tasks. The same does not hold for phonological deficits, which can be found in other disorders, while naming deficits are typical and distinctive for dyslexia.

Secondly, they note that naming deficits in dyslexia have been found consistently across different languages. Conversely, phonological deficits can go unnoticed in languages with a transparent orthography, leading Wolf and colleagues to observe that "when phonological analysis demands placed on young readers are reduced in languages with a more regular orthography, the naming-speed deficit appears as the dominant diagnostic indicator for at-risk readers" (Wolf et al. 2000: 420).

As a consequence, the third evidence is provided by the fact that naming deficits can predict reading difficulties independently from phonological awareness tasks: the studies conducted by Bowers and her colleagues (1991; 1993) revealed that phonological awareness tasks are very reliable at predicting nonword reading, but less effective at detecting word and text reading speed. These factors are, instead, better signaled by naming speed tasks, which have been found independently related to both accuracy and speed of word identification.

On the basis of these arguments, proponents of the Double-Deficit Hypothesis argue that naming speed deficits and phonological deficits are two key characteristics of dyslexia and two separable causes of reading disorders. According to the presence of only one or both deficits, dyslexics can be subdivided in three groups, as reported below.

(i) Phonological subtype: individuals belonging to this group are characterized by poor performance on phonological tasks, word attack and reading comprehension, but they display an intact performance on naming speed tasks.

(ii) Naming speed subtype: these subjects have remarkable problems on naming speed tasks, timed reading, fluency measures and reading comprehension, but their phonological competence is spared.

(iii) Double deficit subtype: these dyslexics are impaired in both phonological and naming speed deficit tasks and in all aspects of reading. Arguably, the presence of both deficits gives rise to the most severe form of reading disability, probably because the co-occurrence of both deficits allows limited compensatory strategies.

Adopting this criterion, Lovett and colleagues (2000) classified a large group composed of 140 dyslexic children aged between 7 and 13 according to the presence of phonological and naming disorders and found that the majority (54,3%) suffered from both deficits, whereas 22,1% had only phonological deficits and 23,6% only naming speed deficits. Interestingly, children classified in the double-deficit subtype showed the worst performance in all measures of reading development and displayed the most severe disorders in all aspects of written language acquisition.

To summarize, the Double Deficit Hypothesis can account for reading and spelling deficits, phonological deficits and rapid naming deficits. However, it has been criticized for both theoretical and methodological problems. Vellutino and colleagues (2004), in particular, challenged the proposal that dyslexics' difficulties can be caused by a general timing deficit, arguing that this argument lacks psychological reality and does not readily generate testable hypotheses. The classification of dyslexics in three subgroups on the basis of phonological awareness and rapid naming tasks has also been criticized for methodological problems. Furthermore, the hypothesis cannot be considered an adequate theory of dyslexia, since it cannot explain the occurrence of grammatical and attention deficits, as those described in Chapter 1. Hence, we have to move towards a new and more comprehensive proposal.

7. The Working Memory Deficit Hypothesis

Observing the deficits manifested by dyslexic children and reviewed in Chapter 1, it appears that difficulties arise proportionately to the increasing complexity of the task that the subjects have to accomplish. This consideration underpins the intuition that dyslexics' problems may be linked to a deficit in their processing abilities or, more specifically, to their working memory resources. As I will review in the following sections, the existence of a noticeable relationship between the deficits exhibited by poor readers and their working memory has been proposed and highlighted by a number of scholars, even though no specific hypothesis about the exact nature of these processing deficits in dyslexia has been formally proposed.

In the following sections, I will introduce the topic, illustrating the more influential models of working memory and devoting special attention to Baddeley's model. I will then review the literature relating working memory skills to language, cognitive development and neurodevelopmental disorders. Finally, I will review the studies suggesting the existence of working memory inefficiencies in dyslexia.

7.1. What is Working Memory?

The concept of Working Memory (WM) was coined in 1960 by Miller and colleagues, who laid the foundation of modern cognitive psychology investigating how the human mind is able to plan and control actions. Specifically, their insight was that there must be "a special place in the mind" devoted to the temporary storage of information, which they call "working memory".

> Particularly if it is a transient, temporary kind of Plan that will be used today and never again, we need some special place to store it. The special place may be on a sheet of paper. Or (who knows?) it may be somewhere in the frontal lobes of the brain. Without committing ourselves to any specific machinery, therefore, we should like to speak of the memory we use for the execution of our Plans as a kind of quick-access, "working memory".
> (Miller et al. 1960: 65)

Working memory was firstly conceptualized as a system deputed to retain and execute plans and goals, which seemed to be located in the frontal lobes. The frontal lobes, in fact, were considered as central components for cognitive processes, especially after the experiments conducted on patients presenting lesions in the prefrontal cortex and exhibiting short-term memory deficits (see Benton 1991 for a review). Moreover, the presence of spared long-term memory processes in patients with impaired short-term memory that had been reported by several studies, suggested that long-term memory (LTM) and short-term memory (STM) should be separated.

One of the first and most accredited models of memory is the one postulated by Atkinson and Shiffrin (1968). According to their proposal, the flow of information is handled by a sequence of three stages, namely a sensory storage, a short-term memory and a long-term memory. The model is exemplified below in Figure 2.1.

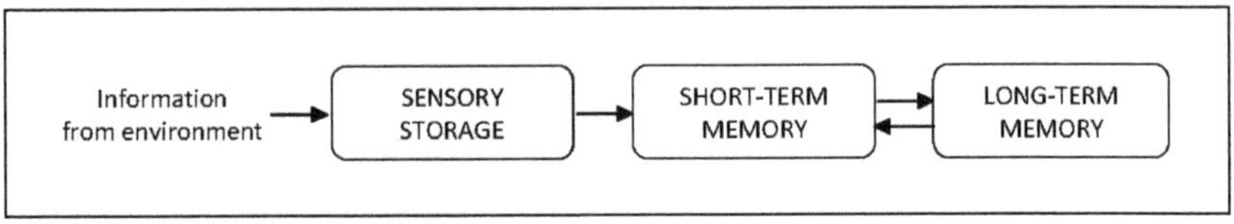

Figure 2.1. Atkinson and Shiffrin's Model of Human Memory.

In Atkinson and Shiffrin's model, information is first processed by sense organs and it flows afterwards into a Short-Term Memory (STM), where it is temporarily maintained through rehearsal operations. Subsequently, STM feeds information into the Long-Term Memory (LTM), which can retain it from minutes to a lifetime. STM is twofold connected to LTM: it allows both the permanent storage of new information in LTM and the retrieval of already stored information from LTM. Given the importance of these functions, STM is considered a central component in cognitive processes and it is viewed by Atkinson and Shiffrin also as a Working Memory, in virtue of its ability to solve problems, direct the information flow and take decisions.

The main difficulty of this model is that it cannot explain why people with impaired STM exhibit a spared LTM, since STM is explicitly considered the only way to access information stored in LTM and to store new lasting information. Baddeley and Hitch (1974) solved this dilemma by arguing that the problem lied in the unitary nature of working memory entailed in Atkinson and Shiffrin's model: they proposed a three-component model of working memory, which became the most influential and well-known model of WM and which I will present and discuss in the following sections.

7.2. Baddeley and Hitch's Original Model of Working Memory

Differently from Atkinson and Shiffrin (1968), Baddeley and Hitch (1974) refer to Working Memory (WM) as a multi-component system, capable of more complex operations than simply temporary storage. Specifically, they propose that temporary memory processes should be seen as the product of a general cognitive mechanism that is responsible for both the storage and the manipulation of information.

In its first formulation, the model was composed by three distinct components: a limited capacity attentional controller, called Central Executive, and two slave subsystems, one performing operations with acoustic and verbal information, dubbed Articulatory (subsequent Phonological) Loop, and the other concerned with visual and spatial information, named Visuo-Spatial Scratchpad (subsequent Sketchpad).

As we will see in the following section, the model has been further implemented by Baddeley (2000), who added a fourth component, the Episodic Buffer, responsible for the integration of the verbal and visual materials stored by the subsidiary systems and retrieved from long term memory, allowing at the same time their manipulation and maintenance.

In this multi-component model, Working memory is defined as the "brain system that provides temporary storage and manipulation of the information necessary for such cognitive tasks as language comprehension, learning and reasoning" (Baddeley 1986). The difference between WM and STM becomes clearer than in Atkinson and Shiffrin's proposal, where the two concepts basically coincide. In Baddeley and Hitch's proposal, in fact, STM refers to the mechanism purely deputed to maintaining information for a limited period of time, whereas WM involves also the capacity to manipulate this information, by performing operations with it. In other words, working memory is a broader concept, as reflected in Baddeley WM model, which comprises two short-term memory stores deputed to the maintenance of stimuli and two other components responsible for the integration, manipulation and coordination of this material.

Baddeley and Hitch's original Working Memory Model is represented in Figure 2.2; the structure and the functions of each component will be described thoroughly in the following paragraphs.

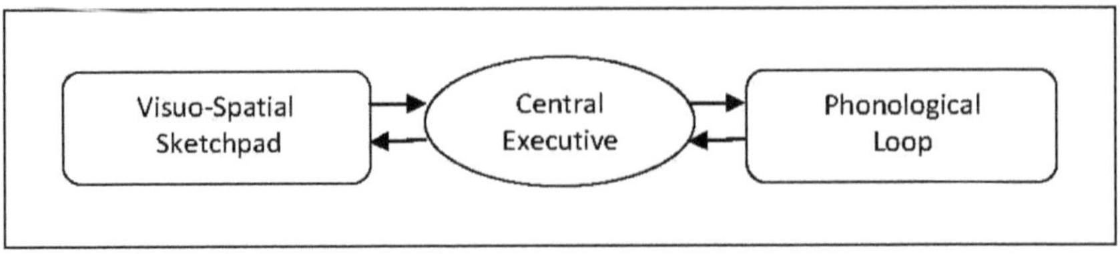

Figure 2.2. Baddeley and Hitch's Tripartite Model of Working Memory.

7.2.1. The Phonological Loop

The Phonological Loop is the most broadly investigated component of working memory; as anticipated above, it is specialized for allowing the temporary retention of verbal material. It includes two independent sub-systems: a Phonological Store, deputed to temporarily store acoustic or speech-based information (its storage capacity lasts about 2 seconds) and an Articulatory Rehearsal Process, which permits to enhance memory performance by refreshing material in the store through subvocal repetition. In other words, phonological memory traces are held in the store over a matter of seconds and they are cyclically refreshed by the subvocal rehearsal system until it is necessary.

To understand how the two mechanisms work, we can imagine a situation in which we need to remember a telephone number until we have dialed it: since the capacity of the store is limited, we are forced to resort to the rehearsal process, repeating mentally (or aloud) the sequence of digits in the right order. This rehearsal process plays a crucial role: if the information is not refreshed, in fact, it decays and fades away.

Besides this limitation in time, the Phonological Loop is also limited in span: when the number of stimuli to be refreshed increases excessively, the first item of the sequence is likely to decay before it is refreshed again. This explains why it is more difficult to remember very long sequences of digits or words.

A second function performed by the Articulatory Rehearsal Process concerns the translation of non-phonological material, such as written words or pictures, in a phonological code, allowing their temporary maintenance in the short-term store.

Furthermore, the Phonological Loop is directly linked to the Central Executive, which can perform operations on the material retained in the store.

The existence and the architecture of the phonological loop is supported by a rich range of laboratory-based findings, such as (i) the phonological similarity effect, (ii) the irrelevant speech effect, (iii) the word-length effect and (iv) the articulatory suppression effect. These effects are typically tested using serial recall tasks, in which the subject is shown a sequence of visually presented items and she is asked to recall them orally in the correct order. The four effects are reviewed below.

(i) **The phonological or acoustic similarity effect**: the phonological similarity effect demonstrates that the Phonological Loop, and in particular the Phonological Store, operate at a phonological level. Experimental data show that the immediate ordered recall of items is poorer when they are phonologically similar, in comparison to when they are different in sound (Conrad 1964; Baddeley 1966). For instance, it is more difficult to recall phonologically similar words such as *cap*, *rat, cat*, *red*, than dissimilar words as *milk*, *toy*, *sun*, *eye*. This effect demonstrates that the basic code involved in the Loop is phonological: similar items have fewer distinguishing cues from an acoustic point of view and are therefore more susceptible to be confounded and forgotten. Further evidence in favor of this specialization comes from the fact that the similarity effect does not appear in presence of similarity of meaning, suggesting that the phonological store supports only a phonological, non semantic, code (Zempleni 2006).

(ii) **The irrelevant speech effect**: a second source of evidence demonstrating that the Phonological Loop operates at the phonological rather than semantic level is the irrelevant speech effect. The available evidence shows that performance on serial recall tasks is disturbed by the presence of irrelevant background speech (Colle and Welsh 1976). This suggests that spoken material has an obligatory access to the Phonological Store, creating an interference with the recall tasks that are being performed. Interestingly, a study on English subjects revealed that this interference arose both when the irrelevant material was presented in English and when it was presented in Arabic, confirming that meaning does not affect performance (see Baddeley 1999). Moreover, it has been shown that the effect is not simply one of distraction: background noise, even though very loud, namely, does not impact on performance. These data suggest that "disruptive spoken material gains obligatory access to the phonological memory store" (Baddeley 1992), whereas noise is filtered out by a mechanism able to distinguish it from spoken material.

(iii) **The word-length effect**: a third source of evidence in favor of the existence of the Phonological Loop and in particular of the Articulatory Rehearsal Process is the word-length effect. It has been shown that the memory span for words is inversely related to their spoken duration (Baddeley et al. 1975; Ellis and Hennelley 1980). In other words, performance in serial recall tasks decreases when the stimuli to be remembered are longer, due to the time-limitations of the rehearsal process. The longer the word, in fact, the longer the time needed to pronounce it and to refresh the sequence of syllables composing it, and hence the more likely traces of earlier words decay. Observing this, Baddeley and colleagues proposed that the effect should disappear if the subject is prevented from rehearsing, for instance in an articulatory suppression task, as discussed below.

(iv) **The articulatory suppression effect**: this effect demonstrates that it is possible to disrupt the subvocal rehearsal process by asking the subject to remember a list of items while uttering at the same time an irrelevant sound, such as the word "the" (Murray 1967; 1968; Baddeley et al. 1984). Articulatory suppression hampers the performance in serial recall tasks, preventing the subject from rehearsing the stimuli she is trying to memorize. As a consequence, the subject is unable to refresh the material and then she has to rely only on the Phonological Store (and maybe on different, visual strategies) to recall the stimuli, with a detrimental impact on general performance. As predicted, articulatory suppression inhibits the word-length effect: since the subject cannot rehearse anymore, the length of the stimuli ceases to be an important variable.

Interesting results also arise when considering the interaction between these effects and the modality of presentation of the stimuli. It has been found, for instance, that articulatory suppression causes a general worsening of the performance but that it interacts differently with the phonological similarity effect and the word length effect depending on the modality of presentation of the items to be remembered. Specifically, the word-length effect is inhibited both with visually (e.g. written words) and orally presented stimuli; the similarity effect, on the other hand, disappears when they are presented as written words and persists under articulatory suppression only when the stimuli are presented orally. These findings highlight two important aspects. First, the disappearance of the word-length effect indicates that it is due to the rehearsal process: when this becomes unavailable, the effect vanishes.

The second consideration concerns the similarity effect, which must be due to the Phonological Store, since it persists under articulatory suppression under the condition that the modality of presentation be oral. Moreover, the disappearance of the effect with written stimuli confirms that the rehearsal mechanism has also the task of translating visual material into a phonological code. In other words, only phonological material has direct access to the Phonological Store, whereas visual material must be first conveniently translated. This translation is operated by the rehearsal process, as demonstrated by the disappearance of the similarity effect with written stimuli under articulatory suppression.

Summarizing, Baddeley and Hitch propose that the Phonological Loop comprises a Phonological Store, deputed to temporarily store phonological information, and an Articulatory Rehearsal Process, which permits to enhance performance by subvocal repetition and which is further concerned with the translation of visual stimuli into phonological material.

A further subdivision within the Articulatory Rehearsal Process has been proposed by Cubelli and Nichelli (1992), who conducted an interesting study to investigate the role of articulation in two anarthric patients. Anarthria is an acquired disorder characterized by a complete loss of the ability to articulate speech which generally results from a brain injury. Despite the inability to vocalize sounds, anarthric patients are generally able to communicate by writing, pointing or typing without committing mistakes.

The goal of the research conducted by Cubelli and Nichelli was to verify whether anarthric patients could rely on a form of covert articulation to enhance their performance in tasks involving phonological memory, and consequently to analyze the relationship between overt articulation and the Articulatory Rehearsal Process.

Specifically, the authors studied two anarthric individuals, a 25-year-old girl, C.M, who presented a locked-in syndrome, characterized by a bilateral pontine lesion, and a 65-year-old man, F. C., who showed a cortical lesion affecting the posterior part of the frontal lobe. Analyzing their performance in a variety of tasks, they found that subvocal articulation can be impaired in different ways, depending on the site of lesion.

Patient C. M., in particular, exhibited a normal phonological similarity effect, both with visually and orally presented stimuli, experiencing more difficulties in tasks requiring recollection of phonologically similar items. Since the Articulatory Rehearsal Process is responsible for the translation of visual into phonological material, the fact that she exhibited the phonological similarity effect even with written words suggests that her rehearsal mechanism was working properly. However, she did not show the word-length effect, performing equally with long and short words, regardless of whether they were presented orally or visually. This result was quite surprising: since the word-length effect depends on the Articulatory Rehearsal Process, her behavior suggests that the latter has to be somehow impaired. The results of the two tasks assessing the phonological similarity effect and the word-length effect, thus, provide conflicting data about the functioning of the Articulatory Rehearsal Process.

A similar conclusion can be drawn analyzing patient F. C.'s performance. Differently from C. M., in fact, he showed normal phonological-similarity effect and word-length effects only with auditory material: the absence of these effects with written words suggests that his Articulatory Rehearsal Process was disrupted, hindering the translation of visual into phonological material. Nonetheless, the occurrence of the word-length effect, even though only with auditorily presented words, should demonstrate that the articulatory rehearsal process is working properly.

Once again, hence, experimental data do not support the internal organization of the Phonological Loop proposed by Baddeley and Hitch. To overcome this problem, Cubelli and Nichelli propose a further distinction within the Articulatory Rehearsal Process, suggesting that it comprises two distinct mechanisms, an Articulatory Rehearsal Process and an Articulatory Recoding Process, concerned with the translation of visual into phonological material. These two processes may be selectively impaired due to a cerebral lesion, as demonstrated by the different behaviours shown by patients C. M. and F. C.

To summarize, the Phonological Loop is composed of two subsystems, served mainly by the left hemisphere: a Phonological Store, deputed to temporarily maintain phonological information, and an Articulatory Rehearsal Process, which has two distinct functions that can be selectively impaired, as shown by Cubelli and Nichelli. Firstly, it enhances memory performance by refreshing the memory traces in the store until it is necessary; secondly, it is concerned with the translation of visually presented items in a phonological code.

7.2.1.1. The Phonological Loop and Language Competence: evidence from language disordered and language gifted people

Despite its capability to account for a wide range of experimental findings, the real function of the Phonological Loop has long been unclear. It is indeed unlikely that it has evolved simply in order for temporarily remembering sequences of numbers or words. An answer for this question is provided by recent studies suggesting that the Phonological Loop plays indeed a fundamental role in human cognition, supporting language learning and, in particular, allowing long-term phonological learning.

Intriguing evidence supporting this hypothesis comes both from acquisitional studies and from lesion studies conducted on people with disorders acquired after brain insults (see Baddeley et al. 1998 for an extensive review). A first source of evidence is provided by the correlation found across early and middle childhood between vocabulary knowledge and both digit span[6] and nonword repetition[7] scores, which are typical tasks employed to measure phonological (also called verbal) STM. Specifically, it has been found that nonword repetition scores at age 4 is highly predictive of vocabulary test scores 1 year later, suggesting that nonword repetition has a causal role in vocabulary development and, consequently, that the Phonological Loop has a strong role in the long lasting acquisition of new words (Gathercole et al. 1992). To further test this assumption, Gathercole and Baddeley (1990) assessed the abilities of 5-year-old children to learn new names of toy animals and found that children with low nonword repetition scores were indeed remarkably less skillful in the task than high-repetition children.

Moreover, it has been found that the relationship linking the Phonological Loop and the Phonological LTM is bidirectional: the Phonological LTM, is namely not only affected by the Phonological Loop but it can influence the functioning of the Loop as well. Gathercole (1995) discovered that children were more accurate at repeating nonwords when they were phonologically similar to existing words, suggesting that their phonological LTM was used to support the repetition of novel strings.

Beyond its supportive function in the learning of one's native vocabulary, the Phonological Loop is fundamental also for the acquisition of a foreign language vocabulary. This has been shown by studies conducted on subjects with acquired brain lesions, as it was the case of the Italian patient P.V. who exhibited a strong phonological deficit after a brain insult. Papagno and colleagues (1991) examined her ability to learn couples of unrelated Italian words (e.g. *cavallo-libro*, 'horse-book') or Italian-Russian pairs (e.g. *rosa-svieti* 'rose'). P.V. was found normal at learning pairs of words in her native language, but highly impaired in learning Russian vocabulary. Similarly, Trojano and Grossi's (1995) patient S.C. was totally unable to learn auditorily presented pairs composed by a word and a nonword. These results confirm that phonological STM deficits strongly hamper the subject's ability to learn new words, whereas her intact repetition of familiar words points to a

6 In digit span tasks the subject is presented with a sequence of digits, either orally or visually, and is asked to orally recall the exact sequence, respecting the correct order of presentation.

7 In non-word repetition tasks the subject is presented with a string of pronounceable but meaningless words and is required to recall the exact sequence.

supportive role of the phonological LTM, consistently with the acquisitional findings reviewed above.

Another source of evidence in favor of the crucial importance of the Phonological Loop as a language-learning device is provided by the studies conducted on subjects suffering from neurodevelopmental disorders (see Gathercole and Alloway 2006 for a review). Individuals with Down syndrome, who present a marked deficit of phonological STM but intact visuo-spatial STM, are remarkably impaired in their ability to acquire new vocabulary. Conversely, people with Williams syndrome, whose spatial cognition is severely disrupted and whose IQ scores are typically delayed, perform normally in verbal tasks and show a very rich vocabulary. Interestingly, Jarrold and Baddeley (1997) found that Down individuals show a very poor digit span in comparison to both Williams syndrome individuals, younger children and subjects with mild learning difficulties matched for verbal mental age.

Children with Specific Language Impairment (SLI) have also been studied, reporting that they have an impaired verbal STM, with nonword repetition skills even identified as a phenotypical marker of the disorder (Bishop et al. 1996, Casalini et al. 2007, Dispaldro et al 2011). Consistently, their vocabulary is significantly poorer even than that of 18–24 months younger children.

Further evidence comes from the studies conducted on polyglots, who manifest a sort of natural talent for acquiring new languages: significantly, their performance in phonological STM tasks is much better than that of non-polyglots (Papagno and Vallar 1995).

As a conclusion, there is strong evidence suggesting that the main function of the Phonological Loop is that of supporting long-term acquisition of new words: the ability to repeat sequences of digits and words is simply a by-product of this more crucial capacity.

7.2.2. The Visuo-Spatial Sketchpad

In Baddeley's model, the Visuo-Spatial Sketchpad is a slave-system deputed to the temporary maintenance and manipulation of visual and spatial information. It is assumed to play an important role in spatial orientation and geographical knowledge, but also in the acquisition of visual semantics, concerning, amongst others, the appearance of objects and the ability to understand complex systems and to use them (Baddeley 2003b).

Like the Phonological Loop, the Visuo-Spatial Sketchpad has a limited capacity, even though its architecture has received less attention in comparison to its verbal equivalent. As illustrated in the preceding section, the Phonological Loop is divided into two subcomponents, a Phonological Store and an Articulatory Rehearsal Process, whereas the presence of a similar subdivision has not been discussed for the Sketchpad. However, the hypothesis that the Sketchpad be concerned with visual and spatial information, without a finer subdivision, has been met with skepticism and perplexity by many scholars.

Indeed, results from neuropsychological studies have provided some evidence in favor of a distinction between two subcomponents, the first dealing with visual material (e.g. the form, appearance and color of an object) and the second with spatial information (e.g. the location of an object in the space). It has been also proposed that another component should be concerned with motor or kinesthetic information (see Logie 1995 for a complete review).

Evidence in favor of such distinction, which has never been formalized in Baddeley's model, comes from the double dissociations found in neuropsychological studies between visual and spatial tasks. A typical task assessing spatial working memory is the Corsi Block task, in which the subject is shown an array of nine blocks and she is asked to repeat a sequence of movements made by the experimenter tapping some of them. In a purely visual task, the subject is shown matrices of cells some of which are filled; the matrix is then removed and the subject is asked to recall the position of the filled cells. Della Sala and colleagues (1999) found that visual and spatial spans are dissociated, with subjects impaired in visual tasks but not in spatial tasks and vice versa.

Moreover, Philips and colleagues (2004) found that individuals with Williams Syndrome, who typically display intact verbal competence and impaired spatial processing, manifest difficulties in processing sentences containing spatial syntactic forms, such as *above* and *below*, whereas they perform normally with complex sentences not involving spatial forms, such as negative and passive sentences. These results led the authors to suggest that the Sketchpad plays a role in sentence processing as well.

To summarize, the Visuo-Spatial Sketchpad is concerned with the storage and manipulation of visual and spatial information. It is mainly controlled by the right hemisphere.

7.2.3. The Central Executive

The Central Executive is the more crucial component of working memory. Despite its importance, as admitted by Baddeley (2003b) himself, it "was initially coinceived in the vaguest possible terms as a limited capacity pool of general processing resources" (89). Actually, it was considered as a sort of homunculus who had the task of deciding how the information provided by the two slave-systems had to be manipulated.

Differently from the two subsystems illustrated above, the Central Executive was initially assumed to be a limited-capacity attentional system without storage capacity, which was linked to both subsystems and to LTM.

Subsequently, Baddeley (1996) proposed that the Central Executive should be fractionated, by individuating its main functions, namely (i) the capacity to focus attention, inhibiting irrelevant stimuli, (ii) the capacity of dividing attention, coordinating performance in dual-tasks, (iii) the capacity of switching attention and (iv) the capacity to create an interface between the two slave-subsystems and LTM.

As far as the first function is concerned, as discussed in Chapter 1, the ability to focus attention is crucial in order for a subject to concentrate on the relevant stimuli, filtering out those that are irrelevant for the undertaken activity. The capacity to divide attention, instead, is crucial for carrying on two different tasks simultaneously. Interesting insights come from the study performed by Baddeley and colleagues (2001), aimed at analyzing the performance of patients affected by Alzheimer Disease (AD). They found that AD patients were significantly more impaired than age-matched controls in dual-task experiments, in which they were asked to perform an auditory digit span task and a pursuit tracking task[8] simultaneously. Since they behaved as accurately as controls when the

8 A *pursuit tracking task* is a typical task tapping the Visuo-Spatial Sketchpad in which the subject is required to match her eye movement with the movement of a visual object.

two tasks were performed separately, pointing to spared Phonological Loop and Visuo-Spatial Sketchpad, their difficulties under dual-task conditions have been ascribed to the Central Executive.

The capacity to switch attention has proven to be more problematic to analyze: studies conducted to investigate this ability have provided controversial results, leaving still open the question whether it is really an executive process (see Baddeley 2002a).

Further problems for Baddeley's (1996) initial proposal for a partition of the Central Executive have been raised concerning the fourth function he individuated, namely the ability to integrate the material store by the two subsystems with the information retrieved from LTM.

A first challenge for the involvement of the Central Executive in the retrieval from LTM came from the results of studies conducted on amnesic patients with impaired LTM who showed anyway an immediate recall for long prose paragraphs. Such prose passages comprised even 25 units, surpassing therefore the capacity of the Phonological Loop and suggesting the presence of a mechanism like "chunking", which could enhance performance (Baddeley 2003b). Such a mechanism should exploit long-term knowledge to package information more efficiently, increasing the storage capacity. This would also explain why it is easier to recall a sequence of digits composed by familiar dates (e.g. 1492 1776 1945) instead of a sequence of digits in random order (Baddeley 2002b). However, the dilemma was precisely that such a mechanism could not be related to the Phonological Loop or to the Visuo-Spatial Sketchpad, whose storage capacity had been proven to be limited. Nor can the Central Executive be held responsible, given that it is not supposed to have a storage capacity. Moreover, the Central Executive should be excluded for another reason: there have been found amnesic patients displaying an excellent immediate recall but a severely impaired delayed recall who have typically preserved intelligence and Central Executive skills. This finding has suggested that immediate recall does not depend on the Central Executive.

A further problem of the original model was its inability to explain how information coming from the two-slave subsystems and from LTM could be integrated and manipulated, given the absence of an appropriate storage mechanism.

To solve these problems, Baddeley (2000) added a fourth component to the original model, the Episodic Buffer, which is assumed to be a storage system able to support a multimodal code and to operate on different kinds of information and which will be described in the following paragraph.

Therefore, the Central Executive maintained only its role of supervision and control. It plays nevertheless a fundamental role in cognitive tasks, thanks to its ability to focus and divide attention. Subjects with impaired Central Executive manifest more difficulties in focusing attention and in filtering out cognitive stimuli, especially in dual-task conditions, where they are required to divide their attention skills while performing two different tasks simultaneously. Moreover, Central Executive skills have proven to be a strong predictor of performance in complex cognitive tasks, such as reading comprehension, problem solving, arithmetics and learning electronics (Baddeley 2003a).

7.2.4. The Episodic Buffer

As anticipated above, the Episodic Buffer has been proposed 26 years after the original formulation of Baddeley and Hitch's model to account for a number of findings showing that a tripartite model could not explain how information coming from the Phonological Loop and the Visuo-Spatial Sketchpad are manipulated and integrated with the material already stored in LTM. In the current model, the Episodic Buffer is supposed to be a storage system supporting a multimodal code which is bidirectionally linked both to the Central Executive and to LTM. As the name suggests, it has a limited capacity and it is able to combine different codes (e.g. phonological, visual and spatial) to form objects or episodes (see Baddeley and Jarrold 2007).

The postulation of the Episodic Buffer solves the problem discussed above and concerning the chunking of information involved in the immediate recall of prose paragraphs. The Buffer can access LTM to facilitate chunking, by aggregating items into larger units (i.e. words into phrases), and it can maintain the information available for immediate recall, thanks to the attentional role played by the Central Executive.

7.3. *Baddeley's revised Model of Working Memory*

In the light of the considerations exposed and discussed in the preceding paragraphs, Baddeley (2000) has proposed a revised model of Working Memory, which is represented below.

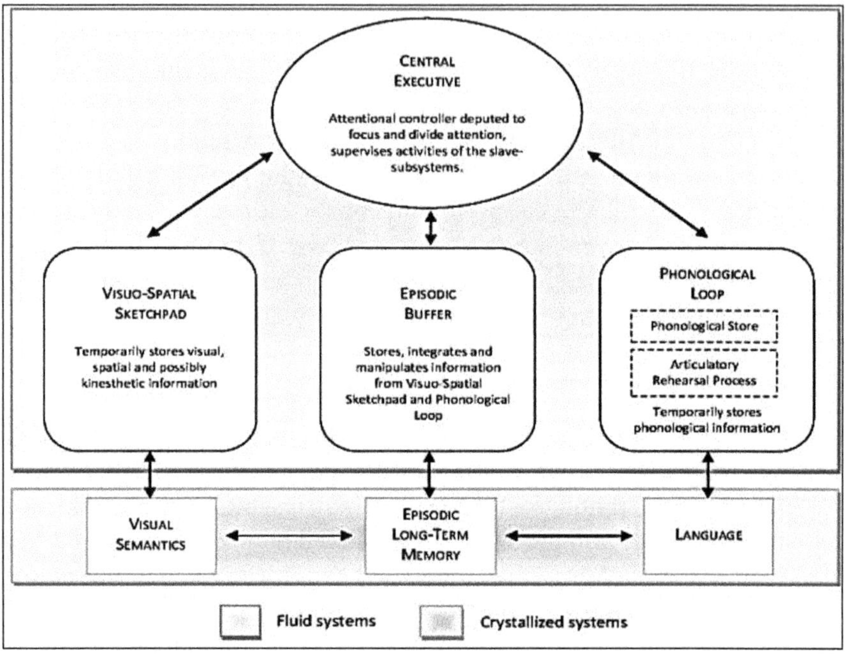

Figure 2.3. Baddeley's Revised Model of Working Memory.

In this new version, an important distinction is made between Fluid and Crystallized System. The Fluid System, which basically corresponds to Working Memory, concerns abilities such as attention, temporary storage and problem-solving, whereas the Crystallized System is able to accumulate long-term information, relying on acquired and specific knowledge.

In Baddeley's revised model of Working Memory, the Central Executive maintains its crucial role of attentional controller, which supervises the activities of three (instead of two) slave subsystems. The Visuo-Spatial Sketchpad temporarily maintains visuo-spatial information, whereas the Phonological Loop, implemented by the Phonological

Store and the Articulatory Rehearsal Process, stores phonological information. The Episodic Buffer, equipped with a storage system, integrates and manipulates the information provided by the other subsystems. In this version of the model, the Episodic Buffer is supposed to receive visuo-spatial and verbal information from the Central Executive, rather than directly from the stores. However, Baddeley and colleagues argue that this initial hypothesis might be contradicted by future experimental findings indicating that the Phonological Loop and the Visuo-Spatial Sketchpad access directly the Episodic Buffer, leading to a reconsideration of the role of the Central Executive.

Interestingly, an explicit bidirectional link is individuated between the subsidiary systems and LTM: the Phonological Loop has a direct access to language, whereas the Visuo-Spatial Sketchpad is connected to visual (nonverbal) semantics, containing information such as colors and shapes of objects and movements of animals together with knowledge about the physical and mechanic world (Baddeley 2002a).

Finally, the Episodic Buffer can access the Episodic LTM[9] to integrate long-lasting stored information with the material provided by the other subsystems.

7.4. *Working Memory and Development*

Human Working Memory undergoes significant changes during life. A number of studies have demonstrated that there is a strong correlation between working memory and age, showing that WM capacity improves steadily until the teenage years, when it starts leveling off, whereas it decreases in older adults (Gathercole et. al 2004; Baddeley 1986; Hulme et al. 1984; 1989; Gathercole and Hitch 1993; Gathercole and Baddeley 1993; Gathercole and Adams 1993).

9 Episodic LTM stores specific facts and events from the past, which can be exploited to react appropriately to similar events or to avoid mistakes. It is generally distinguished from Semantic LTM, which concerns generic knowledge and ideas about the world. In Baddeley's framework the distinction between Episodic Memory and Semantic Memory remains, by his own admission, uncontroversial (Baddeley 2002b).

Specifically, WM performance enhances notably between the ages of 5 and 15 years, improving qualitatively as well as quantitatively (Gathercole 1999).

One crucial developmental change concerns the Phonological Loop. It has been demonstrated that the Phonological Store is in place at about 3 years of age, whereas the Articulatory Rehearsal Process becomes effective only at around 7 years of age: prior to this period, children are not able to refresh information and therefore they can solely rely on the Phonological Store to recall verbal material (Cowan and Kail 1996). As a consequence, they tend to exploit basically the visuo-spatial WM to temporarily memorize materials such as pictures or objects. When spontaneous rehearsal emerges, they abandon these compensatory strategies and rely more heavily on the Phonological Loop to recall verbal material. The use of rehearsal strategies allows therefore the children to remember an increasing amount of phonological information, enhancing their verbal recall performance.

In their experimental study, Gathercole et al. (2004) found that the main components of Baddeley's model of WM are in place by 6 years of age, but that their capacity increases linearly from age 4 to early adolescence. Performance on all WM measures, namely, improves gradually throughout the infancy, approaching adult level around 15 years. Consistently, other studies have demonstrated that performance enhances with age on all WM tests tapping the Phonological Loop, the Visuo-Spatial Sketchpad and the Central Executive. It has been proposed that this improvement arises from increased memory efficiency and from a general enhancement in the speed of cognitive processing which advantages all components of WM (Gathercole et al. 2004; Fry and Hale 2000; Towse, Hitch and Hutton 1998).

To summarize, extensive evidence has shown that WM performance enhances steadily through the childhood years, until early adolescence (age 15), when it starts leveling off, approaching adult levels. On the contrary, WM skills tend to decrease in elderly adults.

7.5. *Working Memory, Cognitive Skills and Neuro-developmental Disorders*

Working Memory has proven to play a crucial role in human cognition: WM skills have been found to correlate significantly with reasoning and comprehension abilities (Baddeley 1999). Moreover, as we will observe in Chapter 4, WM, and in particular the Central Executive, is crucially involved in the execution of all complex activities, ranging from thinking and reasoning, to problem solving and language comprehension.

Strong evidence for the association of WM skills and cognitive abilities is provided by studies conducted on children, where their cognitive profile is compared to their WM skills. It has been found that children who obtained lower scores on WM tasks are more likely to exhibit difficulties in mathematics and in reading acquisition, as well as in the early stages of counting, where they tend to use finger-based counting strategies, differently from their peers with higher WM scores (Geary et al. 2004). Moreover, as discussed above, WM and specifically the Phonological Loop are important for language acquisition.

In agreement with these findings, Gathercole and Baddeley (1990) also found that language-disordered children showed dramatic impairments of the Phonological Loop, performing even worse than control children 4 years younger than them in nonword repetition tasks. Interestingly, however, they displayed the same sensitivity as their peers to both phonological similarity and word length effects, indicating that the Phonological Store and the Articulatory Rehearsal Process are in place and normally functioning and thus suggesting that their difficulties may arise from the Loop's storage capacity or efficiency. Furthermore, it has been found that phonological memory skills offer a critical contribution to reading acquisition and development, supporting the establishment of letter-sound correspondences rules.

Starting from these findings, other authors have suggested that the implication of Working Memory in language competence is even stronger, embracing also syntax, semantics and pragmatics. Ellis and Sinclair (1996), for instance, noted that children who had better verbal WM scores displayed a more proficient grammatical competence and that consistently individuals whose syntactic development is impaired show deficient verbal WM skills.

A further claim in favor of the individuation of different linguistic subcomponents in WM comes from Almor et al. (1999), who hypothesized the existence of a connection between verbal WM and semantics, showing that Alzheimer patients' pronoun processing, in both production and comprehension, reflects the working memory impairment associated with their disease. Analyzing AD patients' spontaneous speech and their performance in processing pronominal expressions, Almor and colleagues discovered that they had remarkable difficulties in comparison to age-matched healthy controls (i.e. they produced more empty speech[10]). Moreover, their comprehension resulted to be highly impaired in assigning the appropriate referent to pronouns. Both groups of participants underwent a battery of working memory tests, to assess whether there was a correlation between WM performance and the interpretation/production of pronominal expressions. Results confirmed that WM performance is associated with referential deficits and led the authors to argue that pronoun processing is highly dependent upon verbal WM skills. In addition, they suggested that pragmatics could be linked to verbal WM as well, following other authors' proposal (Ulatowska and Chapman 1995; Ulatowska et al. 1988) to consider pronoun overuse, typical in AD patients' speech, as a consequence of failing to follow discourse conventions.

Even though this proposal should be assessed with further experiments, it seems plausible, considering that Baddeley himself recognizes the centrality of phonological memory in language tasks.

> Our proposal is that phonological memory makes an important contribution to the development of many complex linguistic abilities in children, and that disordered language development may be a relatively direct consequence of phonological memory impairments. (Gathercole and Baddeley 1990: 358.)

Beyond the importance of WM in language processing, it has been demonstrated that the Central Executive (together with the Episodic Buffer)[11] plays an important role in cognitive activities. As discussed

10 Empty speech can be defined as the overuse of empty words, such as "thing", "do" or "it", which characterizes Alzheimer Patients' speech.

11 An important clarification should be made: Central Executive measures are usually assessed using complex span tasks, in which the subject is asked to carry on

above, one of the major functions of the Central Executive is the ability to focus and switch attention, filtering out irrelevant stimuli. Impairment of the executive functioning has been indeed individuated in children affected by attentional disorders such as the Attentional Deficit with Hyperactivity Disorder (ADHD): specifically, impaired children perform poorly in tasks requiring inhibition of irrelevant stimuli (Gathercole and Alloway 2006). Higher-level interference for the Stroop task (see Chapter 1), for instance, has been found in subjects with a low score in tasks tapping the Central Executive (Kane et al. 2001).

Children with low span in complex tasks, moreover, are more likely to show an inattentive behavior, forgetting the content of instructions, getting lost in complex activities, and abandoning the tasks before completing them.

Furthermore, poor scores on the Central Executive measures have been found highly predictive of literacy and arithmetic problems and appear to provide the most reliable indicators of scholastic failure. Gathercole and colleagues (2006), for instance, found that WM skills are good predictors of children's proficiency in reading and mathematics. In this respect, an interesting study has been conducted by Gathercole and colleagues (2008), who analyzed the behavior of 52 children with low working memory scores, reporting that they displayed shorter attention spans and higher levels of distractibility in comparison to their peers with higher WM scores, together with a failure to plan activities,

---

two different tasks contemporarily. One typical task is the *counting recall task*, in which the subject is asked to count arrays of dots present on a series of cards, and the recall the total number of dots on each of the card seen. As discussed above, the ability to perform dual-tasks is heavily dependent upon the Central Executive, which supervises the activities through attentional processes. However, I think that this kind of tasks does not provide a pure measure of Central Executive skills, given that also the three subsidiary systems, and in particular the Episodic Buffer, are involved. In the *counting recall task*, in fact, both visual and verbal abilities are required and therefore the Episodic Buffer plays a crucial role, allowing the integration and manipulation of multimodal information.

Probably due to the fact that the Episodic Buffer has been only recently introduced, there are not (to my knowledge) tasks tapping directly the Episodic Buffer. Similarly, I think that it is very difficult to develop a task assessing purely Central Executive skills, given the tight relationship between the Central Executive and the three slave subsystems.

monitor the quality of their work and make corrections. Arguably, these difficulties are due to the lower ability of children with poor WM skills to focus and switch attention and to integrate the short-term information provided by the subsidiary systems with acquired knowledge, such as problem-solving strategies, retrieved from LTM (Swanson and Beebe-Frankenberger 2004). Moreover, Gathercole and colleagues (2008) suggested that the limited WM skills of subjects with low spans are unable to satisfy the storage and processing demands of complex cognitive activities, further confirming that working memory plays an important role in supporting reasoning, problem-solving and activity planning.

However, a compensation for the weaknesses affecting one of the WM domains may also occur. In fact, it is possible that an individual suffering from memory impairments affecting one or more components of the WM system be able to enact compensatory strategies, relying more heavily on their unimpaired resources to overcome their difficulties, thanks, for instance, to a high IQ score (Hulme and Roodenrys 1995). Evidence pointing to the activation of compensatory strategies is provided also from neuroscience studies, confirming that, due to its intrinsic plasticity, the neural system serving WM functions allows flexible compensation in cases of disease or disruptions of the circuits (Schlösser et al. 2006).

7.6. Working Memory and Dyslexia

The individuation of Working Memory deficits in children affected by language disorders has suggested that dyslexic children may suffer from WM impairments as well. A number of studies have indeed revealed that dyslexics exhibit remarkably more difficulties in tasks tapping their WM in comparison to age-matched normally achieving children. Different researches have pointed out that dyslexic children perform very poorly in tasks tapping the Phonological Loop, such as the digit span task (see Hulme and Roodneys 1995, Helland and Asbjørnsen 2004). On the contrary, their Visuo-Spatial Sketchpad seems to be normally functioning, whereas impairments have been found in the Central Executive as well (Pickering and Gathercole 2001, Beneventi et al. 2010).

A very complete study is the one conducted by Jeffrey and Everatt (2004), who examined WM skills in 21 dyslexic children (mean age 8 years and 10 months), comparing their performance to that shown by a control group of 40 typically developing children (mean age 9 years and 2 months) and a group composed of 26 children with Special Educational Needs (SEN children), exhibiting problems as dyspraxia[12], emotional/behavioral problems and attention deficits (mean age 9 years and 7 months). Results showed that dyslexics, similarly to children with special educational needs, are remarkably impaired in comparison to controls in phonological measures, whereas they perform normally in visuo-spatial and motor coordination tasks, differently from SEN children. In the Central Executive measures, as well as in the interference tasks, on the contrary, dyslexics showed significant problems, performing even worse than SEN children. These results, therefore, strongly suggest that both the Phonological Loop and the Central Executive are impaired in dyslexia.

The presence of significant impairments at the Central Executive has been reported by Wang and Gathercole (2013), who analyzed WM abilities of 46 children with reading abilities and 45 age-matched controls. Combining two different methods for assessing executive capacity (complex span tasks and dual-tasks) the authors found that poor readers display pervasive deficits affecting their Central Executive. Specifically, problems arise when children are required to combine cognitive demanding tasks, even after performance in simple span test is controlled, leading the authors to propose that the WM deficits exhibited by dyslexics do not simply reflect problems in processing verbal materials, but are strongly related to the functioning of the Central Executive.

WM deficits in dyslexics persist also in adulthood: Ghani and Gathercole (2013) administered a battery of WM tests to 26 postsecondary students with dyslexia and 32 controls, reporting highly significant differences amongst the two groups on all memory measures, comprising verbal short-term memory, verbal working memory, visuo-spatial short-term memory and visuo-spatial working memory. These results

12 Dyspraxia is a specific learning difficulty which affects motor abilities. It generally disturbs planning and organization of movements and coordination skills.

suggest that WM inefficiencies persist also in adult dyslexics who pursue their studies to higher levels.

The proposal that dyslexia is due to a WM deficiency has been put forward by McLoughlin and colleagues (1994) who argued that WM impairments are responsible for all the primary difficulties experienced by dyslexic children. Subsequently, McLoughlin et al. (2002) suggested that dyslexic people have a weakness with low order processing in the Phonological Loop, as shown by their poor performance in tasks tapping verbal WM, and that their Central Executive gets disrupted when it has to support very demanding language tasks. The importance of WM deficits in dyslexia is so crucial for McLoughlin and colleagues that they proposed a new definition of the disorder that individuates in WM problems the cause of the difficulties experienced by dyslexics.

> Developmental dyslexia is a genetically inherited and neurologically determined inefficiency in working memory, the information-processing system fundamental to learning and performance in conventional educational and work settings. It has a particular impact on verbal and written communication as well as on organization, planning and adaptation to change.
> (McLoughling et al. 2002: 19)

However, the authors did not enter into details, avoiding engaging in a precise explanation of the nature of the impairment exhibited by dyslexics and its effects.

A more precise and recent hypothesis claiming that dyslexia is related to a WM impairment has been put forward by Fiorin (2010), whose proposal is formalized in the verbal Working Memory Deficit Hypothesis. According to this hypothesis, dyslexic individuals suffer from a deficit affecting the dynamic dimension of the Phonological Loop. This deficit is also likely to affect the Grammatical Loop, an additional component added by Fiorin to Baddeley's model and assumed to be concerned with storage and manipulation of grammatical representations.

Proceeding step by step, Fiorin started his analysis by observing that the difficulties shown by dyslexics in tasks tapping phonological memory, such as the digit span task, point to a first and fundamental impairment affecting the Phonological Loop. In particular, he proposed that this deficit does not involve the Loop entirely, but only its dynamic component, that is, the Articulatory Rehearsal Process. In his specific implementation of Baddeley's original model, Fiorin suggested that the Phonological Store can be seen as a 'static' dimension, concerned with the temporary storage of phonological material, whereas the Articulatory Rehearsal Process has a dynamic dimension "responsible for accessing the information in order to store it, refresh it, and make it available to other systems (Fiorin 2010, p. 91)".

Referring to Ramus and Szenkovits (2008), who proposed that dyslexics have a specific deficit affecting the access to phonological representations, Fiorin argued that precisely this second, dynamic dimension is affected in dyslexia. This impairment is held responsible for the phonological deficits shown by dyslexics and for their difficulties in tasks requiring phonological representations to be accessed for external computations. Fiorin proposed that dyslexics suffer from an impairment preventing them from normally accessing the phonological representations necessary for external computations. So conceived, the hypothesis constitutes a refined version of the Phonological Deficit Hypothesis and is able to account for the poor phonological awareness shown by dyslexics, as well as for their difficulties acquiring properly reading and spelling skills.

However, Fiorin acknowledged that dyslexics' difficulties are not limited to phonology but also extend to grammar. Therefore, he further implemented his proposal in order to account for grammatical impairments as well, proposing to add a further component to Baddeley's model, a Grammatical Loop. As the Phonological Loop, this subsystem should comprise a 'static' component, deputed to store grammatical information, and a 'dynamic' component, predisposed to access this material in order to refresh it and make it available to other systems for further computation. Fiorin's hypothesis is then able to explain phonological, reading and spelling deficits, arguing that the component deputed to access phonological representation in WM (i.e. the 'dynamic' dimension of the Phonological Loop) is disrupted in dyslexics. In addition, although the author did not explicitly mention naming deficits, the hypothesis can also explain the difficulties exhibited by dyslexics in rapid naming tasks: the 'dynamic' dimension of the

Phonological Loop, in fact, can hinder their capacity to retrieve correctly the phonological form of a visually presented item. Moreover, it can also account for grammatical deficits, postulating the existence of a further component, the Grammatical Loop, which can be disturbed by the impairment affecting the Phonological Loop.

Despite its formal elegance, however, Fiorin's hypothesis faces a potential problem, given that it is not able to explain the attention deficits that have been reported in dyslexic children nor the Central Executive inefficiencies discussed above. Remind, for instance, the poor performance in the Stroop tasks found in the experiment designed by Everatt and colleagues (1997), in which children were asked to name the ink color of words which were printed in a tint different from that denoted by the word itself. Dyslexic children were found significantly more impaired even in comparison to reading-age matched controls in naming the color ink of words, exhibiting thus larger effects of interference. This finding led to suggest that dyslexics are less able to focus attention, inhibiting irrelevant stimuli. Clearly, this impairment cannot be explained by the Verbal Working Memory Deficit Hypothesis, since it is not due to verbal factors. This consideration also holds for the other attention deficits reviewed in Chapter 1, as well as for the results provided by the experiment conducted by Jeffrey and Everatt (2004), reviewed above: this experiment confirms the presence of Central Executive impairments in dyslexia. It seems therefore that Fiorin's hypothesis is in need of further implementation, in order to account also for these deficits.

To address this difficulty, I propose a new hypothesis, which will be presented and discussed in Chapter 4, according to which both the Phonological Loop and the Central Executive are detrimentally impaired in dyslexic individuals, causing the deficits reviewed in (1). Before developing this proposal, however, I decided to perform an additional experiment testing dyslexic children's and age-matched typically developing children's WM, in order to provide further support to the hypothesis claiming that dyslexia is related to a WM inefficiency. The results of the protocol I administered will be presented and discussed in Chapter 3.

8. Summary and Conclusions

In this chapter I presented and discussed the major hypotheses developed to account for developmental dyslexia, analyzing their strengths and weaknesses and focusing in particular on their ability to account for the manifestations of dyslexia reviewed in Chapter 1, that is, reading deficits, spelling deficits, phonological deficits, vocabulary deficits, grammatical deficits and attention deficits.

The first speculations about dyslexia date back to the nineteenth century, when the disorder was initially attributed to a visual deficit, preventing the child from associating the visual form of a word to its spoken form. According to the Visual Deficit Hypothesis, dyslexics are affected by visuo-perceptual deficits responsible for their difficulties in learning to read. Auditory deficits interfering with the child's phonological competence are considered the main cause of dyslexia in the framework of the Auditory Deficit Hypothesis, claiming that dyslexics suffer from a general impairment in sound perception.

Both visual and auditory deficits have been subsumed in the Magnocellular Deficit Hypothesis, claiming that the locus of impairment characterizing dyslexia is the magnocellular system. According to the proponents of this hypothesis, magnocellular impairments cause a reduced sensitivity to rapidly changing stimuli, giving rise to reading and spelling deficits, as well as to poor phonological awareness skills. However, this theory presents important problems: first of all, the results of the studies assessing visual and auditory competence in dyslexics are controversial and cannot be considered conclusive. Moreover, even if we accepted the presence of sensory deficits in dyslexia, these disorders could not explain the occurrence of the grammatical, vocabulary and attention deficits that are typically reported in dyslexia. Therefore, the Visual Deficit Hypothesis, the Auditory Deficit Hypothesis and the Magnocellular Deficit Hypothesis cannot be regarded as adequate frameworks for dyslexia.

The Phonological Deficit Hypothesis, instead, proposes that the underlying cause of dyslexia is poor phonological coding, which causes specific impairments in the representation, storage, manipulation and retrieval of speech sound and is responsible for the phonological, reading and spelling deficits exhibited by dyslexics. However, the main weakness of the Phonological Deficit Hypothesis is that it cannot account for the grammatical, vocabulary and attention deficits that have been detected in dyslexia.

The Double-Deficit Hypothesis attempts to supply to this deficiency, by identifying a naming problem as another core disorder, beyond the phonological deficit, characterizing dyslexia. Supporters of this hypothesis focus, namely, on the deficit experienced by dyslexics in rapid naming tasks, arguing that it is consistent across languages and even more distinctive for dyslexia than poor phonological awareness. In this framework, dyslexics should be divided in three subgroups according to the presence of phonological deficits alone (phonological subtype), naming deficits alone (naming speed subtype) and both deficits (double-deficit subtype). This last subgroup appears to be the most widespread, and arguably correlates with the most severe form of impairment amongst dyslexics. However, the greatest problem of the Double-Deficit Hypothesis is that, similarly to the Phonological Deficit Hypothesis, it does not provide a complete framework able to account for all the manifestation of dyslexia. Both the Phonological Deficit Hypothesis and the Double-Deficit Hypothesis, hence, have to be abandoned in favor of a more comprehensive approach.

Finally, the Working Memory Deficit Hypothesis, proposes a different framework, by identifying WM problems as the core deficit of dyslexia. In particular, we have discussed Fiorin's Verbal Working Memory Deficit Hypothesis, proposing that dyslexia is due to an impairment affecting the 'dynamic' dimension of the Phonological Loop, responsible for the access to phonological material. Dyslexics' poor grammatical competence is also accounted for in Fiorin's model, since the author suggests that a Grammatical Loop should be added to Baddeley's model. This Grammatical Loop, concerned with the temporary storage of grammatical information, is expected to be impaired in dyslexic individuals, causing their grammatical problems. However, this hypothesis does not take in consideration the Central Executive and attention impairments exhibited by dyslexics.

Summarizing, none of the theories exposed in this chapter seems to offer a complete and satisfactory account for the deficits associated with dyslexia, except, to some extent, for the Working Memory Deficit Hypothesis, which needs, however, to be corroborated by more experimental data comparing dyslexics' and controls' WM skills. For this reason, I decided to start my analysis by administering a complete battery of WM tests to a group composed by dyslexic children and a control group composed by age-matched normally achieving children. The results of this protocol will be presented and discussed in Chapter 3. On the basis of these results I will propose a new hypothesis to account for dyslexics' deficits, which will be presented in Chapter 4.

Chapter 3

Working Memory Skills In Developmental Dyslexia

1. Introduction

In Chapter 2 we observed that the most convincing hypothesis formulated about developmental dyslexia is the Working Memory Deficit Hypothesis. However, we have also noted that a complete experimental protocol investigating dyslexic children's WM should be conducted, in order to test their performance in tasks tapping the main components of Baddeley's WM model and to verify if they behave differently from normally-achieving children.

For this reason I decided to administer a WM test battery on a group composed by 21 dyslexic children (mean age 9 years and 3 months) and a group composed by 21 age-matched typically developing children (mean age 9 years and 2 months). To analyze performance in the components of Baddeley's model, I administered the tests developed by Pickering and Gathercole's (2001) in the Working Memory Test Battery for Children (WMTB-C). This battery, which has a high internal validity, has been designed to assess WM skills of children aged between 4.9 and 15.7 years old and it is based on Baddeley and Hitch's WM model. As illustrated in the preceding chapter, Baddeley and Hitch argued that WM is composed by three-main components: the Phonological Loop, a subsidiary subsystem which deals with the temporary storage of phonological material, the Visuo-Spatial Sketchpad, a subsidiary subsystem specialized in the temporary retention of visual and spatial material, and the Central Executive, a limited capacity attentional controller, which supervises the activities of the slave-subsystems and is principally concerned with focusing and dividing attention. As discussed in Chapter 2, this capacity plays a crucial role especially in dual-tasks, that is those tasks that require the subject to simultaneously perform two different operations.

The aim of the experimental protocol that I will present in this chapter was to analyze how dyslexic children perform in comparison to developing children in tasks assessing their WM skills. According to the discussion illustrated in Chapter 2 and on the basis of the studies already conducted on dyslexic children's WM, dyslexics are expected to perform worse than age-matched controls in tasks assessing their WM skills. Specifically, impairments are likely to arise in tasks tapping the Phonological Loop and the Central Executive, whereas the Visuo-Spatial Sketchpad should be relatively spared.

Chapter 3 is organized as follows. I will first describe the general design and procedure, illustrating the nine tasks composing the WMTB-C. I will then present the results both relatively to the entire constructs Phonological Loop, Visuo-Spatial Sketchpad and Central Executive and to the tasks considered separately. Finally, I will present the general discussion and the conclusive remarks.

2. Participants

The experimental protocol was performed on 42 subjects, divided in 2 distinct groups: 21 dyslexic children and 21 age-matched typically developing children. The group of Dyslexic Children (DC) included 21 children (14 males), all native speakers of Italian. At the moment of testing, the group mean age was 9 years and 3 months (SD = 0;11). All children have been chosen from those who had independently received a diagnosis of dyslexia, specifically by the "Centro Audiofonetico" in Trento (in the northern of Italy): in particular, dyslexic children were selected according to different factors: (i) absence of neurological diseases or genetic pathologies, (ii) absence of sensorial diseases, (iii) absence of psychopathological diseases, (iv) IQ > 80 (WISC – R) and (v) fluent and correct reading and writing abilities under 2 SD (Tressoldi et al. Battery, Prove MT).

The group of age-matched control children (AMCC) was composed by 21 primary school children (12 males), all native speakers of Italian. At the moment of testing, the group mean age was 9 years and 2 months (SD = 0;10). Children were selected from those who had no history of reading problems or language disorders. The main features of the two groups are summarized in Table 3.1.

Table 3.1. Children's group data.

Group	Number	Mean Age (SD)
DC	21	9;3 (0;11)
AMCC	21	9;2 (0;10)

3. General Design and Procedure

All subjects have been administered the nine tasks proposed in Pickering and Gathercole's (2001) Working Memory Test Battery for Children.

The WMTB-C comprises 9 tasks designed to assess performance in this three components, 4 testing the Phonological Loop (Digit Recall, Word List Matching, Word List Recall and Nonword List Recall), 2 tapping the Visuo-Spatial Sketchpad (Block Recall and Mazes Memory) and 3 assessing the Central Executive (Listening Recall, Counting Recall and Backward Digit Recall).[1] The complete list of the tasks,

1 An important clarification should be made. In Chapter 2 we observed that a fourth component has been added more recently to the Working Memory Model (Baddeley 2000), with the aim to solve a number of problems mainly raised by converging evidence pointing to the presence of a further storage able to maintain, integrate and manipulate multimodal information. This fourth component is the Episodic Buffer, a subsidiary subsystem which is concerned with the temporary storage, integration and manipulation of information and which supports a multimodal code (see section 2.7.2.4).
Since the WMTB-C was being developed and standardized contemporarily to the introduction of the Episodic Buffer in the original WM model, it does not mention this fourth component, nor it provides tasks specifically designed to assess it.
However, we have already noted that the Central Executive and the Episodic Buffer are intimately linked, since they are both involved in dual-tasks: the Central Executive, indeed, has the fundamental assignment of dividing attention and supervising the activities of the slave-subsystems, mediating the flow of information between the Phonological Loop and the Visuo-Spatial Sketchpad and the Episodic Buffer. Moreover, the Episodic Buffer is involved in the integration and manipulation of this material. For this reason, it is quite possible that the dual-tasks developed in the WMTB-C (namely the Listening Recall, the Counting Recall and the Backward Digit Recall) do not only assess Central Executive

which I all administered to the two groups of children, follows below. Beyond a brief description of each tasks (more detailed information and examples will be provided in the following sections), I reported the component of the WM model assessed in each task.

Since the experiment was conducted in Italian, the tasks involving verbal material (Word List Matching, Word List Recall, Nonword List Recall, Listening Recall) were adapted to Italian, respecting the structure of the original battery.

The tasks were presented in the same order recommended by the authors, established to avoid overtaxing on component of WM in successive subtests and to administer easier tasks before more complex ones, in order to let the child get accustomed to test procedures.

The order of presentation follows below:

1. Digit Recall Task
2. Word Lost Matching
3. Word List Recall
4. Block Recall
5. Nonword List Recall
6. Listening Recall
7. Counting Recall
8. Mazes Memory
9. Backward Digit Recall

Each subtest was preceded by the administration of three practice trials, in order to let the child get acquainted with the task. Practice trails were followed by test trials, administered using a span procedure. Every subtest was composed of a number of blocks (from 6 to 9), each corresponding to a span, and every block was composed of six test trials of the same difficulty level. For instance, Block 1 of the Digit Recall Task was composed by 1 digit, Block 2 was composed by 2 digits and so on.

As recommended by the authors, the administration of the battery followed two main rules:

---

abilities, involving the Episodic Buffer. For future research, it would be interesting to test separately the Central Executive and the Episodic Buffer in order to analyze more precisely their interrelationship and their involvement in dyslexia, as well as in other neurodevelopmental disorders.

(i) **Move On Rule**: when the first four trials of one block are correctly recalled, the fifth and the sixth trials can be omitted and the child is presented with trials of the subsequent block.
(ii) **Discontinuation Rule**: testing must be stopped when the child commits three errors within the same block.

For what concerns scoring, 1 point was assigned to each correctly recalled trial, whereas no points were given to wrongly recalled trials. 1 point was attributed also to each of trials omitted as a consequence of the Move On Rule. No credit, instead, was given for correctly recalled trials after three errors have been committed in a particular block. Finally, the child was attributed a span score corresponding to the last block correctly recalled before the Discontinuation Rule came into force.

Participants were tested individually in a quiet room. The whole test-session lasted 45–60 minutes.

3.1. Tasks assessing the functioning of the Phonological Loop

3.1.1. Digit Recall

The first test to be administered was the Digit Recall, which involved the spoken presentation of sequences of digits. The experimenter uttered a sequence of digits of increasing length (starting from only one digit) and the child was asked to repeat the digits exactly in the same order as they were presented. All digits were uttered in even monotone at the rate of 1 per second.

Since it involves the recall of verbal material, this task taps the Phonological Loop. Both the Phonological Store and the Articulatory Rehearsal Process are engaged, given that the capacity of the Store is just of about 2 seconds (see Chapter 2). The performance of the two groups will therefore reflect the capacity and the efficiency of their phonological storage and rehearsal mechanism.

3.1.2. Word List Matching

In the Word List Matching task, the subject was presented with pairs of word lists. The experimenter uttered a list of increasing length composed of disyllabic and highly frequent words (starting from two words) and immediately after he uttered a second list composed by the same words which could be arranged in the same order as the first list or in a different order. The subject's task was to decide if the words in the second list had been uttered in the same order as in the first list.

The words were uttered in even monotone at the rate of 1 per second. A pause of 2 seconds separated the first list from the second list, so that it was clear for the child when one list ended and the second began.

Since this task is concerned with the recall of verbal information, the performances of the two groups will therefore reflect the capacity and the efficiency of their Phonological Loop.

3.1.3. Word List Recall

In the Word List Recall task, the experimenter uttered a sequence of increasing length (starting from one item) composed by disyllabic and highly familiar words. The child's task was to recall the sequence of words in the same order as it was presented. The words were uttered in even monotone at the rate of 1 per second.

As the Digit Recall and the Word List Matching, this task involves the temporary storage and rehearsal of verbal information and the subject's performance will therefore reflect the functioning and efficiency of her Phonological Loop.

3.1.4. Nonword List Recall

The Nonword List Recall Task involves the oral presentation of sequences of disyllabic nonwords, that is pronounceable but meaningless words (e.g. "lepo"). The experimenter uttered a sequence of nonwords (starting from only one nonword) and the child was asked to repeat carefully the sequence respecting the correct order of presentation.

This task involves the storage and rehearsal of verbal information and therefore it relies on the Phonological Store and the Articulatory Rehearsal Process.

Note that this task can offer a particularly pure measure of the Phonological Loop, since, differently from the other tasks, in this case the child cannot exploit the semantic meaning of the words to recall it, but rather she can rely solely on their phonological forms.

3.2. *Tasks assessing the functioning of the Visuo-Spatial Sketchpad*

3.2.1. *Block Recall*

In the Block Recall task, a block recall board with nine identical blocks was used (see Figure 1). The blocks on the board presented a digit from 1 to 9 printed on the face that only the experimenter, and not the subject, could see.

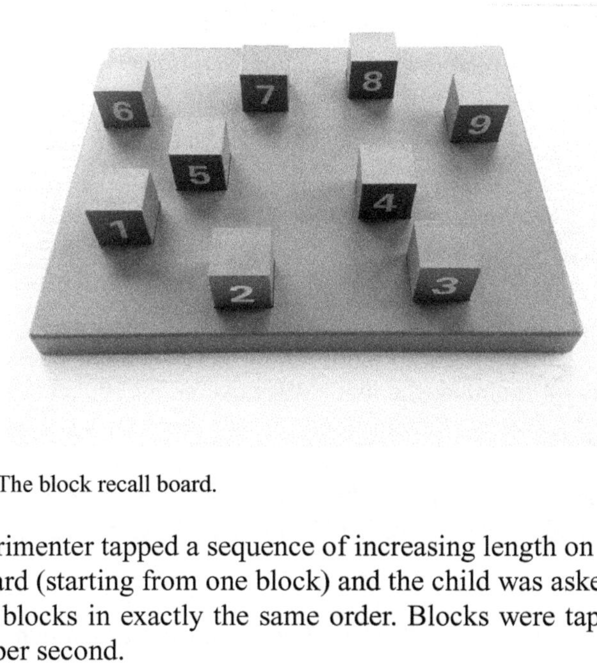

Figure 3.1. The block recall board.

The experimenter tapped a sequence of increasing length on the blocks of the board (starting from one block) and the child was asked to touch the same blocks in exactly the same order. Blocks were tapped at the rate of 1 per second.

This task involves the recall of visual and spatial information and therefore it relies on the Visuo-Spatial Sketchpad. The child's performance will therefore reflect the functioning and efficiency of her Visuo-Spatial Sketchpad.

3.2.2. *Mazes Memory*

As the Block Recall, the Mazes Memory Task was designed to assess the functioning of the Visuo-Spatial Sketchpad. The child was presented with a two-dimensional matrix of increasing size, each size corresponding to the span. She was then shown a route leading from the middle of the maze to the outside, which was marked in red and traced by the experimenter's finger (see Figure 3.2).

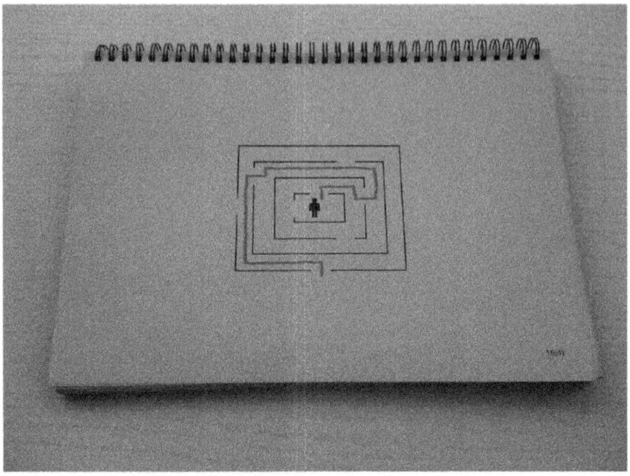

Figure 3.2. An example of the Mazes Memory Task.

In a subsequent moment, the maze was covered and the child was asked to recall the route by drawing it in an identical but blank maze. Each maze was shown to the child for about 3 seconds. This task assesses the visuo-spatial memory of the child; therefore, her performance can be taken as a reliable measure of her Visuo-Spatial Sketchpad's functioning.

3.3. *Tasks assessing the functioning of the Central Executive*

3.3.1. *Listening Recall*

The Listening Recall Task is a dual-task, which requires the contemporary execution of two different tasks.

The task involves the spoken presentation of short sentences, some of which are true (e.g. "knives are sharp") and some of which are senseless and hence false (e.g. "balls are square"). The sequence of sentences presented by the experimenter had an increasing length, starting from only one sentence. The child was asked to perform two operations: she had first to assign a truth value judgment to each sentence by saying "true" or "false" and contemporarily to memorize the final word of the sentence. After the total number of sentences composing each trial (from a minimum of 1 to a maximum of 6) was heard, the child had to recall the final word of each sentence in the same order as it was heard. This task involves the execution of two tasks contemporarily and therefore it relies heavily on the Central Executive. As the reader can note, it is remarkably more difficult than the previous tasks and it requires higher processing costs and WM resources.

3.3.2. Counting Recall

As the Listening Recall, also the Counting Recall is a dual-task, involving the contemporary execution of two different operations, requiring therefore the simultaneous processing and storage of information in WM. In this task, the child was presented with a booklet composed by a series of cards with arrays of dots printed on them, from a minimum of 4 dots to a minimum of 7 (see Figure 3.3).

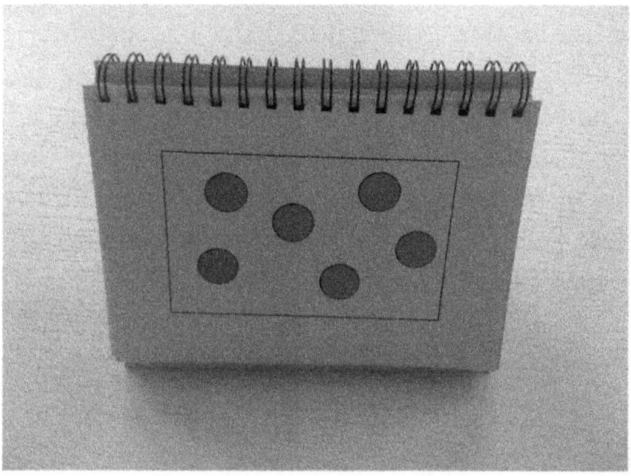

Figure 3.3. The booklet used in the Counting Recall Task.

The series of cards had an increasing length, starting from one card, which corresponded to span 1, to a maximum of 7 cards, corresponding to span 7. The child was asked to count aloud the dots using her finger; once the child had counted all dots of the series of cards, she was asked to say the total number of dots present on each card in exactly the same order as they were seen.

This task involves the execution of two tasks contemporarily, that is counting the dots and remembering the total number of dots printed on each card in the correct order. Being a dual-task, the Counting Recall task relies heavily on the Central Executive, which is concerned with dividing attention and supervising the activities.

3.3.3. Backward Digit Recall

The Backward Digit Recall Task is a dual-task imposing high processing costs on WM and in particular on the Central Executive. In this task, the experimenter uttered a sequence of digits of increasing length (from a minimum of 2 to a maximum of 7) and the child had to recall the digits in the reverse order, starting from the last digit heard and ending with the first.

This task involves the execution of two tasks contemporarily; therefore, it taxes heavily the subject's WM, reflecting in particular her Central Executive capacity. The subject, indeed has to store and recall the sequence of digits in forward order, as the experimenter presented it, and then she has to manipulate it in order to reproduce it in backward order. For this task, then, the Central Executive has a crucial importance, since it has to manage attention and to supervise the activities relative to the maintainance of the information and to the storage of the products of the intermediate computations. Therefore, the Backward Digit Recall Task provides us with a reliable measure for the functioning and efficiency of the Central Executive.

4. Results

In the next sections, I will report the results of the tasks assessing the three main components of Baddeley's Working Memory Model and the statistical analyses run to verify if there were significant differences amongst the two groups of subjects.

4.1. The Phonological Loop

As observed above, the functioning of the Phonological Loop in dyslexic and age-matched typically developing children was assessed by means of four distinct tasks: Digit Recall, Word List Matching, Word List Recall and Nonword List Recall.

All subjects were able to complete practice trials correctly for all four tasks and therefore no one was excluded from the sample. Responses were annotated, and the subject's score was calculated assigning 1 point for each correct answer and no points for wrong answers. Testing was stopped after 3 errors within the same block.

Descriptive statistics are reported in Table 3.2., whereas the performances of the two groups in the four tasks are represented in Graph 3.1.

Table 3.2. Descriptive statistics of the Phonological Loop's measures.

	DIGIT RECALL Mean Score (SD)	**WORD LIST MATCHING Mean Score (SD)**	**WORD LIST RECALL Mean Score (SD)**	**NONWORD LIST RECALL Mean Score (SD)**
DC n°21	22.52 (3.38)	16.90 (7.09)	18.48 (2.71)	11.14 (2.95)
AMCC n°21	26.43 (3.68)	26.95 (8.05)	22.86 (2.78)	16.19 (2.27)

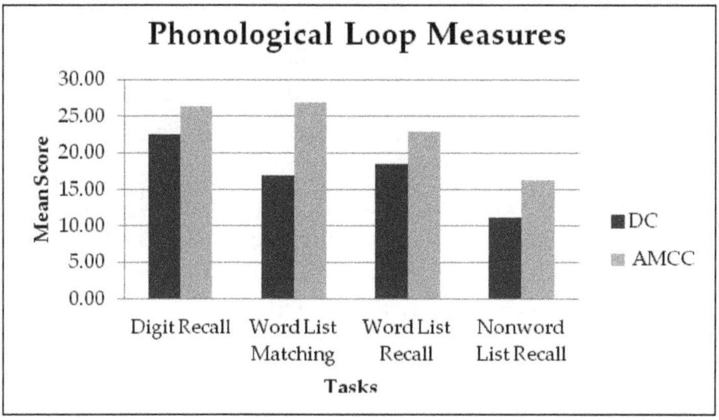

Graph 3.1. Performances of the two groups in the Phonological Loop Measures.

Observing Graph 3.1., it appears immediately evident that DC performed more poorly than controls in all four measures assessing the Phonological Loop.

In the *Digit Recall* task, in which children were asked to repeat a sequence of orally presented digits in the correct order, DC show a lower mean score in comparison to AMCC (22.52 points versus 26.43 points), corresponding to a lower span (3.81, SD = 0.67 and 4.43, SD = 0.59)

Similar results have been reported also for the *Word List Matching* task, in which children were required to compare two lists of words, verifying if the items of the second list were uttered in the same order as the items in the first list. In this task, DC's mean score was quite lower in comparison to that exhibited by AMCC (16.90 versus 26.95 points), corresponding to a significantly lower span (3.48, SD = 1.32 versus 5.52, SD = 1.60).

In the *Word List Recall*, in which subjects were asked to repeat a list of disyllabic and frequent words DC's performance is again worse in comparison to AMCC's performance. Dyslexics show a lower mean score (18,48 versus 22,86) as well as a lower span score (3.00 for DC, SD = 0.54 versus 3.90 for AMCC, SD = 0.70).

The fourth and last Phonological Measure considered was the *Nonword List Recall*, in which subjects were asked to repeat a sequence composed by pronounceable but meaningless words. Again, DC appear to be remarkably more impaired than controls, with a lower mean score (11.14 versus 16.19) and span (1.76, SD = .53 and 2.74 for AMCC, SD = .43). Note that the very low span shown by DC indicates that they cannot recall correctly even two nonwords. Both DC and AMCC show more difficulties in this task in comparison to the *Word List Recall*, that is, they perceive it more difficult to recall correctly nonwords in comparison to words. On average, DC can recall correctly only 1.76 nonwords, whereas they could repeat 3.00 words. Similarly, AMCC can recall 2.74 nonwords in comparison to 3.90 meaningful words. This discrepancy can be ascribed to the fact that in word list recall tasks the subject can rely on semantic cues (i.e. the meaning of the word) to remember and retrieve the correct items, whereas this strategy cannot be exploited with nonwords.

Since, as discussed above, the *Nonword List Recall* task provides a particularly pure measure of the Phonological Loop, the very poor performance displayed by DC confirms even strongly that their phonological memory is impaired.

A statistical analysis was performed on the results reported for the four Phonological Loop measures, to verify if the differences found amongst the groups were significant. The scores on the Phonological Loop tests were subjected to a multivariate analysis of variance (MANOVA) with *Digit Recall*, *Word List Matching*, *Word List Recall* and *Nonword List Recall* as dependent variables and *Group* (DC; AMCC) as fixed factor. A significant effect for *Group* was found ($F(4, 37) = 10.377$, $p < .001$, partial $\eta^2 = .53$) confirming that there were highly significant differences between the mean score of the DC group and the AMCC group. Group was also significantly affected by the tasks separately. *Digit Recall* was highly significant ($F(1, 41) = 12.798$, $p <.001$, partial $\eta^2 = .24$), as well as *Word List Matching* ($F(1, 41) = 18.397$, $p < .001$, partial $\eta^2 = .32$), *Word List Recall* ($F(1, 41) = 26.709$, $p < .000$, partial $\eta^2 = .40$) and *Nonword List Recall* ($F(1 ,41= 38.519$, $p <.001$, partial $\eta^2 = .49$).

These results confirm that there were significant differences amongst the two groups both for the entire construct Phonological Loop and for the tasks separately, demonstrating that dyslexic children performed always significantly worse than age-matched typically developing children.

To summarize, these findings support the evidence that dyslexics manifest marked deficits affecting their Phonological Loop. The *Digit Recall*, the *Word List Matching*, the *Word List Recall* and the *Nonword List Recall* were able to reliably predict the differences amongst the two groups. Since all four tasks require both temporary storage and rehearsal of verbal information, the results demonstrate that the Phonological Store and the Articulatory Rehearsal Process are both impaired in developmental dyslexia.

4.2. *The Visuo-Spatial Sketchpad*

The functioning of the Visuo-Spatial Sketchpad was assessed by means of two tasks, namely the *Block Recall* and the *Mazes Memory*, in dyslexic children and in typically developing children. All subjects were able to complete practice trials correctly in both tasks and therefore no one was excluded from the sample. Responses were annotated, assigning 1 point for each correct answer and no points for wrong answers; both the total score and the span were annotated.

Descriptive statistics are reported in Table 3.3., whereas the performances of the two groups in the four tasks are represented in Graph 3.2.

Table 3.3. Descriptive statistics of the Visuo-Spatial Sketchpad's measures.

	BLOCK RECALL Mean Score (SD)	**MAZES MEMORY Mean Score (SD)**
DC n°21	25.90 (4.79)	20.81 (7.18)
AMCC n°21	27.76 (3.88)	19.71 (6.24)

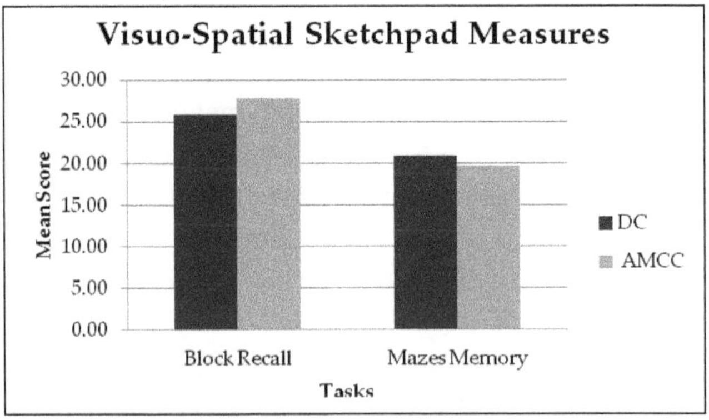

Graph. 3.2. Performances of the two groups in the Visuo-Spatial Sketchpad Measures.

In the *Block Recall* the subjects were asked to recall a sequence of blocks tapped by the experimenter on a Block Recall Board by touching each block in the correct order. In this case DC's performance is only slightly lower than AMCC's performance: DC perform as well as AMCC, showing a similar mean score (25.90 versus 27.76) and mean span (4.23 for DC, SD = .83 versus 4.48 for AMCC, SD = .65).

Similar results have been obtained in the *Mazes Memory* task, in which subjects were presented with a maze and were asked to recall the route from the middle of the maze to the outside as it was shown by the experimenter, by drawing it on a blank maze. Again, results show that dyslexics perform as well as their peers, showing a similar mean score (20.81 for DC versus 19.71 for AMCC) and mean span (4.33 for DC, SD = 1.35 versus 4.26 for AMCC, SD = 1.05).

A statistical analysis was performed on the results reported for the two Visuo-Spatial Sketchpad measures, to verify if the differences found amongst the groups were significant. The scores on the Visuo-Spatial Sketchpad tests were subjected to a multivariate analysis of variance (MANOVA) with *Block Recall* and *Mazes Memory* as dependent variables and *Group* (DC; AMCC) as fixed factor. No significant effect for *Group* was found ($F (2, 39) = 1.897$, $p = .164$, partial $\eta^2 = .09$) confirming that the two groups of children did not perform differently in the Visuo-Spatial Sketchpad tasks. No significant differences were found also considering the two tasks separately. *Block* Recall, in fact, was not significant ($F (1, 41) = 36.214$, $p = .176$, partial $\eta^2 = .05$), as well as *Mazes Memory* ($F(1, 41) = 12.595$, $p = .601$, partial $\eta^2 = .01$).

Summarizing, these data show that DC and AMCC performed similarly in tasks involving their visuo-spatial memory, suggesting that their Visuo-Spatial Sketchpad is unimpaired.

4.3. The Central Executive

The functioning of the Central Executive was assessed by means of three tasks, namely the Listening Recall, the Counting Recall and the Backward Digit Recall.

All subjects were able to complete practice trials correctly in both tasks and therefore no one was excluded from the sample. Responses were annotated, assigning 1 point for each correct answer and no points for wrong answers; both the total score and the span were annotated.

Descriptive statistics are reported in Table 3.4., whereas the performances of the two groups in the four tasks are represented in Graph 3.3.

Table 3.4. Descriptive statistics of the Central Executive's measures.

	LISTENING RECALL Mean Score (SD)	**COUNTING RECALL Mean Score (SD)**	**BACKWARD DIGIT RECALL Mean Score (SD)**
DC n°**21**	10.76 (3.78)	17.14 (4.02)	8.95 (3.29)
AMCC n°**21**	14.48 (3.45)	23.10 (4.74)	13.76 (3.56)

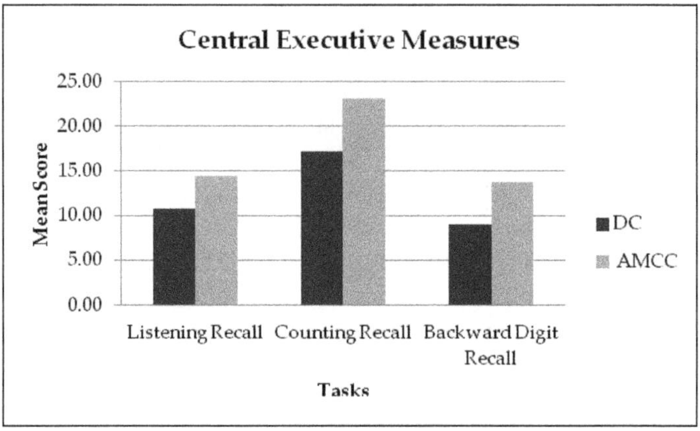

Graph 3.3. Performances of the two groups in the Central Executive Measures.

Observing Graph 3.3. it appears evident that dyslexics underperform in comparison to controls in all three measures assessing the Central Executive.

In the *Listening Recall*, a task in which subjects were asked to execute two tasks simultaneously, evaluating a series of truth or false sentences and recalling the last word of each sentence in the correct order, DC display remarkably more difficulties in comparison to their peers, with a lower mean score (10.76 versus 14.48) and a lower mean span (1.67, SD = 0.70 versus 2.43, SD = 0.67). Note that the very low span shown by DC indicates that they could not even recall correctly the final word of two sentences, whereas controls performed much better.

Similar findings have been reported for the *Counting Recall*, another complex task requiring the subject to count the number of dots presented on a series of cards and to recall the total number of dots of each card in the correct order. Again, DC underperform in comparison to their peers, with a lower mean score (17.14 versus 23.10) and a lower mean span (2.76, SD = 0.70 versus 3.70, SD = 0.81). This suggest that they are remarkably more impaired than typically developing children in the Counting Recall Task, indicating that they suffer from an impairment affecting the Central Executive.

The third and last measure assessing the Central Executive was the *Backward Digit Recall*. In this task, subjects were presented with a sequence of digits and they were asked to recall the sequence in reverse order. Once again DC underperform in comparison to their peers, with a very low mean score (8.95 versus 13.76) and mean span (2.43, SD = 0.67 versus 3.22, SD = 0.62), showing that they are outstandingly more impaired than controls.

A statistical analysis was performed on the results reported for the three Central Executive measures, to verify if the differences found amongst the groups were significant. The scores on the Central Executive tests were subjected to a multivariate analysis of variance (MANOVA) with *Listening Recall*, *Counting Recall* and *Backward Digit Recall* as dependent variables and *Group* (DC; AMCC) as fixed factor. A significant effect for *Group* was found ($F(3, 38) = 8.908$, $p < .001$, partial $\eta^2 = .41$) confirming that there were highly significant differences between the mean score of the DC group and the AMCC group. Group was significant affected also considering the tasks separately. *Listening Recall* was highly significant ($F(1, 41) = 11.036$, $p < .001$, partial $\eta^2 = .22$), as well as *Counting Recall* ($F(1, 41) = 19.217$, $p < .001$, partial $\eta^2 = .33$) and *Backward Digit Recall* ($F(1, 41) = 20.637$, $p < .001$, partial $\eta^2 = .34$).

These results confirm that there are significant differences amongst the two group both for the entire construct Central Executive and for the tasks separately, showing that dyslexic children underperform in comparison to control children. To summarize, then, these findings confirm that dyslexics suffer from marked deficits affecting their Central Executive, as evidenced by their poor performance in the *Listening Recall*, the *Counting Recall* and the *Backward Digit Recall* tasks.

5. General Discussion

Dyslexic children's and age-matched typically developing children's Working Memory Skills were tested with the aim of evaluating the hypothesis according to which dyslexics suffer from the memory deficits exposed in Chapter 2. We administered the Working Memory Test Battery for Children, developed by Pickering and Gathercole in order to assess children's WM skills. The battery comprised 9 tasks assessing the three main components of Baddeley's model, namely 4 tasks testing Phonological Loop (i.e. *Digit Recall*, *Word List Matching*, *Word List Recall* and *Nonword List Recall*), 2 tasks testing the Visuo-Spatial Sketchpad (i.e. *Block Recall* and *Mazes Memory*) and 3 tasks testing the Central Executive (i.e. *Listening Recall*, *Counting Recall* and *Backward Digit Recall*).

Results provided strong support in favor of the hypothesis that dyslexia is related to a WM inefficiency, confirming that dyslexic children are indeed highly impaired in comparison to control children in all Phonological Loop and Central Executive measures. Conversely, their Visuo-Spatial Sketchpad is unimpaired and well-functioning, as demonstrated by the fact that no significant differences have been found between the two groups of children.

Specifically, it has been proven that dyslexics exhibit remarkable difficulties concerning their phonological memory when asked to recall sequences of digits, words and nonwords, and when required to compare the order of the words presented in two lists. Since these tasks require both temporary storage and rehearsal of verbal information, results demonstrate that the Phonological Store and the Articulatory Rehearsal Process are both impaired in dyslexics.

The greatest difference between DC and AMCC is found in the *Word List Matching* task, in which dyslexics scored remarkably lower than their peers. This particularly high difference can be explained by observing that the *Word List Matching* taxes more heavily the capacity of the Phonological Loop, in comparison to the other phonological measures. The sequence of items to be remembered is namely much longer, given the presentation of two lists instead of only one.

Nonetheless, all the phonological memory tasks proposed in this protocol have been found able to reliably predict the difficulties associated with dyslexia.

The same considerations also hold for the tasks assessing the Central Executive, namely the *Listening Recall*, the *Counting Recall* and the *Backward Digit Recall*: in all of these measures DC exhibited a very poor performance in comparison to AMCC. In this case, the worst performance is registered in the Counting Recall task, where children are asked to count aloud arrays of dots printed on a series of cards and to recall the total number of dots present on each card. In this task, DC scored 5.95 points less than AMCC, corresponding to a span of 0.93 items.

As discussed above, the difficulty experienced by dyslexics in Central Executive tasks is arguably due to the processing load imposed by the request to perform two tasks simultaneously.

Nevertheless, it is important to notice that all the three tasks assessing the functioning of the Central Executive involve the verbal dimension; one could then hypothesize that dyslexics' impaired Phonological Loop could have contributed to their poor performance. To dispel this doubt it would be extremely interesting to test dyslexics' and controls' performance using dual tasks based on visuo-spatial, rather than verbal, material. However, results from existing experiments, as the ones reviewed in Chapter 2 testing the control of attention and the effects of interference, have already demonstrated that Central Executive functioning is remarkably compromised in dyslexics. As a consequence, we should expect that dyslexics experience difficulties also in visuo-spatial Central Executive measures, in spite of their good visuo-spatial competence.

The results reported for the two tasks assessing the Visuo-Spatial Sketchpad, in fact, have revealed that DC behave as well as AMCC and that their ability to temporarily store visual and spatial information is spared. Analyzing their performance in non-verbal Central Executive tasks, then, could further confirm that their difficulties are actually due to Central Executive impairments. If dyslexics' Central Executive is damaged or not properly functioning, in fact, it should be expected that they manifest difficulties in all kinds of dual-tasks, independently of the nature of the stimuli presented.

To summarize, results demonstrate that dyslexic children suffer indeed from a Working Memory deficit, affecting their Phonological Loop and Central Executive, whereas their Visuo-Spatial Sketchpad is spared.

These findings, which are consistent with the results of previous studies, provide further evidence in favor of the hypothesis according to which dyslexics' working memory skills are impaired.

6. Summary and Conclusions

In this chapter I have presented and discussed the results of an experimental protocol administered to analyze dyslexics' and age-matched typically developing children's performance in a series of working memory tasks. Results have demonstrated that dyslexics suffer from remarkable impairments affecting their Phonological Loop and Central Executive, but leaving their Visuo-Spatial Sketchpad completely spared. These data, obtained with the administration of the WMTB-C, indicate then that dyslexics exhibit highly significant deficits in comparison to their peers in the execution of phonological memory tasks and also in dual tasks imposing a great load on their Central Executive.

In conclusion, the results obtained with the administration of the WMTB-C, strongly support the hypothesis claiming that dyslexia is linked to a working memory inefficiency, affecting dyslexics' phonological competence and their performance in demanding tasks, such as dual-tasks.

Based on this robust result, I will propose in Chapter 4 an original hypothesis arguing that the WM deficit exhibited by dyslexics can be held responsible for all the manifestations of dyslexia reviewed in Chapter 1.

Chapter 4

The Phonological and Executive Working Memory Deficit Hypothesis

1. Introduction

In Chapter 2 I have presented and discussed the hypotheses proposed by McLoughlin (1994; 2002) and Fiorin (2010), which suggest that developmental dyslexia is related to a Working Memory Deficit.

As discussed in Chapter 3, the administration of the Working Memory Test Battery for Children, developed by Pickering and Gathercole precisely with the purpose of assessing children's WM, has provided further interesting results in favor of the hypothesis that dyslexics suffer from WM deficits. In particular, dyslexic children have been found remarkably impaired in comparison to their peers in all the measures assessing the functioning of the Phonological Loop and the Central Executive. Instead, no significant differences have been found between dyslexics and controls in the measures assessing their Visuo-Spatial Sketchpad.

Taking into consideration these experimental data, I will present in this chapter an original proposal that is able to account for all the manifestations of dyslexia reviewed in Chapter 1, pointing to a disruption of dyslexics' verbal and executive Working Memory skills. Implementing Fiorin's hypothesis, indeed I will argue that dyslexics suffer from both a phonological memory impairment and an inefficiency affecting their executive functions, which leads to a disorder in their ability to carry out complex tasks that are particularly demanding in terms of processing resources.

However, before presenting the hypothesis, I would like to set Working Memory in a broader perspective, with the intent of showing that it represents a fundamental ingredient of human cognition. Specifically,

I will argue that WM plays a crucial role in both reasoning and language comprehension, two aspects that are essential for our discussion on developmental dyslexia.

I will then present the Capacity Constrained Comprehension Theory, which has been developed by Just and Carpenter (1992; 2002) to account for linguistic deficits in individuals whose Working Memory skills are particularly poor. After dealing with these matters, I will present my proposal, that I call the Phonological and Executive Working Memory Deficit Hypothesis, and I will demonstrate how it is able to account for the deficits discussed in this book.

2. Working Memory and Human Cognition

It is now generally acknowledged that Working Memory has a fundamental importance in human cognition and that it is crucially involved in the execution of all complex activities, ranging from thinking and reasoning, to problem solving and, much interestingly for our discussion, to language comprehension.

Although Baddeley and Hitch's (1974) and Baddeley's (2000) Working Memory models have been criticized for being too simplistic and not readily falsifiable, their proposals offer a good starting point for the conceptualization of WM, providing evidence for a dissociation between the visuo-spatial and the verbal components and for the existence of a system capable of controlling and supervising operations.

Beyond its short-term storage capacity, in fact, it is widely recognized that WM is equipped with a pool of operational resources that executes the actual computations required, temporarily maintaining their intermediate and final products (Just and Carpenter 1992, 2002). The efficiency of an individual's WM system determines therefore her ability to perform complex operations, as demonstrated by a study conducted by Kyllonen and Christal (1990) that examined the correlation between WM abilities and reasoning, measured with tests of fluid intelligence. The authors tested 2144 adults and they found that WM skills were highly correlated to reasoning as well as to processing speed[1], demonstrating therefore that WM skills constitute the core of human cognition.

In their comprehensive review of the literature concerning the relationship between WM, fluid intelligence and processing speed, Fry and Hale (2000) noticed that these three components are strongly correlated in children as well. Specifically, they observed that WM, fluid intelligence and processing speed tend to develop in concert following a similar course and that children's processing speed increases with age. As they grow up, indeed, children become able to process information more quickly, while adult levels are reached in middle adolescence. Interestingly, this developmental trend is very similar to that reported for WM skills and reviewed in Chapter 2.

An explanation for the correlation between WM and reasoning skills is provided by Just and Carpenter (2002), who propose an account based on the notion of capacity, arguing that the greater is the capacity of an individual's WM and the more information she can handle simultaneously for problem solving. Importantly, they identify an individual's WM with the functioning of her Central Executive, leaving aside the two modality-specific subsystems, namely the Phonological Loop and the Visuo-Spatial Sketchpad, since they are supposed to serve only for storage. As we will discuss in the following section, this assumption is also shared by Caplan and Waters, who identify the Central Executive as the "workhouse and mastermind of human cognition" (Caplan and Waters 1999: 77).

As mentioned above, a key concept in Just and Carpenter proposal is that of *capacity*, intended as the maximum amount of activation available in WM to support both storage and processing functions. Very briefly, an item is said to be activated when it crosses a minimum threshold value, becoming available in WM, and it can be used to perform the requested computations. An individual able to maintain higher levels of activations can then rely on greater processing resources to perform tasks, and consequently she will show greater reasoning abilities and speed. Conversely, an individual with a lower WM capacity can rely on lower activation resources and therefore she is forced to reallocate the activated elements, resulting in a worse and slower performance.

1 Processing speed can be defined as the speed at which an individual is able to perform and complete a task.

Similarly, when the task's demands are particularly high and exceed the general capacity of the system, "some of the activation that is maintaining old elements will be deallocated, producing a kind of forgetting by displacement" (Just and Carpenter 2002: 132). In other words, when an individual has to perform a very difficult operation or a complex reasoning, both storage and computations may be degraded, with the consequence that the processing slows down and that some partial results may be forgotten, giving rise to errors.

In Just and Carpenter framework, then, individual differences do not depend on the architecture of the system, but rather on its capacity: a person whose WM capacity is higher will be more skilled in making inferences and in problem solving, thanks to her ability to maintain in WM all the necessary representations at once. Importantly, a significant consequence of this proposal is that individual differences arise when subjects are presented with processing demanding tasks. It is very likely, indeed, that all subjects perform similarly in easy tasks.

Another important proposal put forward by Just and Carpenter is that different processing domains rely on different pools of activation resources whose capacities are not necessarily correlated with each other: it follows, for instance, that an individual with a good verbal competence and high comprehension skills is not necessarily equally skilled in visuo-spatial complex tasks. Notice that this specification permits to explain why each individual can present strengths in one domain and weaknesses in another domain, and why patients affected by neurodevelopmental disorders can exhibit impaired processing at certain levels and normal performance in other cognitive areas.

To summarize so far, in Just and Carpenter's account Working Memory skills, which coincide with the Central Executive functions, are supposed to be intimately linked to reasoning abilities and processing speed. However, individual differences concerning performance in distinct processing domains are also predicted, since specific cognitive abilities rely on specific and independent pools of resources. Note that their Capacity Constrained Comprehension Theory gives rise to precise predictions: if an individual's verbal WM is particularly poor, in fact, she is expected to show a slower and more impaired performance in those tasks which are particularly demanding. Conversely, a subject exhibiting a greater verbal WM capacity is predicted to perform faster and more efficiently. These predictions have been tested by Just and Carpenter, whose theory has been indeed applied successfully to language comprehension, providing interesting results that will be exposed in the following section.

3. Working Memory and Language Comprehension

Just and Carpenter (1992; 2002) discussed specifically the role of Working Memory in language comprehension, presenting a theory, the *Capacity Constrained Comprehension Theory*, based on the concepts of capacity and activation introduced above. In their proposal, the information generated by computations or retrieved from long-term memory, is activated in WM during the comprehension process. Once the relevant information is activated (i.e. once it surpasses a certain threshold), it becomes available in WM and it can be used to perform the requested computations.

However, processing resources are needed to maintain the activation level: if the resources available are lower than the amount required to perform the task, then some of the information may be forgotten. As a consequence, the individual might need to process the sentence another time, causing a slowdown of the processing. Or, again, she might misinterpret the utterance.

Difficulties can arise, in particular, when the number of processes required to understand a sentence exceeds the general capacity of the system. Just and Carpenter emphasize that many of the processes required for the comprehension of an utterance occur in parallel, that is, they are executed simultaneously, generating partial products which are to be maintained and further manipulated in order to obtain the final meaning. Storage demands in WM are generally minimized by means of the tendency to interpret each new phrase as soon as possible when it is entered in the computation.

To better understand this proposal, let us analyze first a simple sentence, as that reported in (1), and then a more complex utterance, as the relative sentences in (2) and (3).[2]

(1) The girl caressed the cat.

In this case, the processor identifies *the girl* as the grammatical subject of the sentence and therefore it generates the expectation that a verb will occur. This expectation is satisfied as the verb *caressed* is encountered: at this point, the parser can establish the subject-verb dependency between *the girl* and *caressed*. Once this relation is established, it is not necessary to maintain the subject activated in memory any longer. Moreover, the verb *caressed* generates the expectation that an object will soon occur. Again, the expectation is satisfied by the presence of the object *the cat*. While syntactic dependencies are being computed, the human processor can further calculate other semantic and pragmatic features in order to assign the appropriate meaning to the sentence.

The processing is arguably more loaded when the subject has to compute a sentence like (2) and even more when it is presented with a sentence like (3).

(2) The boy scared the cat that the girl caressed.
(3) The boy that the cat that the girl caressed scared laughed.

As discussed in Chapter 1, the processing of relative sentences is remarkably demanding. The activated elements, in fact, are to be maintained in memory until the syntactic dependencies have been established. While computing a sentence like (3), in particular, most individuals are likely to experience problems assigning the appropriate thematic roles and establishing who did what to whom.

In Just and Carpenter, as well as in Gibson (1991; 1998), this happens because the amount of resources available is exceeded by the computational demands of the sentence. Specifically, the capacity of the system is not sufficient to maintain activated all the items encountered while parsing the sentence. As a consequence, the processing

2 Cf. with the processing of relative sentences discussed in Chapter 1. The model proposed by Gibson (1991, 1998) shares the assumptions of the approach proposed by Just and Carpenter and reviewed in this paragraph.

slows down and some information may be forgotten. Formally, Just and Carpenter argue that "if the activation propagation on a given cycle of production firings would exceed the activation maximum, then both the activation propagated and the activation used for maintainance are scaled back proportionally to their current use" (Just and Carpenter 2002: 133).

The main consequence of this proposal is that language comprehension is supposed to be constrained by an individual's WM capacity. The authors suggest, in fact, that the amount of activation available to each individual varies depending on her WM capacity: a subject WM capacity, then, might determine the amount of resources that she can rely on, influencing therefore both the accuracy and the speed of her language comprehension skills.

In order to test this proposal, Just and Carpenter analyzed the performance of people with higher and lower WM skills on a range of different tasks. WM capacity was generally assessed by means of the Reading Span Task (Daneman and Carpenter 1980), in which the subject is asked to read a set of unrelated sentences and to recall, at the end of the series, the last word of each utterance in the correct order. Notice that the Reading Span Task is very similar to the Listening Span Task that I administered and discussed in Chapter 3, and that it determines the efficiency of the subjects' Central Executive. In fact, it requires the individual to perform two tasks simultaneously, involving both storage and processing functions. Just and Carpenter administered a series of experimental protocols to high-span and low-span subjects[3] to verify if there were significant differences amongst the groups, consistently with the predictions raised by their proposal. Specifically, they tested garden path sentences, ambiguous sentences and object relative clauses. Each experiment will be briefly reviewed in the following sections.

3 The spans of the Reading Span tests typically range from 2 to 5.5 words for sentences such as "When at last his eyes opened, there was no gleam of triumph, no shade of anger". High span subjects have spans of four words or more, whereas low span subjects have spans of less than three words. Medium span subject, instead, have spans of three and three and a half words (Just and Carpenter 1992).

3.1. The comprehension of garden path and ambiguous sentences

Garden path sentences are utterances that can be easily misunderstood, because of a local ambiguity, which leads to an improper parsing. A typical garden path sentence is the one reported in (4).

(4) Fat people eat accumulates.

Individuals generally tend to analyze *fat* as an adjective modifying the noun *people*. Therefore, they process *eat* as the main verb of the sentence, establishing a syntactic dependency between *fat people* and *eat*, but they get stuck when they encounter the verb *accumulates*. They are then forced to reread the sentence, recognizing that *people eat* is actually a reduced relative clause and that *accumulates* is the main verb of the sentence. In other words, they have been "led down the garden path" due to the local ambiguity of *fat*, which can be interpreted as a noun or as an adjective. The ambiguity, in fact, disappears in (5):

(5) The fat that people eat accumulates.

Just and Carpenter tested a specific type of garden path sentences, following the proposal by Ferreira and Clifton (1986) who ideated a task in which readers had the possibility to avoid being led down the garden path resorting to nonsyntactic information. Consider (6):

(6) The defendant examined by the lawyer shocked the jury.

Sentence (6) is temporarily ambiguous, due to local ambiguity of the verb *examined*, which can both be the main verb of the sentence and the verb of a reduced relative clause. However, since *the defendant* is a plausible agent of the verb *examined*, the parser is more likely to interpret it as the main verb of the sentence. However, the interpretation of the verb can change radically if *the defendant* is replaced with an inanimate object, as *the evidence* in (7):

(7) The evidence examined by the lawyer shocked the jury.

While parsing (7), the reader can resort to nonsyntactic information to avoid being led down the garden path, observing that *the evidence* is an inanimate object and that therefore it cannot be interpreted as the agent of the verb *examined*. If the subject makes this reasoning, than she will interpret *examined* as the verb of a reduced relative clause.

Just and Carpenter examined reading times of high-span and low-span subjects asked to read and understand sentences like (6) and (7). Interestingly, they found that only people with a high WM span are sensitive to the nonsyntactic cue provided in sentences like (7), which indicates that *examined* should be interpreted as the verb of a reduced relative clause, given that *the evidence* cannot be its subject. Specifically, only high-span readers show a faster processing when the grammatical subject was inanimate, whereas no time differences are found between (6) and (7) in low-span subjects. This finding is strongly consistent with the predictions made by Just and Carpenter's hypothesis: only people with high WM span have an amount of available resources that is sufficient to carry on a nonsyntactic analysis contemporarily to the syntactic parsing. Subjects with a lower span, instead, lack the resources to execute both analyses simultaneously and this prevents them from using the nonsyntactic cue to parse the sentence and to avoid being led down the garden path.

Similar results have been found with ambiguous sentences like the one reported below.

(8) The experienced soldiers warned about the dangers before the midnight raid.
(9) The experienced soldiers spoke about the dangers before the midnight raid.

The verb *warned* in (8) is locally ambiguous, since it is interpreted both as the main verb of the sentence and as the verb of a reduced relative clause.

However, Just and Carpenter found that only high-span subjects asked to read the target sentences were sensitive to this ambiguity, as demonstrated by their reading times, which were longer than that shown by low-span subjects. According to the authors, the slowing down of their processing is due to the fact that they are maintaining in memory both possible representations of the ambiguous sentence. The low-span readers, instead, show faster reading times while reading sentences like (8), whereas the differences between the two groups of subjects disappears with unambiguous sentences. This demonstrates that low-span readers represent just one, the most likely one, of the alternatives, which turned then to be the correct one.

Again, these different tendencies are consistent with the hypothesis proposed by Just and Carpenter: people with a lower WM capacity do not have enough resources to maintain both representations, and tend to immediately abandon the less likely one. On the contrary, individuals with a greater WM capacity can rely on an amount of resources that is sufficient to satisfy the additional demand of maintaining simultaneously two representations instead of only one.

3.2. The comprehension of object relative clauses

We have already observed that the comprehension of object relative clauses is particularly demanding, since it forces the subject to maintain the elements activated in memory longer in comparison to subject relative clauses (cf. Chapter 1). Just and Carpenter measured and confronted the reading times showed by high-span subjects and low-span subjects asked to read sentences like the ones reported in (10) and (11).

(10) The reporter that attacked the senator admitted the error.
(11) The reporter that the senator attacked admitted the error.

Arguably, (10) is easier to understand, since while analyzing (11) the subject has to maintain both *the reporter* and *the senator* activated in memory, demanding thus more processing resources.

The authors found that low-span subjects show longer reading times in comparison to high-span subjects and that they display even a less accurate performance. When asked to answer comprehension questions about these sentences, in fact, they respond correctly only in 64% of the cases, versus the 85% of the high-span subjects.

Summarizing, despite they spend more time processing the sentence, low-span readers are less accurate and commit more errors than high-span subjects. Again, then, the finding is consistent with Just and Carpenter's proposal.

3.3. *Further evidence in favor of the Capacity Constrained Comprehension Theory: extrinsic memory load and distance effects*

Another way to test the Capacity Constrained Comprehension Theory proposed by Just and Carpenter consists in manipulating the experimental context, adding to the comprehension task the request to maintain contemporarily an extrinsic memory load.

Specifically, subjects were asked to retain a sequence of digits or words during sentence comprehension. In their proposal, this additional verbal load is supposed to impose an extra burden on the individual's WM, since further costs are needed to maintain it in memory while computing the sentence meaning.

King and Just (1991) found that the additional task of remembering a series of words affects significantly the comprehension of subject and object relative clauses. Specifically, the general accuracy decreases drastically as the request to perform this additional task is introduced, suggesting that both tasks compete for the same WM resources and that this reduces the total capacity of the system.

Finally, the analysis of distance effects has provided interesting results, too. The concept of distance refers to the gap occurring between two pieces of information that are to be related. A crucial part of language comprehension is that of establishing relationships between elements in the discourse. Clearly, it is more difficult to correlate two constituents that are distant from each other, since in this case the individual is forced to maintain the first item in WM for a longer period, increasing then the probability of forgetting and resulting in a lower accuracy. Establishing a relation between two pieces of information is indeed possible only if earlier material is still activated in memory and available for further computations.

Consistently, Daneman and Carpenter (1980) found that high-span subjects are able to maintain information activated longer in comparison to low-span subjects and that their greater capacity allows them to retrieve more accurately the appropriate antecedent of a pronoun. Examining these results, Just and Carpenter observe that WM capacity is crucially involved also in the construction of a coherent discourse interpretation.

To summarize, the experiments conducted on high-span and low-span subjects testing the interpretation of garden path and ambiguous sentences, the comprehension of relative clauses, and the effects of adding an extrinsic memory load and of increasing the distance between two elements to be related, provide strong evidence in favor of the Capacity Constrained Comprehension Theory. This suggests that the WM capacity of an individual constrains severely her comprehension skills, determining her ability to generate inferences, to represent simultaneously the different readings of ambiguous sentences and to establish relationships between distinct pieces of information.

3.4. Is there a general verbal Working Memory or a specific and independent WM for language comprehension?

In the preceding sections we have observed that Working Memory plays a crucial role in the comprehension of language. As anticipated in Chapter 2, the importance of WM in language had been grasped already by Baddeley, even though he did not analyze language comprehension in detail. Actually he simply mentioned that the Phonological Loop seems to be involved in the acquisition of language.

Another important step in this direction has been made by Just and Carpenter, who developed the Capacity Constrained Comprehension Theory precisely to account for the involvement of WM in linguistic computation. Specifically, we have observed that they identified the Central Executive as the component crucially involved in language processing and that they formulated a proposal based on the notion of capacity. Moreover, they provided strong evidence confirming that an individual with a greater WM capacity has more resources available to perform computations and that, as a consequence, she can process language faster and more efficiently in comparison to an individual with a lower WM capacity.

These results demonstrate on the one side that if the Phonological Loop is involved in the acquisition of vocabulary, influencing also the individual's phonological awareness, the Central Executive is the component responsible for language comprehension. The Phonological Loop, in fact, cannot account for syntactic, semantic and pragmatic computations, but rather it provides only a phonological analysis of the sentence to be interpreted.

As mentioned above, one important consequence of this approach is that the effects of an impaired Central Executive functioning are expected to be more evident with linguistically complex sentences. A low-span subject may actually nevertheless have an amount of resources sufficient to compute easier structures and her impairment may therefore be manifested only in more demanding tasks.

Although the importance of WM in language comprehension is not challenged, a debate has arisen concerning the question whether there is a unitary verbal WM, deputed to compute also non-linguistic but verbal material, or instead a WM specific for linguistic processing.

The first proposal, shared by Just and Carpenter (1992; 2002), Fedorenko and colleagues (2006) and Gordon and colleagues (2002), argues that both linguistic and non-linguistic but verbally-mediated processing rely on a general resource pool dedicated to verbal WM.

The second account, instead, as proposed by Caplan and Waters (1996; 1999), claims that there is a verbal WM specialized for linguistic computations and another verbal WM deputed to the computation of verbal but non-linguistic material. Specifically, they suggest that the WM system involved in interpretive processes (i.e. syntactic and semantic computations) is a separate subsystem within verbal WM. This proposal raises the specific prediction that the addition of verbal material to be remembered should not interfere with the interpretation of a sentence, given that they rely on different pools of resources. According to the authors, in fact, the request of maintaining in memory a sequence of words or digits does not involve interpretive processes and it should not affect syntactic and semantic computation. However, this prediction has been disconfirmed by the results of the experimental protocols performed by Gordon and colleagues (2002) and, more recently, by Fedorenko and colleagues (2006; 2007). Fedorenko, Gibson and Rohde (2007), in particular, developed an interesting experiment, asking subjects to process syntactically complex sentences while performing a secondary task. In the first condition, this additional task had a verbal but non-linguistic nature, involving arithmetic integration processes; specifically, the subject was required to read a set of relative clauses and, simultaneously, to sum a sequence of numbers. The sentence was divided into four regions and it was presented on a computer screen in four fragments (e.g. “The janitor / who frustrated the plumber / lost the key / on the street”), whereas the numbers for the addition task were presented simultaneously above each fragment (e.g. “12 / +4 / +5 / +4”). Both the sentence and the addition presented varied in complexity; the amounts of time required by the subject to read each fragment of the sentence and to perform the respective addition were recorded. In the second condition, the secondary task was a spatial-rotation task, in which the subject was shown a circle with a colored sector. In correspondence of each of the four fragments of the sentence, the subject was instructed to imagine adding each sector to the preceding ones, remembering the angle obtained by the combined sectors. For the reader’s convenience, an example of this secondary task is reported below.

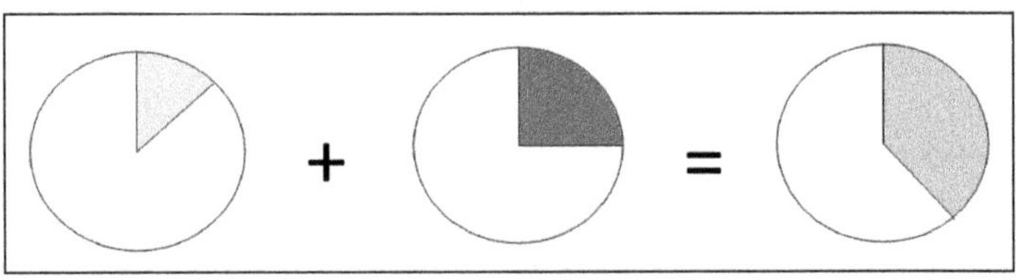

Figure 4.1. An example of the experiment developed by Fedorenko, Gibson and Rohde (2007).

As the arithmetic addition task, the spatial rotation task involves the integration of an incoming element into the original representation. Although the kind of processing required is similar, the spatial rotation task does not rely on verbal WM and therefore it should not affect performance in the reading task, differently from the arithmetic integration task, which instead should interfere with reading speed. Results are indeed consistent with both predictions: a strong interaction has been found in the first condition, where subjects had to compute the additions, indicating that this task relied on the same pool of resources as the linguistic task. Conversely, a significantly weaker interaction has been observed in the second condition, where participants had to perform the spatial rotation task. On one side these findings show once again that verbal WM and visuo-spatial WM are independent from each other, whereas on the other side they provide evidence against the hypothesis by Caplan and

Waters that linguistic computations are served by a specific and separate subsystem within verbal WM. Conversely, results support the view that both linguistic and non-linguistic but verbally mediated processes rely on verbal WM.

To summarize so far, in these sections we have observed that Working Memory, and especially the Central Executive, is crucially involved in the comprehension of language, as well as in other complex activities. In the following paragraph I will propose that a Central Executive impairment, together with a Phonological Loop impairment, can be held responsible for the manifestations of dyslexia reviewed in Chapter 1.

4. The Phonological and Executive Working Memory Deficit Hypothesis

As discussed both in Chapter 2 and in the present chapter, Working Memory is the brain system which has the function to (i) temporarily store information, (ii) manipulate this information in order to perform cognitive tasks (iii) and to temporarily maintain the outcomes of intermediate computations. A number of studies have provided evidence for the existence of a distinction between the storage of verbal material and that of visuo-spatial (and possibly kinesthetic) material, which in Baddeley's and Hitch's model are handled respectively by the Phonological Loop and the Visuo-Spatial Sketchpad. Experimental results seem to indicate that a similar subdivision can be found also within the Central Executive, which is the system deputed to control attention, to supervise the activities and to perform the computations necessary to carry out cognitive tasks. Specifically, the experiment by Fedorenko and colleagues reviewed above strongly indicates that the processing of verbal material relies on the same pool of WM resources, independently from its linguistic or non-linguistic nature, whereas the processing of visuo-spatial material is served by a separate pool.

Moreover, we have observed that the Capacity Constrained Comprehension Theory proposed by Just and Carpenter (1992; 2002), consistently with a huge amount of experimental results, show that people with a lower verbal WM capacity will likely exhibit a slower and less accurate performance in those tasks requiring a complex processing and, therefore, a greater amount of WM resources.

As observed in Chapter 1, it seems that dyslexics are remarkably impaired in comparison to their peers just in demanding and complex tasks, besides their well-known phonological impairments. For this reason, I propose that their deficits arise from a specific impairment affecting their Working Memory, and in particular, resorting to Baddeley and Hitch's terminology, their Phonological Loop and their Central Executive. As confirmed by the experimental results reported in Chapter 3, as well as by those reported in Chapter 2, the functioning of the Phonological Loop and of the Central Executive are severely compromised in dyslexics, who underperform in comparison to controls in all measures tapping their phonological memory and executive functions. In my hypothesis, formulated below, these impairments are to be considered responsible for the deficits manifested by dyslexic individuals.

(12) *The Phonological and Executive Working Memory Deficit Hypothesis*
Dyslexic individuals suffer from a limitation affecting their Working Memory and hampering in particular their phonological memory and their executive functions. As a consequence, this impairment disrupts their phonological competence, as well as their performance in complex tasks that are particularly demanding in terms of Working Memory resources.
On the contrary, dyslexics can rely on a spared visuo-spatial memory, to which they can resort for the accomplishment of compensatory strategies.

The Phonological and Executive Working Memory Deficit Hypothesis yields, therefore, the very specific prediction that dyslexic individuals are likely to underperform in all those tasks which involve a fine phonological competence and which are particularly demanding in terms of processing resources. Similarly to what predicted by the Capacity Constrained Comprehension Theory, I propose that their more limited or less efficient WM compromises their performance in complex tasks that require an amount of processing resources that overcomes their actual capacity. As a consequence, they display a less accurate and slower performance. Conversely, dyslexics are predicted to behave normally in easier and less demanding tasks.

Based on these premises, then, the Phonological and Executive Working Memory Deficit Hypothesis is able to account for all the deficits typically associated with dyslexia and reviewed in Chapter 1, which, indeed, share the common and crucial features of either necessitating a precise phonological analysis (as phonological awareness tasks) or a complex and costly processing (as linguistic comprehension tasks) or both (as reading and spelling). In the following sections we will discuss in detail how this hypothesis can explain reading and spelling deficits, poor phonological competence, vocabulary and rapid naming deficits, grammatical problems and attention disorders.

4.1. How the hypothesis explains reading and spelling deficits

In Chapter 1 we have observed that dyslexic children suffer from marked reading impairments, as evidenced by their slow, inaccurate and effortful reading. Their error patterns typically seem to reflect a poor capacity to visually discriminate similar graphemes and a tendency to substitute similar looking words. Remarkable difficulties arise in particular when they are asked to read nonwords or very long words, whereas they perform better with highly frequent and shorter words. Moreover, we have noted that deficits appear to be more marked in those children whose mother-tongue has an opaque orthographic system like English.

Analyzing the Dual-Route Model of reading developed by Coltheart (1985), we have observed that dyslexic children appear to rely more heavily on the lexical route, which processes familiar words that are already stored in the semantic system, as evidenced by their better performance with frequent words. In the lexical route, in fact, stimuli are processed as indivisible units and their phonological form is thus accessed directly. Problems are more marked, instead, when dyslexics are forced to use the sublexical route, which breaks down the string in its minimal components, resorting to a set of orthographic-phonological conversion rules to retrieve the pronunciation of each unit. This route is obligatorily used to read nonwords and less familiar words, whose phonological form is not stored in the semantic system. The deficits shown by dyslexics in nonword reading tasks suggest that their sublexical route is not functioning properly, pointing to a difficulty at establishing the correct relationships between graphemes and phonemes. Similarly, we have noted that Frith's (1986) model of learning to read predicts that the deficits exhibited by dyslexics are caused by a failure to successfully master the conversion rules that are normally acquired in the alphabetic stage, suggesting that they are not able to perform the requested phonological analysis.

In both models, then, it is predicted that dyslexics' deficits are due to a phonological weakness preventing them from acquiring the orthographic-phonological conversion rules. This weakness can be explained by the Phonological and Executive Working Memory Deficit Hypothesis, if we consider that Working Memory is crucially involved in phonological analyses as well as in complex tasks. Reading and spelling are namely not only activities that necessitate a good phonological competence, but they are also complex tasks that require a considerable amount of processing resources.

Let us analyze, for instance, the process required to read a stimulus in a transparent language like Italian using the sublexical route. In this case, the child has to: (i) decompose the string, (ii) identify each grapheme, (iii) retrieve and apply the appropriate grapheme-phoneme conversion rule for each grapheme composing the stimulus and (iv) maintain the intermediate products activated in memory in order to blend phonemes together as long as the stimulus has been completely processed. Arguably, this process protracts longer with longer words, hence the minor difficulty experienced by dyslexics with shorter stimuli. Things can be further complicated in presence of irregular clusters, such as the Italian *gn* cluster in a word like *sogno* ('dream'). In this case, the child cannot operate the normal grapheme-phoneme conversion rule that would assign to the grapheme "g" the phoneme /g/ and to the grapheme "n" the phoneme /n/. Rather she has to retrieve the orthographic-phonological conversion rule according to which the cluster "gn" is to be translated into a single phoneme, namely /ɲ/. Arguably, then, reading becomes even more demanding in presence of irregular words, as evidenced by the greater difficulties experienced by dyslexics in these cases. Consequently, it is not hard to believe that children have even more troubles at learning to read in a language like English, where there are more possible mappings between graphemes and phonemes. Conversely, the child's task is facilitated in the presence of highly familiar words, whose phonological forms have already been stored and can be retrieved directly through the lexical route.

Once we have established that reading is indeed a complex and resource-demanding activity, it appears clear that a normally functioning Working Memory constitutes a fundamental prerequisite for the proper acquisition of the correspondences between graphemes and phonemes. Those children who suffer from WM limitations, i.e. by hypothesis dyslexic children, will arguably show more difficulties in learning to read in comparison to normally achieving children that can rely on a more efficient WM, exhibiting a slower and less accurate reading. Fortunately, these difficulties tend to disappear, or at least to diminish, as the child starts to automatize the process, relying more heavily on the lexical route and therefore bypassing the harder and more laborious processing involved by the sublexical route. However, difficulties reappear as soon as they are presented with nonwords, as indicated by the fact that even adult dyslexics, whose reading competence has achieved a satisfactory level, have troubles in reading novel or non-existing stimuli.

To summarize, then, the difficulties in learning to read experienced by dyslexics can be ascribed to an impairment affecting both their phonological memory and executive functions (i.e. Phonological Loop and Central Executive in Baddeley and Hitch's terminology).

A similar argument can be put forward to explain spelling difficulties, which often co-occur with reading deficits in developmental dyslexia. As observed in Chapter 1, the mastery of phoneme-grapheme conversion rules is essential for the appropriate acquisition of spelling skills. Typical misspellings shown by dyslexic children concern omissions of consonants in complex clusters, omissions of double consonants, confusion of similar graphemes or phonemes and incorrect translations of irregular spellings, especially in languages whose orthographic system is opaque, as English. As in reading, children's difficulties increase when they have to spell longer and less frequent words or nonwords, whereas they perform better with shorter and familiar words, suggesting that they can rely on already stored orthographic forms to retrieve the correct spelling of familiar words. An impaired phonological analysis, then, affects detrimentally the child's spelling abilities.

Furthermore, spelling is a complex task too, requiring the subject to perform a sequence of steps, applying phonological-orthographic conversion rules and maintaining in memory the products of intermediate computations. Arguably, then, WM is crucially involved in this activity: errors and slowness increase proportionately to the processing costs required to perform the task, that is, with longer, unfamiliar and irregular words. The typical misspellings reported above, then, can be interpreted as the consequence of a cognitive overload: the elements that are more frequently forgotten, in fact, are often "redundant" items, such as double consonants or silent graphemes.

Summarizing, then, we can maintain that dyslexics' reading and spelling deficits are caused by their limited phonological memory and executive functions, as argued by the Phonological and Executive Working Memory Deficit Hypothesis.

4.2. *How the hypothesis explains phonological deficits*

In Chapter 1 we have reviewed a number of studies demonstrating that phonological deficits are very widespread amongst dyslexic people. 100% of dyslexics exhibit, in fact, a very poor phonological awareness, as assessed by metalinguistic tasks. Typical phonological awareness tasks require the subject to identify the initial, final or middle sound of words, to detect and produce words that rhyme, to decompose words into syllables and sounds, to blend syllables and sounds into words and to delete or substitute syllables or sounds in words. A compelling body of evidence, indeed, has confirmed that dyslexics perform very poorly in phonological tasks and that their phonological awareness is significantly low, suggesting that they meet difficulties in analyzing the internal structure of words.

Moreover, poor phonological competence in developmental dyslexia persists across ages, as proved by the fact that it is displayed both by children and by adults, and across different languages. As argued, amongst others, by Ramus and Szenkovits (2008), as well as by Ramus and Ahissar (2012) and Ramus et al. (2013), the deficient phonological ability displayed by dyslexics seems to be caused by a specific deficit affecting the access to phonological representations, which are in themselves intact and fully specified. This proposal is perfectly in line with the Phonological and Executive Working Memory Deficit Hypothesis, which argues that dyslexics exhibit an impairment affecting their phonological memory. As emphasized by Fiorin (2010) in his Verbal Working Memory Deficit Hypothesis, in fact, the Phonological Loop is precisely concerned with the abstract representations of the sounds composing language and it plays a crucial role in accessing those representations.

Since it has been demonstrated that the Phonological Loop is remarkably impaired in dyslexic children, it is reasonable to propose that this impairment is responsible for the deficits they exhibit in phonological awareness tasks.

4.3. How the hypothesis explains vocabulary and naming deficits

Another deficit typically reported in dyslexic individuals concerns their vocabulary development and their performance in rapid naming tasks, in which they are required to rapidly name pictures of colors, objects or alphanumeric characters (see Chapter 1). Specifically, we have noted that dyslexic children's vocabulary is often underdeveloped in comparison to that of age-matched controls and that they display significant length and frequency effects, remembering better short and frequently used words.

Again, this deficit can be captured by the Phonological and Executive Working Memory Deficit Hypothesis: as demonstrated by Baddeley and colleagues, in fact, WM, and in particular the Phonological Loop, has the fundamental function of supporting the long lasting acquisition of new words (see Chapter 2). Dyslexics' poorly functioning Phonological Loop may then hamper their vocabulary learning, affecting even more evidently the acquisition of long and infrequent words. Arguably, this deficit affects also the learning of foreign language vocabulary, causing the difficulties often exhibited by dyslexic children in acquiring a second language.

Beyond their poor vocabulary knowledge, dyslexics have been found remarkably impaired in rapid naming tasks across ages and languages: both children and adults are namely much slower at picture naming than chronological age-matched unaffected individuals and even than reading age-matched controls. Interestingly, the greatest difficulties appear when they are asked to quickly name pictures of objects in comparison to alphanumeric characters or colors. These results suggests that the retrieval is slower in dyslexic individuals and that slowness increases proportionately to the number of possible responses.

This lexical access deficit can be viewed as consequence of a poorly functioning WM. As shown by Baddeley, WM is intimately linked to Long-Term Memory: in his model, specifically, the connection relating the Phonological Loop and language indicates that the Loop is also engaged in the retrieval of the words that are already permanently stored. The impairment affecting dyslexics' WM could then hamper their ability to retrieve the words stored in LTM, mainly resulting in a general slowing down of the process. Moreover, the greatest difficulty reported when subject are asked to quickly name objects in comparison to alphanumeric characters and colors can be interpreted as a consequence of the greater amount of resources required. There is, in fact, a limited number of colors, digits and letters, whereas the number of possible alternatives increases radically in the case of objects, enhancing proportionately also the processing costs of the operation performed.

4.4. How the Phonological and Executive Working Memory Deficit Hypothesis explains grammatical deficits

In Chapter 1 we have observed that dyslexics' linguistic difficulties are not confined to the domains of phonology and vocabulary, showing that they extend to grammar as well. Specifically, we have noted that dyslexic children are remarkably impaired in comparison to controls in the interpretation of tough sentences, pronouns, relative clauses, passive sentences and grammatical aspect and that they exhibit morphosyntactic deficits as well. In this paragraph I will argue that these deficits appear to reflect a processing difficulty affecting dyslexic individuals, as predicted by the Phonological and Executive Working Memory Deficit Hypothesis. Specifically, I will refer to the Capacity Constrained Comprehension Theory developed by Just and Carpenter and discussed above, suggesting that individuals with a lower Working Memory Capacity[4] are more likely to manifest deficits in the interpretation of those sentences which are particularly demanding in terms of processing resources. We have observed, in fact, that difficulties arise when the processing cost of the operations to be performed exceeds the general capacity of the system: if the parser is not able to process or maintain activated all the items necessary for the actual comprehension of the sentence, then the processing will slow down and some information, as the intermediate products of previous computations, may be forgotten.

According to the Phonological and Executive Working Memory Deficit Hypothesis, then, dyslexics are likely to manifest a less accurate performance or even to get stuck when asked to carry out demanding operation and to interpret linguistically complex sentences. Bearing this in mind, we can now try to provide an explanation to the grammatical deficits reported by dyslexic children, considering the results of the experiments presented in Chapter 1.

4.4.1. The Interpretation of Tough Sentences

Let us consider first the interpretation of tough sentences, reexamining the examples discussed in Chapter 1 and reported below.

(13) a. The snake is glad to bite.
b. The snake is hard to bite.
c. The snake is horrible to bite.

As we have noted, both acquisition studies and the experiments conducted by Byrne (1981) have revealed that O-type constructions, such as (13b), are more difficult to interpret for both young children and dyslexics, who show instead a normal performance with S-type sentences,

4 As Just and Carpenter do, I will use the label Working Memory (WM) to refer to Baddeley and Hitch's Central Executive.

like (13a). Moreover, both groups of children manifest the tendency to interpret utterances like (13c), which are ambiguous between the two types of interpretations, as S-type constructions, differently from typically developing children matched for chronological age with dyslexic children. Arguably, the discrepancy between the two types of constructions can be ascribed to processing factors: in (13a), in fact, *the snake* is both the grammatical subject of the utterance and the logical subject of the action of biting. The parser is then simply required to compute the dependency between the subject *the snake* and the verb *to bite*. In (13b), instead, *the snake* is the object of the action of biting. The interpretation of the sentence, then, involves the computation of two, instead of only one, syntactic dependencies: the role of the subject, in this case, is carried by a silent (i.e. not phonetically realized) pronoun, traditionally indicated, in the syntactic literature, as PRO. Therefore, the parser must compute first the dependency between PRO and the verb *to bite* and then the dependency between the verb and the object *the snake*.

Therefore, O-type constructions are more difficult to interpret than S-type constructions and more demanding in terms of processing resources. The greater difficulty experienced by dyslexics and young children, together with the higher tendency to interpret ambiguous sentences as S-type constructions, suggests then that their processing resources are more limited. This is consistent both with the Capacity Constrained Comprehension Theory, claiming that individuals with a lower WM capacity are expected to manifest deficits with complex constructions, and with the Phonological and Executive Working Memory Deficit Hypothesis, arguing that dyslexics suffer precisely from a WM limitation.

4.4.2. The interpretation of pronouns

In Chapter 1 we have observed that dyslexic children are remarkably more impaired than age-matched typically developing children in the interpretation of pronouns, performing as younger children. Waltzman and Cairns (2002) found that they are impaired in the comprehension of sentences like (14), accepting as grammatical a sentence like (14b) in a context in which Anna admires herself, in violation of Principle B of the Binding Theory.

(14) a. Anna_j admires her_i.
b. *Anna_j admires her_j.

Discussing this finding, we have adopted Grodzinsky and Reinhart (1993)'s proposal according to which the interpretation of sentences like (14) involves the computation of Rule I, reported below, which is very demanding in terms of processing resources.

(15) Rule I
α and β cannot be covalued in a derivation D, if
a. α c-commands β
b. α cannot bind β in D, and
c. The covaluation interpretation is undistinguishable from what would be obtained if α binds β.
[To check c, construct a comparison-representation by replacing β, with a variable bound by α].

According to Grodzinsky and Reinhart the computation of Rule I is necessary to determine if a sentence like (14b) is grammatical or not, and it is very costly in terms of memory resources. In order to apply Rule I, in fact, an individual has to perform three different steps: in this case, for instance, she has first to verify if *her* is c-commanded by *Anna* and secondly if it can be bound by *Anna*. Once ascertained that the pronoun is c-commanded by the DP, she has to construct a comparison-representation to establish if the two readings, obtained respectively by covaluation and binding, are equivalent or not. This third step is supposed to be the most expensive, since it requires the subject to construct, maintain in memory and compare two distinct representations. This operation, known as Reference Set Computation, is arguably very demanding in terms of WM capacity (see Chapter 5). Specifically, Grodzinsky and Reinhart argue that young children lack the resources necessary to carry out this task. Arguably, this is due to the fact that their WM is still developing.

As young children, dyslexics seem to be unable to compute Rule I, committing more errors than their peers. In the framework of the Phonological and Executive Working Memory Deficit Hypothesis, this is due to the fact that their low WM capacity prevents them from performing cognitively complex operations, like the Reference Set Computation, consistently with what predicted by the Capacity Constrained Comprehension Theory.

This hypothesis permits also to explain the results reported by Fiorin (2010) who tested sentences that were ambiguous between the bound-variable and the coreferential reading, as (16).

(16) Every friend of Francesco painted his bike.
Binding: For every x, if x is a friend of Francesco, then x painted **x**'s bike
Coreference: For every x, if x is a friend of Francesco, then x painted **Francesco**'s bike

Fiorin found that dyslexics, unlike control children, displayed a constant tendency to assign the same interpretation to ambiguous sentences, and he proposed that this tendency was a consequence of their limited processing resources. Dyslexics' propensity to stick to the same interpretation can be seen as a strategy adopted to avoid the expensive process of resolving the ambiguity of the sentence by applying Rule I and, thus, deriving both possible representations.

Once again, these results can be accounted for by the Phonological and Executive Working Memory Deficit Hypothesis.

4.4.3. The Interpretation of Relative Clauses

As discussed above, the Capacity Constrained Comprehension Theory predicts low-span individuals to manifest considerable deficits in the interpretation of object relative clauses. The comprehension of this kind of sentences requires the subject to maintain two DPs (instead of only one as it happens with subjects relatives) activated in memory in order to establish the appropriate syntactic dependencies. Interestingly, it has been found that, similarly to the low-span subjects tested by Just and Carpenter, dyslexics have troubles with object relative clauses, as the one reported in (17b).

(17) a. The lion hugs the bear that rolls the ball.
b. The bear that the lion hits rolls he ball.

To compute the syntactic dependencies of (17a) the parser has to keep in memory only one DP at once: *the lion* is maintained until the verb *hugs* is encountered and then *the bear* has to be maintained until *rolls* is found. To interpret (17b), instead, the parser needs to maintain both *the bear* and *the lion* simultaneously activated in memory in order to establish their relations to the verbs *hits* and *rolls.* Arguably, then, the computation of (17b) is more costly: people with a lower WM capacity are then supposed to be more impaired than people with higher processing resources available to perform the operation. The fact that dyslexic children underperform in comparison to age-matched typically developing children while computing object-relative clauses is then compatible with the Phonological and Executive Working Memory Deficit Hypothesis, arguing that they lack the processing resources required to interpret this kind of syntactic structures. Conversely, they do not manifest problems with the interpretation of simpler structures like (17a), whose lower demand of resources can be successfully handled by their WM.

4.4.4. The Interpretation of Passive Sentences

In Chapter 1 we have discussed the results of the experimental protocol administered by Reggiani (2010) to test the interpretation of passive sentences in dyslexic children. Results have demonstrated that dyslexics are remarkably more impaired than age-matched controls in the interpretation of reversible non-actional passives, like that reported in (18), performing at the same level of younger preschool children.

(18) Winnie the Pooh is seen by the bees.

Specifically, sentence (18) was judged grammatical in a context in which Winnie the Pooh saw, without being seen, some bees. To explain this result, Reggiani argued that dyslexics' poor performance is caused by a processing deficit. The interpretation of passive clauses such as (18), in fact, requires the subject to handle both the non-canonical word order typical of passive sentences and the use of a psychological non-actional verb like *to see*. Performing like younger children, dyslexics appear then to show the so-called Maratsos Effect, which arises precisely when these two ingredients are to be computed at once.

Along these lines, Reggiani suggests that the computation of passive sentences constructed with non-actional psychological verbs constitutes a too difficult task for both dyslexic and control children, whose

WM capacity is not large enough to cope with this kind of operation. This would entail, again, that results can be accounted for by the Phonological and Executive Working Memory Deficit Hypothesis.

4.4.5. The Interpretation of Grammatical Aspect

The interpretation of grammatical aspect in dyslexic children has been tested by Fiorin (2010). As discussed in Chapter 1, he tested the interpretation of the Italian past tenses *Imperfetto*, which encodes the imperfective aspect, and *Passato Prossimo*, which encodes the perfective aspect, in sentences like those reported below:

(19) a. IMPF: Marco mangiava il gelato.
'Marco ate-IMPF the ice-cream'.
b. PP: Marco ha mangiato il gelato.
'Marco ate-PP the ice-cream'.

Dyslexics displayed a significantly poorer behaviour in comparison to age-matched normally achieving children when asked to interpret sentences encoding the imperfective aspect, accepting (19a) as a correct description of a picture that portrays Marco having already finished eating the ice-cream. Conversely, they interpreted as well as controls sentences like (19b).

To explain these results, Fiorin argued that the association of IMPF sentences with ongoing situations is very expensive, since it requires the subject to perform a complex reasoning, computing a conversational implicature. Specifically, she has to reason that if the speaker had wanted to refer to a complete situation, she would have used a PP sentence, since it would be more informative: whereas IMPF sentences can be used both for complete and ongoing situations, in fact, PP sentences can only describe complete events. Therefore, the speaker's choice to use the less informative IMPF construction indicates that the PP would have not been appropriate and that the complete situation is to be discarded in favor of the ongoing situation. As we will discuss in Chapter 5, Reinhart (1999; 2006) showed that the computation of conversational implicatures is costly in terms of processing resources, since it involves a Reference Set Computation, requiring the subject to construct and compare the two alternative interpretations of the sentence.

Consistently with the Capacity Constrained Comprehension Theory, the Phonological and Executive Working Memory Deficit Hypothesis can explain dyslexics' difficulties, arguing that they lack the WM resources necessary to accomplish this task. Their better performance with PP constructions further confirms that their difficulties arise in presence of structures that are costly in terms of the involved processing resources, whereas they perform normally with less demanding structures.

4.5. How the hypothesis accounts for morphosyntactic deficits

The presence of morphosyntactic deficits in dyslexic children has been reported in the experiments administered, amongst others, by Joanisse and colleagues (2000), Jiménez and colleagues (2004) and Rispens (2004). Results showed that dyslexics' morphosyntactic competence is highly impaired in comparison to that displayed by both chronologically age-matched and reading age-matched normally achieving children. Specifically, problems arose when children were asked to apply morphosyntactic rules, such as those concerning the formation of past tenses and plurals.

Again, findings seem to evidence a disruption in dyslexic children's ability to apply rules: similarly to what happened in the acquisition of the grapheme-phoneme conversion rules necessary for correctly reading and spelling, dyslexics appear to be slower and more impaired than typically developing children in acquiring and applying morphosyntactic rules.

In the Phonological and Executive Working Memory Deficit Hypothesis, this impairment can be interpreted as a consequence of dyslexics' poorer Working Memory: the lack of an appropriate amount of cognitive resources hampers their speed and efficiency in the acquisition and application of rules. However, this does not mean that dyslexics will never be able to apply those rules, but simply that their ability will develop more slowly. As soon as the rules get automatized, in fact, the amount of processing resources required to apply them is expected to decrease noticeably.

4.6. How the hypothesis accounts for attention deficits

In Chapter 1 we have observed that dyslexics tend to exhibit an inattentive behaviour, characterized by lacks of concentration, high levels of distractibility and short attention spans. We have noted that attention is the ability required to direct the necessary resources to a task, focusing on the relevant information and filtering out irrelevant material. Experimental protocols specifically designed to detect the presence of attention deficits in dyslexics have revealed that they are more impaired than typically developing children in tasks testing their attention and their resistance to interference, as the Stroop Task. In this task, in particular, dyslexic children manifest remarkably higher levels of interference in comparison to controls when asked to name the ink color of words printed in a tint, which was different from that denoted by the word itself.

The attention deficits displayed by dyslexic individuals can be accounted for by the Phonological and Executive Working Memory Deficit Hypothesis, which claims that, beyond a phonological memory impairment, dyslexics suffer from a limitation affecting their executive functions. Remember that first Baddeley and Hitch (1974) and then Baddeley (1996; 2000) argue that a fundamental function of the Central Executive consists in controlling attention, an ability which plays an essential roles in all cognitive tasks, and especially in those situations in which more tasks have to be performed simultaneously.

Since dyslexics' Central Executive functioning has been found impaired, it appears evident that the attention deficits reported represent a direct consequence of this impairment. Moreover, the inattentive behaviour frequently displayed by dyslexic children is a further effect of their poor executive functioning, which is responsible for their tendency to forget the content of instructions, to lose the focus of the task and to abandon an activity before having completed it, together with their difficulty in shifting attention from one task to another and in organizing their activity.

5. Summary and Conclusions

In this chapter I have presented the Phonological and Executive Working Memory Deficit Hypothesis, arguing that people affected by developmental dyslexia suffer from an impairment hampering the efficiency and the capacity of their phonological memory and executive functioning. Moreover, I have proposed that these deficiencies can be held responsible for the manifestations of dyslexia discussed in Chapter 1: specifically, I suggested that dyslexics' difficulties are caused either by a phonological impairment, which can be traced back to an impaired Phonological Loop, or by the excessive complexity of the task. Adopting the perspective put forward by Just and Carpenter (1992; 2002) in their Capacity Constrained Comprehension Hypothesis, I argued that dyslexics' more limited WM (or Central Executive) capacity prevents them from performing those tasks whose cognitive demands exceed their processing resources. Specifically, I suggested that they lack the cognitive resources necessary to carry out complex and demanding tasks, determining a general slowness and worsening of their performance. On the contrary, as predicted, they perform normally in those tasks for which they have a sufficient amount of resources available.

An important consequence of this hypothesis, claiming that individual abilities are determined by the individual's Working Memory capacity, is that different degrees of severity are supposed to arise. It is not expected, in fact, that all dyslexic individuals will perform in the same manner, as their behavior is essentially dependent on their individual cognitive capacities. Dyslexics with a less severe WM limitation, for instance, are likely to manifest less marked difficulties in complex tasks in comparison to dyslexics with a more severe deficit. Arguably, then, the severity of the disorder is determined by the general damage affecting the system. This permits to explain the great differences and variability found within the dyslexic population.

Another interesting aspect of this hypothesis, thus, is that it can account for individual differences without assuming that they are determined by a difference in the underlying architecture of the system.

Furthermore, an important qualification should be made: the majority of the data discussed in this book concerns experiments that have been administered on dyslexic children. As we have observed in the preceding chapters, however, children's Working Memory is not yet fully developed, since individuals' WM is expected to increase until adolescence. This means that their performances are predicted to enhance with age, and that their deficits are likely to become more attenuated or even to disappear as their WM's development completes. However, this does not imply that they will catch up completely with their peers in every aspect: conversely, dyslexics are supposed to keep showing a more limited WM in comparison to normally achieving individuals, although it is very likely that it will go unnoticed in everyday activities. The impairment, in fact, will be evident only when they will be engaged in relatively complex tasks whose computation exceeds the general processing capacity of the system, without interfering with the execution of simple, or relatively simple, activities.

Moreover, it is important to remember that compensation is allowed: it has been proven, indeed, that individuals can bypass their difficulties by resorting to a better functioning system to overcome the poor functioning of another system (see Chapter 2). As evidenced by Hulme and Roodenrys (1995), in fact, memory problems "may not have devastating consequences for cognitive development in the presence of adequate compensatory resources" (392). An individual with a high IQ score, thus, can be able to learn new strategies to bypass her difficulties, achieving anyway a good and satisfactory performance. An interesting example in this respect is provided by the reading strategies shown by those dyslexics who learn to read relying more heavily on the lexical route in order to bypass their impaired sublexical route.

To conclude this chapter, once ascertained that dyslexics' difficulties arise in particular in demanding task, I decided to further test the Phonological and Executive Working Memory Deficit Hypothesis by assessing dyslexics' linguistic ability in the comprehension of complex constructions. With this purpose, I developed and administered three experimental protocols assessing linguistic aspects that have proven to be particularly challenging in terms of processing resources, like the computation of scalar implicatures, the comprehension of negative sentences and the reference assignment to both zero and phonetically realized pronouns. The results of these experiments will be presented and discussed respectively in Chapter 5, Chapter 6 and Chapter 7.

Chapter 5

The Computation of Scalar Implicatures in Developmental Dyslexia

1. Introduction

In this chapter I will present and discuss the results of an experimental protocol that I performed to test how dyslexic children interpret sentences involving the computation of a scalar implicature. As we will observe in the first sections of this chapter, supporters of the Pragmatic Approach to the computation of implicatures have argued that drawing a scalar inference is a costly operation, very demanding in terms of processing resources. Assessing the computation of scalar implicatures in dyslexic children, therefore, can be useful to test the Phonological and Executive Working Memory Deficit Hypothesis, under the proposal that dyslexics' difficulties are caused by a processing limitation hampering their performance in complex and demanding tasks.

In the experimental protocol that I will present in this chapter, dyslexics' performance has been compared to that shown by age-matched typically developing children, younger preschool children and control adults. The protocol comprised five distinct experiments testing the interpretation of pragmatically infelicitous sentences with the quantifier *some* or the disjunction operator *or* (Exp. 1), the interpretation of the quantifiers *some* and *most* (Exp. 2) and of the frequency adverbs *sometimes* and *often* (Exp. 3) in contexts requiring the computation of scalar implicatures. The processing of disjunction has been further tested both in contexts involving the computation of the implicature and in downward entailing contexts, where scalar inferences do not arise (Exp. 4). Finally, a felicity judgment task has been administered to test the computation of the implicature generated by *or* with a different methodology aiming at decreasing the processing load of the task (Exp.5). In line with the predictions, results showed that dyslexic children are dramatically impaired in all tasks requiring the computation of scalar inferences, displaying a performance which is very similar to that exhibited by children three and five years younger than them. These data provide therefore strong evidence in favor of the Phonological and Executive Working Memory Deficit Hypothesis.

Before presenting the experimental protocol, I will briefly introduce the topic, explaining what scalar implicatures are and in which contexts they arise; I will also discuss the two main approaches developed to account for implicatures' computation and argue that experimental data support the Pragmatic Approach, proposing that implicatures' calculation is a costly operation.

2. What are Scalar Implicatures?

One of the most intriguing aspects regarding language is that sentences often convey far more than their strict literal meaning and that hearers can, without any difficulty and almost unconsciously, go beyond what speakers say retrieving the real meaning of their utterances.

Consider for instance the dialogue reported below:

(1) Anna: Would you like a piece of cake?
(2) Lisa: I am on a diet.

From this dialogue we can easily deduce that Lisa does not want the piece of cake that Anna is offering her, even though the sentence she uttered does not literally say this. Actually, Lisa did not utter that she did not want a piece of cake: she *implicated* it. The term *implicature* was coined by Paul Grice, who defined it as a message that goes beyond what the speaker literally says. The main idea behind this is that we first consider the literal meaning of the utterance and then, if it turns out to be inadequate for the communicative goals, we make a hypothesis about what the speaker may have intended to say, computing an implicature.

A fundamental role in this mechanism is carried out by the so-called Cooperative Principle, formulated by Grice, which states: "Make your conversational contribution such as is required, at the stage at which it occurs, by the accepted purpose or direction of the talk exchange in which you are engaged" (Grice 1975). According to this principle, then, speakers tend to use meaningful and appropriate utterances to further the conversation, assuming that their interlocutors are doing the same. Grice postulated four principles specifying how to be cooperative, namely the Conversational Maxims, reported in (3).

(3) *The Maxims of Conversation*
   (i) *Quality*: Make your contribution true.
      Do not say what you know that is false.
      Do not say that for which you lack adequate evidence.
   (ii) *Quantity*: Make your contribution as informative as is required.
      Do not make your contribution less or more informative than required.
   (iii) *Relation*: Be relevant.
   (iv) *Manner*: Be perspicuous.
      Avoid obscurity of expression.
      Avoid ambiguity.
      Be brief, avoid unnecessary wordiness.
      Be orderly.

According to Grice's original framework, the hearer looks for implicatures when one of the conversational maxims is violated.

In a conversational exchange as the one reported above, the Maxim of Relevance is violated, since Lisa does not seem to reply to Anna's question, answering *yes* or *no*. However, given that we suppose that Lisa wants to be cooperative, we are led to infer that she is trying to be cooperative (i.e. to provide an answer to Anna's question), even though her utterance seems to violate the Maxim of Relation. On these grounds, considering that eating cakes and being on a diet are incompatible actions, we are led to infer that Lisa must have intended that she does not want a piece of cake, given the fact that she is on diet.

In the Gricean framework, the implicature generated by Lisa's utterance reported in (2) is dubbed "Relevance Implicature", since it is triggered by the violation of the Relation Maxim. Lisa's sentence, is actually an infringement of this maxim, given that it does not seem to constitute an appropriate answer to Anna's question, which would have rather required a yes-no response. As a consequence, Lisa's violation of the Relation Maxim generates a conversational implicature, leading the addressee to go beyond what the speaker literally said and to draw an inference about what she really *intended* to say.

In this framework, a Scalar Implicature (SI henceforth) can be defined as a quantity implicature (related to the Quantity Maxim), based on the use of an informationally weak term in an implicational scale. An implicational scale can be defined as a set of ordered alternatives, in which the assertion of a lower-ranking alternative implicates that the higher-ranking one does not hold.

Classical examples of scales include:

(i) Quantifiers (some<many<most<all)
(ii) Connectives (or<and)
(iii) Adverbs (sometimes<often<always)
(iv) Modals (may<should<must; possibly<necessarily),
(v) Verbs of completion (start<finish)
(vi) Verbs of ranking (think<believe<know)
(vii) Numerals (one<two<three…).

What characterizes the information scales reported above is the presence of one-way semantic entailment relations (i.e. *all* entails *some* as *and* entails *or*, but not vice versa). Consider the example in (4), where the scalar quantifier *some* is used:

(4) Anna ate some of the candies that were on the table.
(5) ALTERNATIVE: Anna ate all of the candies that were on the table.
(6) IMPLICATURE: Anna didn't eat all of the candies that were on the table.

Computing a sentence like (4), people generally infer the meaning in (6), assuming that Anna ate some *but not all* of the candies that were on the table, even though the logical meaning of *some* is *more than one (and possibly all)*. This happens because we reason that the speaker would have had a more informative alternative, namely the one reported in (5), to say that Anna ate *all* of the candies that were on the table, using the universal quantifier *all* instead of the weaker existential quantifier *some*. Nonetheless, given that the speaker is supposed to be cooperative, her choice to utter the less informative sentence in (4) leads the hearer to infer that the alternative and stronger utterance in (5) does not hold. Consequently, the addressee computes the implicature in (6), narrowing down the logical meaning of *some*, and thus excluding the possibility that Anna ate all the candies.

A similar reasoning underpins the interpretation of a sentence containing the disjunction operator *or*, as the one reported in (7).

(7) Every child received a chocolate or a candy.
(8) ALT: Every child received a chocolate and a candy.
(9) IMPL: Every child did not receive both the chocolate and the candy.

Interpreting the sentence in (7) people compute the implicature in (9), inferring that every child received or a candy or a chocolate, *but not both*. Nevertheless, from a logical point of view, the disjunction operator *or* would have an inclusive meaning, i.e. it results in true assertions whenever one or more, and thus possibly all, of its operands are true. In ordinary language, instead, disjunction receives an exclusive interpretation, as reported in (9), where the possibility that both its operands are true is excluded. By hypothesis, this narrowing of the logical meaning of disjunction is determined by the computation of an implicature. Interpreting (7), in fact, the addressee reasons that if the speaker had wanted to say that children received both sweets, she should have uttered the more informative utterance in (8), as demanded by the Quantity Maxims. Assuming that the speaker is trying to be cooperative and to conform to the Maxims of Conversation, the hearer infers that the stronger alternative in (8) is not true, and hence she computes the implicature in (9). Therefore, disjunction is given an exclusive interpretation.

However, it has been reported that scalar implicatures do not arise in every type of context. As it will be discussed in the following section, there are indeed specific contexts in which scalar inferences do not arise.

2.1. *The interpretation of scalar expressions in downward entailing contexts*

A distinctive property of SIs is that they do not always occur when a scalar terms is introduced in the discourse; there are namely some contexts in which SIs are not computed, as downward entailing contexts.

A context is defined as *downward entailing* (DE) if and only if it licenses inferences from sets to subsets.[1] On the contrary, a non-downward entailing context, or upward entailing (UE) context, licenses inferences from sets to supersets. To better understand this concept, consider the contrast reported below between the affirmative sentence in (10) and the negative sentence in (11).

(10) John bought a car.
$\nrightarrow$ John bought a red car.
(11) John didn't buy a car.
$\rightarrow$ John didn't buy a red car.

As exemplified in (10), affirmative sentences are non-DE contexts, since they do not permit to license inferences from sets to subsets: asserting that John bought a car, in fact, does not necessarily imply that John bought a *red* car. Conversely, an inference from the set of cars to the subsets of red cars can be licensed by negative contexts, which are DE-context, as shown in (11), where the fact that John didn't buy a car necessarily entails that John didn't buy a red car.

As noted first by Gazdar (1979) and then by Horn (1989), scalar implicatures do not seem to arise in negative sentences, which are DE contexts. Consider for instance the negative counterpart of the sentence discussed in (4), as reported below.

(12) Anna did not eat some of the candies that were on the table.
(13) ALT: Anna didn't eat all of the candies that were on the table.
(14) IMPL: It is not true that Anna didn't eat all of the candies.

Interpreting a sentence like (12) we generally infer that Anna ate only one, or possibly none of the candies that were on the table. However, if

1 Chierchia (2004) defines formally downward entailing contexts, arguing that a function is said to be DE iff f(A) entails f(B), whenever $B \subseteq A$.

we computed the implicature in (14), negating the stronger alternative in (13), we would infer that Anna indeed ate all of the candies, which is clearly distinct from the interpretation that we intuitively attribute to (12).

Beyond negative sentences, there are other DE contexts in which scalar implicatures do not arise, such as antecedents of conditional sentences, embedded sentences and restrictions of quantifiers. Consider, for instance, the interpretation attributed to the disjunction operator *or* when it occurs in the restriction of the quantifier *every*, as in (15).

(15) Every child who received a candy or a chocolate is happy.

Recall the example in (7), where disjunction occurred in an UE context and received an exclusive interpretation by means of the computation of a scalar implicature. In this case, instead, the scalar term *or* occurs in the restriction of the quantifier *every*, which is a DE context, and the implicature is suspended, since disjunction is attributed an inclusive or logic interpretation: the sentence is indeed an appropriate description of a context in which also children who received *both* the chocolate and the candy are happy.

The fact that scalar implicatures do not arise in some contexts has generated a still ongoing debate. As I will discuss in the following section, the Structural Approach claims that implicatures are computed by default and that they have to be removed in DE contexts. Conversely, the Pragmatic Approach maintains that scalar inferences are added only when the context demands it: in DE environments the computation of implicatures is simply not required.

3. The computation of scalar implicatures: the Structural and the Pragmatic Approach

In the preceding sections, we have observed that the computation of a scalar implicature is achieved through a subtle reasoning: assuming that the speaker will conform to the Conversational Maxims trying to be cooperative, the fact that she used a weak term instead of its stronger alternative makes the hearer infer that the informationally stronger sentence does not hold. This consideration leads to the exclusion of the stronger alternative and, as a consequence, to the computation of an implicature. However, we have also noted that implicatures are not necessarily associated to scalar terms and, more particularly, that they do not arise in downward entailing contexts.

Considering these peculiarities of scalar inferences, two main approaches have been formulated to account for their computation: on the one side there is the Structural Approach proposed by Chierchia (2004) and Levinson (2000), whereas on the other side there is the Pragmatic Approach defended by Carston (1998), Recanati (2003), Sperber and Wilson (1995).[2]

In the structural view, also known as "Default view", SIs are supposed to be generated automatically and by default. In Levinson (2000), specifically, SIs are defined as default inferences, that is inferences which are associated automatically to each scalar term and which can be removed when the context demands it, as in DE environments. Analogous conclusions are advocated by Chierchia (2004), who proposes that the cancellation of implicatures in these contexts is due to the application of a general rule that he names Strength Condition. Very briefly, Chierchia argues that every scalar term is provided by the grammar with two values, a plain value and a scalar or strengthened value, which is automatically computed by exploiting its alternatives. However, this mechanism is governed by the Strength Condition, whose formulation[3] is reported below.

(16) Strength Condition
a. The strengthened value of a scalar term α cannot be weaker than its plain value;
b. A value α is said to be stronger than a value β if and only if α entails β.

2 A detailed discussion of the existing literature about the computation of scalar implicatures goes beyond the goals of this book. For more exhaustive information see Levinson (2000), Chierchia (2004), Breheny and colleagues (2006).

3 Cfr. Reinhart (2006).

The Strength Condition predicts that the scalar value of the term cannot become weaker than its plain value: when the computation of an implicature leads to a weakening instead of a strengthening of the original information content, the inference is removed. According to Chierchia, it is precisely the application of the Strength Condition to be responsible for the removal of scalar inferences in DE contexts.

To understand how the Strength Condition works, consider the sentences discussed in the previous sections and reported below for convenience, where disjunction occurs respectively in an upward entailing context, as in (17) and in the restriction of the quantifier *every*, a downward entailing context, where implicatures do not arise, as in (20).

(17) Every child received a chocolate or a candy.
(18) Every child (λx (x received a chocolate or a candy)
(19) Every child (λx (x received a chocolate or a candy and ¬x received a chocolate and a candy)
(20) Every child who received a chocolate or a candy is happy.
(21) Every child (λx (x received a chocolate or a candy) (x is happy)
(22) Every child (λx (x received a chocolate or a candy and ¬x received a chocolate and a candy) (x is happy)

According to Chierchia, grammar provides the disjunction operator *or* with a plain value (i.e. corresponding to the inclusive interpretation: the chocolate or the candy *and possibly both*) and a strengthened value (i.e. corresponding to the exclusive interpretation: the chocolate or the candy *but not both*). However, the scalar value must be stronger than the plain value; otherwise, the implicature is to be filtered out. In the case of (17), the scalar value represented in (19) is indeed stronger than the plain value in (18), given that (19) entails (18). In the case of (20), instead, it is actually the other way around, since the scalar value in (22) does not entail but it is rather entailed by the plain value in (21). Therefore, the strengthened value of the scalar term *or* turns out to be weaker than its plain value and the Strength Condition filters out the implicature. Adopting this framework, Chierchia and colleagues are able to derive the reason why scalar implicatures do not arise in downward entailing contexts, by arguing that implicatures are always and automatically associated to scalar terms but they are deleted when the Strength Condition fails to apply.

An important consequence of this approach concerns the computational costs required by implicature computation in upward entailing and downward entailing contexts. Given that scalar inferences are supposed to arise automatically, their computation should be almost costless, whereas, on the contrary, their cancellation in DE contexts should be more expensive in terms of processing costs, since the relevant interpretation would require a further step.

Radically different predictions are made by the Pragmatic Approach[4], also known as "Context-Driven Account", according to which scalar implicatures are context-dependent, that is, they do not arise automatically, but their generation is rather determined by the context. Supporters of this view, hence, argue that implicatures are computed only when the context demands it; specifically, they distinguish two kinds of contexts: lower-bound and upper-bound contexts. Consider the examples below, taken from Levinson (2000) and Breheny and colleagues (2006).

(23) A: "Is there any evidence against them?"
B. "Some of their identity documents are forgeries."
(24) A. "Were all their documents in order?"
B. "Some of their identity documents are forgeries."

The conversational exchange in (23) represents a typical example of lower-bound context, where the implicature (i.e. some *but not all* of their documents are forgeries) is not computed. In this case, in fact, it would be irrelevant for A to know if *all* their documents are forgeries, as it is enough to know that *at least some* of them are. In (24), an upper-bound context, instead, the question uttered by A is different and although the answer provided by B is identical to that in (23), it receives a distinct interpretation through the computation of the implicature. In this second case, in fact, it is highly relevant for A to know whether *all* or *only some* of the documents are forgeries: hence, the computation of the implicature is necessarily required. Comparing (23) and (24), then, it is possible to observe how the context determines the generation of implicatures, which are irrelevant for the discourse purposes

4 Cfr. The Pragmatic or Context-Driven Approach is also supported by the Relevance Theory (Sperber and Wilson 1986; Carston 1998).

in lower-bound context but relevant in upper-bound contexts. In this framework, DE contexts can be considered as lower-bound contexts, in which scalar inferences do not arise simply because their computation would be irrelevant for the discourse purposes: in these contexts, in fact, the communicative goals are already satisfied by the plain value of the scalar term, without any need to generate an implicature.

It should be evident that such an approach makes different predictions with respect to the Structural Approach, for what concerns the processing costs of scalar terms interpretation in upward entailing and downward entailing contexts. The generation of implicatures, in fact, is supposed to be an expensive operation being "a product of attentional processing, requiring effort beyond that devoted to automatic, default processes" (Breheny et al. 2006: 439). Conversely, the interpretation of scalar terms occurring in lower-bound and DE contexts is predicted to be easier and effortless, since no inference is generated in these cases. In other words, a processing effort is expected in UE contexts, but not in DE contexts.

To summarize, the Structural Approach and the Pragmatic Approach lead to opposite predictions for what concerns the cognitive costs demanded for the interpretation of scalar terms, as reported in a schematized form below.

Table 5.1. Predictions of the two approaches to SIs computation.

PROCESSING COSTS	CONTEXTS WHERE SIs ARE COMPUTED	CONTEXTS WHERE SIs ARE NOT COMPUTED
STRUCTURAL APPROACH	Effortless	Costly
PRAGMATIC APPROACH	Costly	Effortless

3.1. *Experimental studies assessing Scalar Implicatures' computation*

In the previous section we have observed that the structural and the pragmatic approach lead to opposite predictions for what regards the processing costs related to the interpretation of scalar terms. These predictions have been assessed by means of experimental studies conducted both on children and adults, whose results will be discussed in this section. As we will observe, data provide strong support in favor of the Pragmatic Approach, confirming that the computation of implicatures is indeed a cognitively demanding task, which imposes a great load on the subject's processing capacities.

3.1.1. The computation of Scalar Implicatures in children: acquisitional data

Amongst the first studies conducted in the acquisitional field to test the computation of scalar implicatures in young children there are the works by Smith (1980) and Brain and Rumain (1981), who tested respectively the interpretation of quantifiers and connectives. Specifically, Smith (1980) found that preschool children, aged between 4 and 7 years old, manifest a great tendency to accept infelicitous sentences such as the one reported in (25), treating the quantifier *some* as equivalent to the quantifier *all* and failing therefore to compute the scalar implicature. Older children and adults, conversely, tend to reject this kind of sentences, judging them inappropriate.

(25) Some elephants have trunks.

Similarly, Brain and Rumain (1981) showed that children tend to interpret disjunction inclusively, considering *or* as compatible to *and* (i.e. A or B and possibly both), whereas adults favored the exclusive interpretation, computing the implicature (i.e. A or B but not both).

These findings were replicated by Noveck (2001), who reported that young children are less prone than older children and adults to derive scalar implicatures and that they tend to treat scalar terms logically rather than pragmatically. Beyond the quantifier *some*, the author tested the interpretation of modals, asking subjects to judge the appropriateness of sentences like (26) in a context in which it would have been more appropriate to utter (27).

(26) There might be a parrot in the box.
(27) There must be a parrot in the box.

Young children manifested a strong preference for the logic interpretation both with quantifiers and modal verbs, leading Noveck to deduce that the logical meaning is the one associated by default to the scalar terms, whereas the stronger interpretation is achieved only later, presumably because it requires high processing resources.

The same tendency to treat scalar terms logically rather than pragmatically has been reported by Chierchia and colleagues (2001) and Gualmini and colleagues (2001), who found that preschool children manifest greater difficulties in comparison to older children and adults when asked to interpret the disjunction operator *or* in sentences that involve the computation of an implicature. Significantly, instead, children display an adultlike behavior when disjunction occurs in a downward entailing environment, where the implicature does not arise. In accordance with Noveck, the authors claim that the difficulties experienced by children might stem from a limitation in their processing capacity, rather than from an absence of linguistic competence. Chierchia and colleagues, in fact, propose that SIs computation imposes considerable demands in terms of processing resources and that children's impairments are due to a processing limitation, that is, to the fact that their working memory is not yet fully developed. Specifically, they suggest that the interpretation of a scalar term requires the subject to maintain in memory and compare the two alternative representations of the target sentence, constructed respectively with the plain value and the strengthened value of the scalar term.

In order to test this hypothesis, which they call Processing Limitation Hypothesis, Chierchia and colleagues applied a new experimental technique, the Felicity Judgment Task, which involves the explicit presentation of the two alternative descriptions of the context under consideration. In this kind of task, the subject is told that she will have to choose out of two sentences the one that best describes the context, focusing on the *appropriateness* of the target sentences. For instance, in a context in which every farmer cleaned both a horse and a rabbit, the subject has to choose the most appropriate out of the two utterances reported below:

(28) Every farmer cleaned a horse and a rabbit.
(29) Every farmer cleaned a horse or a rabbit.

In this case, hence, the computational load of the task gets significantly reduced: since the alternative sentences are explicitly presented, the subject does not need to construct them, but her task is simply to compare them and to choose the one which is the most appropriate description of the context under consideration. Results provided support in favor of the Processing Limitation Hypothesis: children, in fact, show a correct performance, strongly suggesting that the difficulties showing up in previous experiments had been determined by the complexity of the task, and specifically by the need to construct and then to compare the two alternative representations of the context.

Summarizing, then, acquisitional studies suggested that young children exhibit remarkable difficulties when they are asked to interpret sentences requiring the computation of a scalar implicature. Unlike older children and adults, in fact, they tend to assign a logical interpretation to scalar expressions, failing to compute the implicature. Their performance enhances significantly when the computational load of the task is reduced, as in the Felicity Judgment Task, suggesting that their difficulties are due to a processing limitation. Interestingly, however, children do not manifest problems in the interpretation of scalar terms occurring in downward entailing contexts, where implicatures are not computed. This result speaks against the structural approach put forward by Levinson and Chierchia, according to which scalar implicatures are computed automatically and deleted in DE context (see section 5.3). As discussed above and summarized in Table 5.1, the Structural Approach predicts that a SIs computation is almost costless in upward entailing contexts and more expensive in downward entailing contexts; therefore, children should have manifested even more difficulties in DE contexts, instead of performing adultlike.

Results of the studies conducted in the acquisitional field, then, provide support to the Pragmatic Approach, confirming that the computation of SIs is indeed an expensive operation in terms of processing resources, which exceeds young children's processing capacities.

3.1.2. The computation of Scalar Implicatures in adults: experimental data

Beyond the acquisitional results reviewed above, experimental studies conducted on adults have provided interesting data as well, confirming that the computation of scalar implicatures requires a considerable amount of processing resources. Noveck and Posada (2003) developed an interesting experiment aiming at assessing adult's reaction times in the interpretation of scalar items; participants were asked to give a truth value judgment to underinformative sentences such as the one discussed above and reported in (30) for convenience.

(30) Some elephants have trunks.

Interestingly, the authors found that those adults who rejected the sentence, computing the implicature, showed longer response times in comparison to those subjects who accepted the sentence. Specifically, individuals who computed the implicature showed more than double latencies, confirming thus that drawing scalar inferences is linked to a processing effort. Moreover, the authors found that subjects who accepted the underinformative sentences showed faster response times also with control items, suggesting that adults tend to adopt two different strategies: those who accept sentences like (30) tend to interpret scalar items literally and to perform quicker, whereas those who reject these utterances follow a more complex reasoning, which leads precisely to the computation of implicatures.

The same result was found by Bott and Noveck (2004), who confirmed that reaction times increase when subjects generate the scalar inference; specifically, the authors showed that subjects give significantly more "true" responses, accepting sentences like (30) and avoiding SIs computation, when they are limited to 900 millisecond to answer, in comparison to when they had 3 seconds time. A similar finding is reported by Katsos, Breheny and Williams (2005), who asked subjects to read short texts such as those presented below:

(31) John was taking a university course and working at the same time. For the exams he had to study from short and comprehensive sources. Depending on the course, he decided to **read the class notes or the summary.**

(32) John heard that the textbook for Geophysics was very advanced. Nobody understood it properly. He heard that if he wanted to pass the course he should **read the class notes or the summary.**

Notice that the final sentence "read the class notes or the summary" can receive two different interpretations, depending on the context generated by the preceding sentence. In (31), indeed, disjunction is interpreted exclusively, and thus with the computation of an implicature, whereas in (32) it receives an inclusive interpretation. The authors found that, as in previous experiments, reading times were significantly longer in the condition where scalar inferences had to be computed, suggesting that they were generated only in those cases.

All these outcomes support a model in which scalar implicatures are costly inferences that impose a high processing load on working memory, in accordance with the predictions made by the pragmatic approach. This hypothesis is supported also by Reinhart (1999; 2006), who argues that scalar implicatures are expensive in terms of processing resources since they require a reference-set computation. Her proposal will be briefly presented in the following section.

3.2. The Reference-Set Computation

As observed above, a sentence containing a scalar term, like (33), is ambiguous because the disjunction operator *or* could receive both a logical and a pragmatic interpretation. To solve this ambiguity one has to compare the sentence with an alternative utterance constructed with the conjunction *and*, which is indeed a stronger and more informative scalar term, as in (34).

(33) Alice ate meat or fish.
(34) Alice ate meat and fish.

This procedure is dubbed "Reference-Set Computation" by Reinhart (1999), who proposes that the resolution of ambiguous sentences forces the subject to (i) create a set of alternatives, (ii) compare the different representations and (iii) choose the most appropriate one. Although this kind of operation is available to the human computational system, it is highly expensive in terms of processing resources, since it requires the subject to construct and maintain in memory more representations of the same sentence. For this reason, Reinhart observes that Reference-Set

Computation applies "only as a "last resort", when the output of core syntax operations are insufficient for the interface" (Reinhart 2006: 2). In other words, ambiguities are seen as imperfections of the system, which require a peculiar and expensive kind of operation, as the Reference-Set Computation, in order to be solved. Crucially, the great load that this kind of operation imposes on working memory can be generally carried out by adults, whereas it results too difficult for young children, whose computational resources are still developing.

As the reader may have observed, this proposal is consistent with the experimental results discussed above and showing that young children manifest remarkable difficulties in the interpretation of sentences involving the computation of an implicature and that they tend to avoid this computation by adopting a logical reading of scalar expressions. Furthermore, Reinhart's proposal is also able to explain why implicatures arise only in certain contexts, as demonstrated by the contrast between (31) and (32) discussed above. In those cases in which the computation of an implicature would not lead to an advantage, Reference-Set Computation is simply not applied.

Summarizing, Reinhart argues that the derivation of scalar implicatures requires a Reference-Set Computation, which permits to compare the target sentence with a set of alternative utterances. Given that this operation is quite expensive in terms of processing resources, it imposes a great burden on Working Memory, as demonstrated by the longer response times shown by adults and by the difficulties exhibited by young children, whose cognitive resources are still developing. Reinhart's proposal, then, is in line with the Pragmatic Approach discussed above, which considers SIs computations a highly expensive task.

For this reason, it can be interesting to investigate dyslexic children's ability to compute scalar implicatures, comparing their performance to that shown by age-matched typically developing children, adults and younger children. If the Phonological and Executive Working Memory Deficit Hypothesis is correct, dyslexics are expected to manifest, in fact, more difficulties in the interpretation of sentences requiring the computation of an implicature in comparison to controls, due to their more limited amount of processing resources. To test this prediction I developed an experimental protocol aiming at assessing dyslexics' ability to draw scalar inferences. The results will be presented and discussed in the following sections.

4. Experimental Protocol

The experimental protocol comprises five distinct studies. Experiment 1 was a statement evaluation task assessing the subject's sensitivity to pragmatic infelicitous utterances with the disjunction operator *or* and the quantifier *some*. Experiment 2 was a truth value judgment task testing the comprehension of the quantifiers *some* and *most* in contexts involving the computation of a scalar implicature. Experiment 3 was a truth value judgment task assessing the interpretation of the frequency adverbs *sometimes* and *often* again in contexts involving SIs computation. In Experiment 4, again a truth value judgment task, I tested the interpretation of the disjunction operator *or* both in contexts requiring the computation of an implicature and in downward entailing contexts, where implicatures are not computed. Finally, Experiment 5 was a felicity judgment task assessing the interpretation of disjunction. As anticipated above, Chierchia and colleagues (2001) applied this experimental methodology with the aim of facilitating the subject's task, reducing the computational load by explicitly presenting the two alternative representations of the utterance. In this case, therefore, the subject has simply to compare the two utterances and to choose the most appropriate one, without the need of constructing them. As a consequence, the processing load required to perform the task decreases radically. Assuming that dyslexics' difficulties are caused by a WM limitation, dyslexics are expected to perform better in this kind of task, approaching their peers' performance.

Experiments 1, 2 and 5 have been administered to 4 groups of subjects: a group of dyslexic children, a group of age-matched typically developing children, a group of adults and a group of younger preschool children. Experiments 3 and 4, instead, have been conducted on 3 groups of subjects: a group of dyslexic children, a group of age-matched typically developing children and a group of younger children attending to the first class of the primary school.

4.1. Experiment 1: a statement evaluation task

This task is partly based on Noveck's (2001) experiment that tested the interpretation of pragmatically infelicitous sentences with the form "Some X [verb] Y". In my experiment both the interpretation of sentences containing the quantifier *some* and the disjunction operator *or* are examined.

4.1.1. Participants

The experimental task was performed on 72 subjects, divided in 4 distinct groups: 18 dyslexic children, 18 age-matched typically developing children, 18 control adults, and 18 younger children.

The group of Dyslexic children (DC) included 18 children (11 males), all native speakers of Italian. At the moment of testing, the group mean age was 9 years and 9 months (SD = 1;5). All children have been chosen from those who had independently received a diagnosis of dyslexia, specifically by the "Servizio di Neuropsichiatria Infantile" in Rovereto (TN): in particular, dyslexic children were selected according to different factors: (i) absence of neurological diseases or genetic pathologies, (ii) absence of sensorial diseases, (iii) absence of psychopathological diseases, (iv) IQ > 80 (WISC – R) and (v) fluent and correct reading and writing abilities under 2 SD (Tressoldi et al. Battery, Prove MT).

The group of age-matched control children (AMCC) comprehended 18 primary school children (5 males), all native speakers of Italian. At the moment of testing, the group mean age was 9 years and 8 months (SD = 0;10). Children were selected from those who had no history of reading problems or language disorders.

The group of control adults (CA) was composed by 18 adults (6 males), all native speakers of Italian with no history of reading or language disorders. At the moment of testing, the group mean age was 26 years and 7 months (SD = 13;8).

The group of younger children (YC) included 18 preschool children (7 males), all native speakers of Italian with no reports of language problems. At the moment of testing the group mean age was 5 years and 4 months (SD = 0;8). The main features of the four groups are summarized in Table 5.2.

Table 5.2. Group data of the subjects who took part in Exp. 1.

Group	Number	Mean Age (SD)
DC	18	9;9 (1;5)
AMCC	18	9;8 (0;10)
CA	18	26;7 (13;8)
YC	18	5;4 (0;8)

4.1.2. Design and Procedure

A sentence evaluation task, similar to that developed by Noveck and colleagues (2001), was administered. Participants were told that they were going to be presented with a series of statements and that they simply had to say whether or not they agreed with each by pressing a smiling face for a correct sentence or a crying face for a wrong sentence. The task comprised 8 target sentences, subdivided in two experimental conditions: in the first condition (Condition A, Quant_P.I.), pragmatically infelicitous sentences were tested, with the quantifier "*some*" used to describe a situation where the quantifier "*all*" would have been more appropriate. Similarly, in the second condition (Condition B, Disj_P.I.), subjects had to accept or reject target sentences constructed with the disjunction operator *or* used in an infelicitous way. The target sentences, 4 for each condition, were interspersed with 16 felicitous utterances, 8 false and 8 true, where the quantifier *some* and the disjunction operator *or* respectively were used in an appropriate way. There were two different models; target sentences and fillers were presented randomly. Examples of both target sentences and fillers follow below.

(i) Condition A, Quant_P.I.: Pragmatically infelicitous "some" sentences
Alcuni pesci vivono nell'acqua
'Some fishes live in water'

(ii) Condition B, Disj_P.I.: Pragmatically infelicitous "*or*" sentences
Le persone hanno gli occhi o la bocca
'People have the eyes or the mouth'

(iii) Filler, Quant_F_True.: Felicitous and true "*some*" sentences
Alcuni bambini portano gli occhiali
'Some children wear glasses'

(iv) Filler, Quant_F_False: Felicitous and false "*some*" sentences
Alcuni fiocchi di neve sono fucsia
'Some snowflakes are fuchsia'

(v) Filler, Disj_F_True: Felicitous and true "*or*" sentences
Le ragazze possono indossare la gonna o i pantaloni
'Girls can wear trousers or skirts'

(vi) Filler, Disj_F_False: Felicitous and false "*or*" sentences
I cavalli hanno la coda o le ali
'Horses have the tail or the wings'

Notice that if the subject rejects the sentence tested in Condition A, this means that she has computed the implicature, excluding the stronger sentence with *all* (i.e. "All fishes live in water") and obtaining the false statement "some *but not all* fishes live in water". Conversely, if the subject does not compute the implicature, she will treat *some* as compatible with *all*, thereby accepting the infelicitous sentence. Similarly, if she accepts the sentence tested in Condition B (i.e. "People have the mouth or the eyes", it means that she did not compute the implicature, considering it as equivalent to its stronger alternative "People have the mouth *and* the eyes".

4.1.3. Results

All subjects included in the four groups gave the correct answer to the vast majority of the fillers and therefore nobody was excluded from the sample. Descriptive statistics are reported in Table 5.3, whereas the error rates shown by the four groups of participants are reported in Graph. 5.1.

Table 5.3. Descriptive statistics of Exp. 1.

	Group	N	Mean Error Rate	Std. Deviation
QUANT_P.I.	DC	18	0.59	0.10
	AMCC	18	0.20	0.09
	CA	18	0.20	0.07
	YC	18	0.65	0.10
DISJ_P.I.	DC	18	0.61	0.10
	AMCC	18	0.22	0.07
	CA	18	0.12	0.07
	YC	18	0.66	0.09

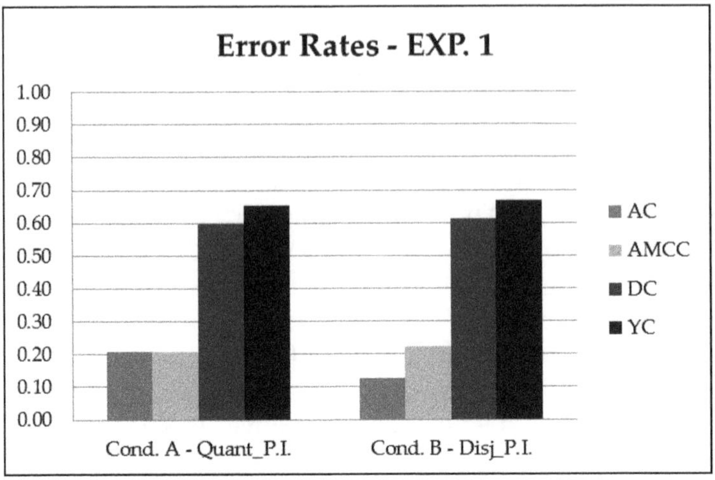

Graph. 5.1. Mean Error Rates of the four groups in Exp. 1.

Graph 5.1 represents the error rates displayed by each group respectively in Condition A (Quant_P.I.) and in Condition B (Disj_P.I.). As the graph shows, it is possible to distinguish two different behaviors amongst the four groups: dyslexic children display a very poor performance in both conditions, as well as younger children. Conversely, age-matched control children and adults show a much more correct performance.

A statistical analysis was conducted on these data, to verify if there were statistically significant differences between the performances of the four groups of participants. A one-way ANOVA was conducted (α-level= 0.05), with 'Group' (DC; AMCC; CA; YC) selected as the dependent factor. For what concerns Condition A "Quant_P.I.", 'Group' is highly significant, revealing that there are highly significant differences amongst the four groups of subjects and that the error rates are significantly affected by the group to which subjects belong (F (3, 68) = 6.440, p <.001, $\eta 2$ = .22.).

Levene's test for homogeneity of variances resulted non significant: p >.05. Therefore, a subsequent post hoc comparison test for equal variance assumed (Tukey HSD), with a α-level of 0.05 showed that DC's performance differs significantly from AMCC's and CA's one (p < .05), whereas DC do not perform differently from YC (p = 1.000); AMCC's and CA's scores do not differ significantly, too (p = 1.000). Interestingly, there is instead a statistically significant difference between YC and AMCC ($p < .01$).

Similar results have been found for Condition B "Disj_P.I.", where disjunction was used in an infelicitous context: 'Group' is highly significant, showing that there are significant differences amongst the groups (F (3, 68) = 9.777, $p < .001$, $\eta 2 = .30$). Levene's test for homogeneity of variances resulted significant ($p < .05$); therefore, a subsequent post hoc comparison test for equal variance not assumed (Dunnett T3), with a α-level of 0.05 showed that DC's performance differs significantly from AMCC's ($p < .05$) and CA's ($p < .01$) performance. Conversely, DC do not behave differently from YC ($p = .969$), whereas AMCC's and CA's show a similar performance ($p = .924$). As in Condition A, there is a statistically significant difference between AMCC and CA ($p < .01$).

Summarizing, DC show a significantly poorer performance in comparison to AMCC and CA in both conditions, while, interestingly, they behave similarly to YC, five years younger than them. AMCC, instead, show an adultlike performance in both conditions. In other words, dyslexics and preschool children tend to interpret scalar expressions logically rather than pragmatically, avoiding to compute scalar implicatures and treating *some* as equivalent to *all* and *or* as compatible with *and.*

4.1.4. Discussion

Results show that dyslexic children tend to accept pragmatically infelicitous sentences, behaving as preschool children, five years younger than them, and differently from age-matched typically developing children, who display instead an adultlike behaviour. Data show clearly, indeed, that dyslexic children perform more poorly than age-matched typically developing children when asked to evaluate sentences containing the quantifier *some* and the disjunction operator *or* used in an infelicitous way. Specifically, they treat weaker scalar terms as compatible with their stronger alternatives: *all* as compatible with *some* and *or* as compatible with *and.*

These results are consistent with the Phonological and Executive Working Memory Deficit Hypothesis, arguing that dyslexic children suffer from a processing limitation, which affects significantly their performance in those tasks that are especially demanding in terms of WM resources. From this perspective, what renders underinformative sentences difficult to reject is the need to compute a scalar implicature and, in particular, to process the necessary Reference-Set Computation, requiring the subject to construct an alternative sentence with the stronger scalar term and to compare it with the given infelicitous sentence. Moreover, the poor performance shown by younger children in comparison to control children can be explained by remembering that working memory develops with age and that, consequently, older children can rely on more efficient processing resources.

4.2. Experiment 2: the interpretation of quantifiers

The goal of this experiment was to investigate how dyslexic children interpret sentences containing the quantifiers *some* and *most* and involving the computation of a scalar implicature. Consistently with the Pragmatic Approach, sentences involving SIs' computations are expected to be more difficult for dyslexic children and younger children, whose processing abilities are more limited.

4.2.1. Participants

Experiment 2 was performed on 58 subjects divided in three groups: 20 dyslexic children, 20 age-matched typically developing children and 18 younger children attending to the first class of the primary school.

The group of dyslexic children (DC) included 20 children (12 males), all native speakers of Italian. At the moment of testing, the group mean age was 9 years and 12 months (SD = 0;11). All children have been chosen from those who had independently received a diagnosis of dyslexia, specifically by the "Dipartimento di Neuropsichiatria Infantile" at the ULSS20 (Local Public Health and Social Authority) in Verona, Italy. Diagnostic criteria included: (i) absence of neurological diseases or genetic pathologies, (ii) absence of sensorial diseases, (iii) absence of psychopathological diseases, (iv) IQ > 80 (WISC – R) and (v) fluent and correct reading and writing abilities under 2 SD (Tressoldi et al. Battery, Prove MT). The group of age-matched control children (AMCC) was composed by 20 primary school children (6 males), all native speakers of Italian. At the moment of testing, the group mean age was 9 years and 10 months (SD = 0;11). Children were selected from those who had no history of reading problems or language disorders.

The group of first class children (FCC) was composed by 18 children (9 males), all native speakers of Italian with no history of reading or language disorders. At the moment of testing, the group mean age was 6 years and 9 months (SD = 0;2). The main features of the three groups are summarized in Table 5.4.

Table 5.4. Group data of the subjects who took part in Exp. 2.

Group	Number	Mean Age (SD)
DC	20	10;0 (0;11)
AMCC	20	9;9 (0;11)
FCC	18	6;9 (0;2)

4.2.2. Design and Procedure

A truth value judgment task was performed. Subjects were shown some pictures on a computer screen that portrayed a short story involving three, five or seven characters performing some actions. The experimenter introduced the participants with a puppet, Little Red Riding Hood, who had the task to explain what was happening in the picture. The subject was told that Little Red Riding Hood was not always able to describe properly what was happening in the story. Therefore, the subject's task was to decide if Little Red Riding Hood described the picture appropriately or not by pressing a smiling face for the right answer and a crying face for the wrong answer.

The task comprised 8 target sentences, subdivided in two experimental conditions: in the first condition (Condition A, "Some_P.I."), the quantifier "*some*" was used to describe a situation where the quantifier "all" would have been more appropriate. Similarly, in the second condition (Condition B, "Most_P.I."), subjects had to accept or reject target sentences constructed with the quantifier "*most*" used in an infelicitous way. The target sentences, 4 for each condition, were interspersed with 10 felicitous utterances, 5 false and 5 true, where the quantifiers "*some*", "*most*" and "*every*" were used in an appropriate way. An example of each of the two experimental conditions is reported below.

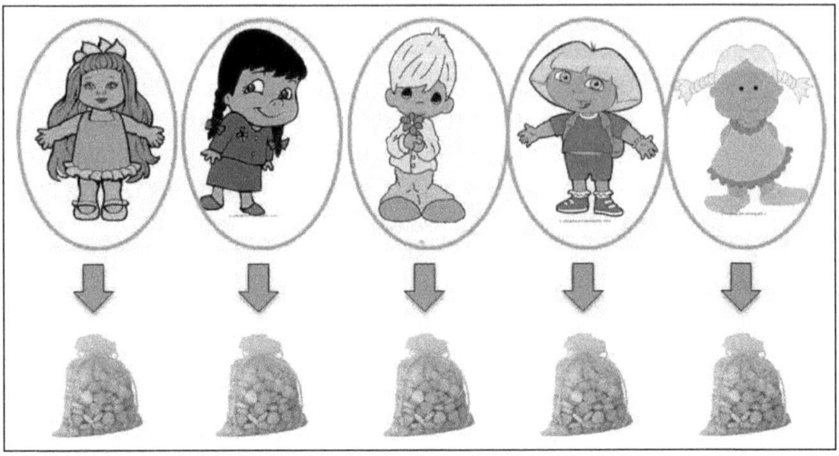

Figure 5.1. An example of Condition A "Some_P.I.".

(35) Sperimentatore: Questi sono cinque bambini. La loro maestra ha deciso di regalare un sacchettino di caramelle a chi ha fatto bene i compiti. Vediamo chi ha ricevuto le caramelle. Il primo bambino ha ricevuto le caramelle, anche il secondo le ha ricevute, anche il terzo, il quarto e perfino il quinto ha ricevuto le caramelle. Cappuccetto, cos'è successo a questi bambini?
Cappuccetto: Alcuni bambini hanno ricevuto le caramelle.

('Experimenter: These are five children. Their teacher decided to give a sack of candies to the children who did their homework well. Let's see which children received the candies. The first child received the candies, also the second child received them, also the third child, the fourth and even the last child received the candies. Little Red Riding Hood, what happened to these children?
LRRH: Some children received the candies.')

Observe that in this case the sentence uttered by Little Red Riding Hood is false, since all children, and not only *some* of them, received the candies. Therefore, the logical meaning of *some* has to be narrowed down computing the implicature. Conversely, if subjects do not compute it, they will treat *some* as compatible with *all* and will accept the utterance.

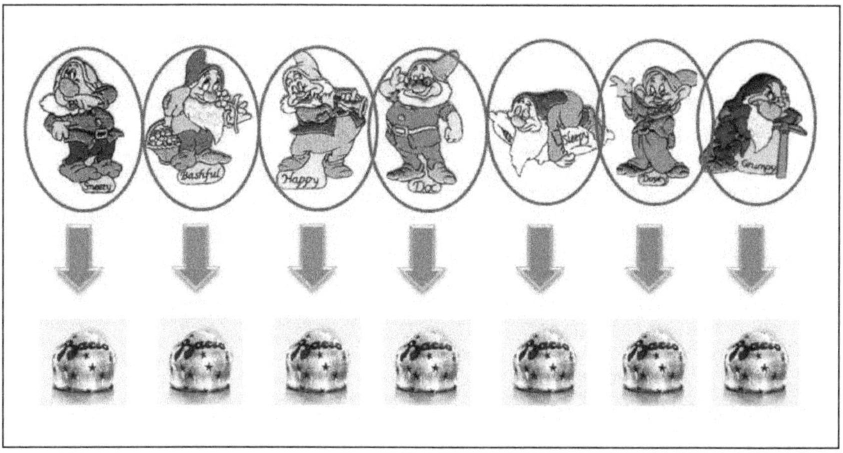

Figure 5.2. An example of Condition B "Most_P.I.".

(36) Sperimentatore: Questi sono i sette nani: Eolo, Mammolo, Gongolo, Dotto, Pisolo, Cucciolo e Brontolo. Siccome sono molto golosi, tutti i nani mangiano qualcosa di dolce. Vediamo un po': Eolo mangia un cioccolatino, Mammolo mangia un cioccolatino, Gongolo mangia un cioccolatino, anche Dotto, Pisolo, Cucciolo e perfino Brontolo mangia un cioccolatino. Cappuccetto, cosa hanno fatto questi nani?
Cappuccetto: La maggior parte dei nani ha mangiato un cioccolatino.

('Experimenter: These are the Seven Dwarves: Sneeze, Bashful, Happy, Doc, Sleepy, Dopey and Grumpy. Since they are all very greedy, they want to eat something sweet. Let's see what they eat: Sneeze eats a chocolate, Bashful eats a chocolate, Happy eats a chocolate, also Doc, Sleepy, Dopey and even Grumpy eats a chocolate. Little Red Riding Hood, what did these dwarves do?
LRRH: Most dwarves ate a chocolate.')

Again, the sentence is judged false only if the implicature is computed and the stronger alternative with *all* is excluded.

4.2.3. Results

All subjects included in the three groups gave the correct answer to the vast majority of the fillers and nobody was excluded from the sample. Descriptive statistics are reported in Table 5.5, whereas the error rates shown by the four groups of participants are reported in Graph. 5.2.

Table 5.5. Descriptive statistics of Exp. 2.

	Group	N	Mean Error Rate	Std. Deviation
Sometimes_P.I.	DC	20	0.46	0.45
	AMCC	20	0.08	0.23
	FCC	18	0.65	0.40
Most_P.I.	DC	20	0.53	0.46
	AMCC	20	0.13	0.30
	FCC	18	0.93	0.18

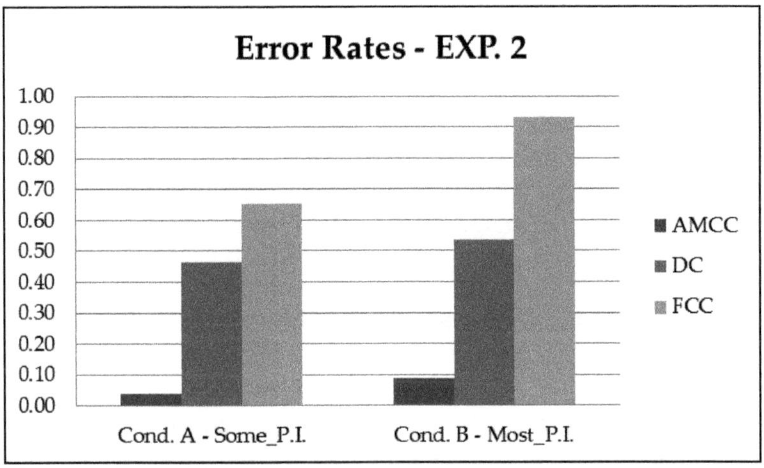

Graph 5.2. Mean Error Rates of the three groups in Exp. 2.

Graph 5.2 represents the error rates displayed by the three groups respectively in Condition A (Some_P.I.) and in Condition B (Most_P.I.).

Looking at the graph, it appears immediately clear that dyslexics underperform in both conditions in comparison to age-matched control children, whereas their performance is more similar to that of first-class children. DC, in fact, exhibit a very poor performance, as well as FCC), whereas AMCC show a very correct behavior.

A one-way ANOVA was conducted (α-level= 0.05), with 'Group' (DC; AMCC; FCC) selected as the dependent factor. For what concerns Condition A "Some_P.I.", 'Group' is highly significant, revealing that the error rates were significantly affected by the group to which subjects belonged (F (2, 55)= 11.333, p < .001, η**2** = .29). Levene's test for homogeneity of variances resulted significant: p= .000. Therefore, a subsequent post hoc comparison test for equal variance not assumed (Dunnett T3), with a α-level of 0.05 shows that DC's performance differs significantly from AMCC's one (p < .01). On the contrary, DC's do not perform differently from FCC (p = .441), whereas FCC show a significantly poorer behavior in comparison to AMCC's (p < .001).

Similar results have been reported for Condition B "Most_P.I.", where the quantifier "*most*" was used in an infelicitous context: 'Group' is highly significant, showing that there are significant differences amongst the groups (F (2, 55) = 2.983, p < .001, η**2** = .48). Levene's test for homogeneity of variances resulted significant (p < .001); therefore, a subsequent post hoc comparison test for equal variance not assumed (Dunnett T3), with a α-level of 0.05 showed that DC's performance differs highly significantly from AMCC's performance (p < .01). In this condition, FCC show a significantly poorer behavior both in comparison to DC (p < .01) and AMCC (p < .001).

Summarizing, in both conditions dyslexic children underperform in comparison to age-matched typically developing children, committing significantly more errors. Conversely, they behave similarly to first-class children, three years younger than them, when asked to interpret the quantifier "*some*". With the quantifier "*most*", instead, first-class children exhibit a poorer performance, with a very high error rate.

4.2.4. Discussion

Results indicate that dyslexics are remarkably more impaired than controls in computing the meaning of sentences requiring the computation of a scalar implicature. Specifically, they tend to accept the quantifiers *some* and *most* as equivalent to the stronger *all*. Control children, instead, seem to handle the computation of scalar implicatures effortlessly, as evidenced by their very low error rates. Finally, first-class children manifest the same tendency shown by dyslexic children, with the exception of the strikingly high error rate in Condition B, which involved the interpretation of the quantifier *most*. In this case, their difficulties appear to be related to the semantics of *most*, which may be not completely clear to them.

Again, these results are consistent with the Phonological and Executive Working Memory Deficit Hypothesis, suggesting that both dyslexics and younger children lack the processing resources necessary to accomplish a Reference-Set Computation and to compute scalar implicatures.

4.3. Experiment 3: the interpretation of frequency adverbs

The third experiment aimed at testing dyslexic children's interpretation of sentences containing the Italian frequency adverbs "*a volte*" ('sometimes') and "*spesso*" ('often') and involving the computation of a scalar implicature. Consistently with the pragmatic approach, sentences involving SIs' computations are expected to be more difficult to be processed for dyslexic children and younger children.

4.3.1. Participants

The experiment was performed on the same 58 subjects who took part in Experiment 2, whose main features are summarized in the table reported below for convenience.

Table 5.6. Group data of the subjects who took part in Exp. 2.

Group	Number	Mean Age (SD)
DC	20	10;0 (0;11)
AMCC	20	9;9 (0;11)
FCC	18	6;9 (0;2)

4.3.2. Design and Procedure

As in Experiment 2, a truth value judgment task was performed. Subjects were shown some pictures portraying a short story that involved only one character performing an action a certain number of times during the week. At the end of the story a puppet, Little Red Riding Hood, tried to explain what happened; the subject's task was to give a truth value judgment about her utterance.

The task comprised 8 target sentences, subdivided in two experimental conditions: in the first condition (Condition A, "Sometimes_P.I."), the frequency adverb *"sometimes"* was used to describe a situation where the quantifier "*always*" would have been more appropriate. Similarly, in the second condition (Condition B, "Often_P.I."), the subject had to accept or reject target sentences constructed with the frequency adverb "*often*" used in an infelicitous way. The target sentences, 4 for each condition, were interspersed with 10 fillers, 5 false and 5 true, where the frequency adverbs "*sometimes*", "*often*" and "*always*" were used felicitously. An example of each condition is reported below.

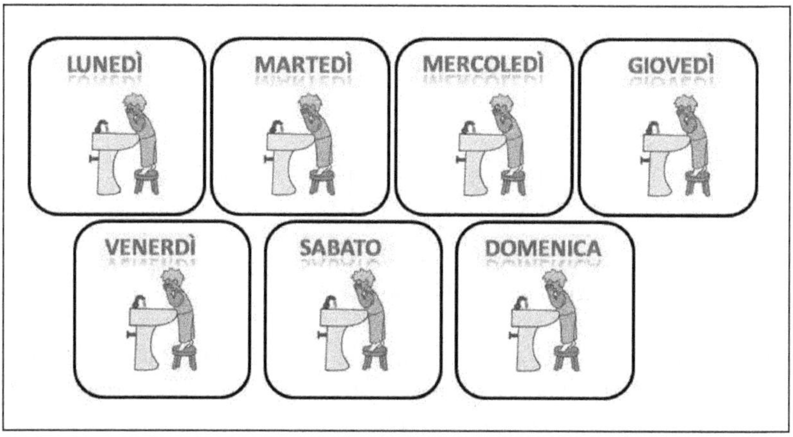

Figure 5.3. An example of Condition A "Sometimes_P.I.".

(37) Sperimentatore: Questo bambino si chiama Luca. Vediamo cos'ha fatto Luca appena alzato questa settimana. Lunedì si è lavato il viso, anche martedì si è lavato il viso, anche mercoledì, giovedì, venerdì e anche sabato si è lavato il viso. Cappuccetto, cos'ha fatto Luca appena sveglio questa settimana?
Cappuccetto: A volte Luca si è lavato il viso.

('Experimenter: This boy is Luca. Let's see what Luca did last week after getting up. On Monday he washed his face, on Tuesday he washed his face too, also on Wednesday, Thursday, Friday,

Saturday and Sunday he washed his face. Little Red Riding Hood, what did Luca do after having gotten up last week?
LRRH: Sometimes Luca washed his face.')

Notice that the sentence uttered by the puppet is false, since Luca washed his face *always* and not only sometimes. Nonetheless, if the subject does not compute the implicature, she will accept the utterance, treating *sometimes* as equivalent to *always*.

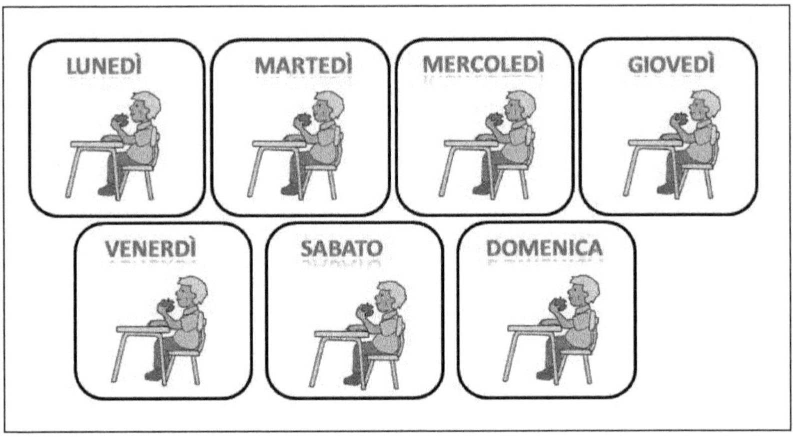

Figure 5.4. An example of Condition B "Often_P.I.".

(38) Sperimentatore: Questo bambino si chiama Andrea. Vediamo cos'ha fatto Andrea questa settimana durante il pomeriggio. Lunedì ha fatto merenda, anche martedì ha fatto merenda, anche mercoledì, giovedì, venerdì, sabato e perfino domenica ha fatto merenda. Cappuccetto, cos'ha fatto Andrea nel pomeriggio questa settimana?
Cappuccetto: Spesso Andrea ha fatto merenda.

('Experimenter: This boy is Andrea. Let's see what Andrea did last week during the afternoon. On Monday he had a snack, on Tuesday he had a snack too, also on Wednesday, Thursday, Friday, Saturday and even on Sunday he had a snack. Little Red Riding Hood, what did Andrea do in the afternoon last week?
LRRH: Often Andrea had a snack.')

Again, the sentence is judged true only if the implicature is not computed and *often* is treated as compatible to *always*. Otherwise, the utterance has to be rejected.

4.3.3. *Results*

All subjects included in the three groups gave the correct answer to the vast majority of the fillers and nobody was excluded from the sample. Descriptive statistics are reported in Table 5.7, whereas the error rates shown by the four groups of participants are reported in Graph 5.3.

Table 5.7. Descriptive statistics of Exp. 3.

	Group	N	Mean Error Rate	Std. Deviation
Sometimes_P.I.	DC	20	0.32	0.46
	AMCC	20	0.01	0.05
	FCC	18	0.31	0.39
Often_P.I.	DC	20	0.47	0.10
	AMCC	20	0.05	0.22
	FCC	18	0.59	0.43

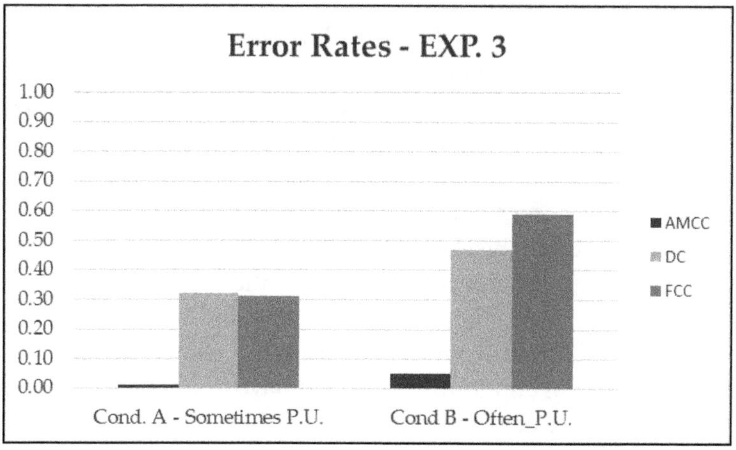

Graph 5.3. Mean Error Rates of the three groups in Exp. 3.

Graph 5.3. displays the error rates shown by the three groups respectively in Condition A (Sometimes_P.I.) and in Condition B (Often_P.I.). Looking at the graph, it appears immediately clear that dyslexics perform very poorly in comparison to age-matched control children, represented by the red bar, whose performance is generally correct. Conversely, dyslexics' behavior resembles again that of first-class children.

A one-way ANOVA was conducted (a-level= 0.05), with 'Group' (DC; AMCC; FCC) selected as the dependent factor. In Condition A "Sometimes_P.I.", 'Group' is highly significant, revealing that the error rates are significantly affected by the group to which subjects belong (F (2, 55) = 5.091, $p < .01$, $\eta 2 = .16$). Levene's test for homogeneity of variances resulted significant: $p < .001$. Therefore, a subsequent post hoc comparison test for equal variance not assumed (Dunnett T3), with a α-level of 0.05 confirmed that DC's performance differs significantly from AMCC's one ($p < .05$). On the contrary, DC show the same performance of FCC (p= 1.000), whereas FCC display a significantly poorer behavior in comparison to AMCC ($p < .05$).

Similar results have been reported for Condition B "Often_P.I.", where the quantifier "*most*" was used in an infelicitous context: 'Group' is highly significant, showing that there are significant differences amongst the groups (F (2, 55) = 10.172, $p < .001$, $\eta 2 = .27$). Levene's test for homogeneity of variances resulted significant: $p < .001$. Therefore, a subsequent post hoc comparison test for equal variance not assumed (Dunnett T3), with an α-level of 0.05 shows that DC's performance differs highly significantly from AMCC's performance ($p < .01$). In this condition, FCC show a behavior similar to that of DC ($p = .743$) but significantly poorer than that of AMCC ($p < .001$).

Recapitulating, dyslexic children's interpretation of frequency adverbs occurring in sentences that involve the computation of a scalar implicature is impaired. As in Experiments 1 and 2, their performance is significantly different from the performance shown by age-matched typically developing children, who do not have trouble with this kind of task. Conversely, dyslexics' behavior resembles that of first-class children, who are three years younger than them.

4.3.4. Discussion

Results suggest that dyslexics and first-class children display a marked tendency to compute the frequency adverbs *sometimes* and *often* as if they were compatible to their stronger alternative *always*. This indicates that they tend to avoid the computation of the scalar implicature necessary to reject the target sentences. Control children, instead, show a very correct performance.

Again, these results are in line with the predictions made by the Phonological and Executive Working Memory Deficit Hypothesis, which argues that dyslexics' and younger children' more limited processing resources hinder their performance in demanding tasks.

4.4. Experiment 4: The interpretation of disjunction

Aim of this experiment was to test dyslexic children's interpretation of sentences containing the disjunction operator *or* both in non-DE contexts, where the computation of a scalar implicature is required, and in DE contexts, where conversely the implicature does not arise. Consistently with the pragmatic approach, a higher error rate is expected in non-DE contexts.

4.4.1. Participants

The experiment was performed on the same 72 subjects who took part in Experiment 1, whose main features are reported in the table below for convenience.

Table 5.8. Group data of the subjects who took part in Exp. 4.

Group	Number	Mean Age (SD)
DC	18	9;9 (1;5)
AMCC	18	9;8 (0;10)
CA	18	26;7 (13;8)
YC	18	5;4 (0;8)

4.4.2. Design and Procedure

A truth value judgment task was administered. The subject was shown some pictures on a computer screen that portrayed a short story involving some characters that perform some actions. The experimenter introduced the subject with a puppet, Little Red Riding Hood, who had the task to explain what happened in the short story. The subject was told that the puppet could not always describe correctly what happened in the story; thus, the participant's task was to decide whether the puppet said the truth about what happened in the story or whether she lied.

The task involved 10 experimental items intertwined with 5 fillers; there were two different experimental conditions: in the first condition ("non-DE context") the sentence contained the disjunction operator *or* in a non-downward entailing context, where scalar implicatures have to be computed. In this condition, therefore, the disjunction operator *or* should be given an exclusive interpretation. In the second condition ("DE context"), instead, the disjunction operator *or* occurred in a DE-context, specifically in the restriction of the quantifier *every*. Therefore, implicatures do not arise and disjunction should receive an inclusive interpretation.

Consistently with the Pragmatic Approach, higher difficulties are expected for dyslexics and younger children in the first condition, where the computation of a scalar implicature is required. Conversely, no problems are predicted for the second condition, which does not involve implicatures computation.

Examples of both conditions are reported below.

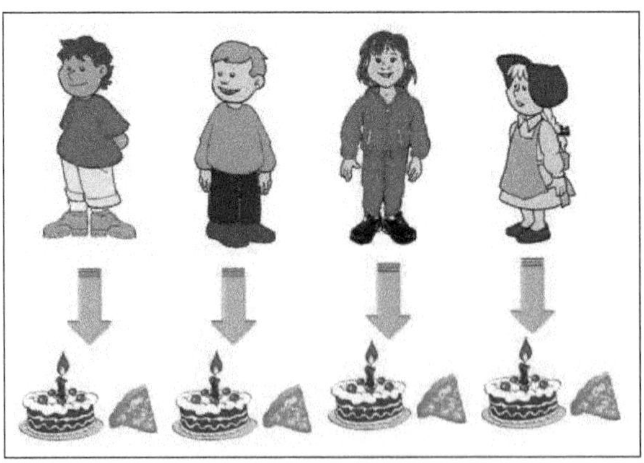

Figure 5.5. An example of Condition A – non DE contexts.

(39) Sperimentatore: “Guarda questi bambini, Marco, Gianni, Anna e Lisa. Sono stati invitati ad una festa di compleanno, dove c’erano molte cose buone da mangiare, come pasticcini, torta, pizza e patatine. Vediamo cosa hanno mangiato: Marco ha mangiato sia la torta che la pizza, anche Gianni ha mangiato sia torta che pizza, anche Anna e Lisa hanno mangiato sia torta che pizza. Chiediamo a Cappuccetto Rosso se ha capito cos’è successo nella storia. Cappuccetto, cos’è successo?
Cappuccetto: “Ogni bambino ha mangiato torta o pizza”.

(‘Experimenter: “Look at this children, Marco, Gianni, Anna and Lisa. They have been invited to a birthday party; at the party there were many delicious things to eat, as pastries, cake, pizza and chips. Let’s see what they have eaten: Marco ate both cake and pizza, also Gianni ate both cake and pizza, and also Anna and Lisa ate both cake and pizza. Let’s ask Little Red Riding Hood if she understood what happened in the story. Little Red Riding Hood, what happened?”
LRRH: “Every child ate cake or pizza’”.)

Notice that in this condition, the disjunction operator *or* occurs in an upward entailing context, where the scalar implicature has to be computed. Therefore, the sentence uttered by the puppet must be judged false. If the implicature is not computed, instead, disjunction is given a logical and thus inclusive interpretation and the utterance is considered correct.

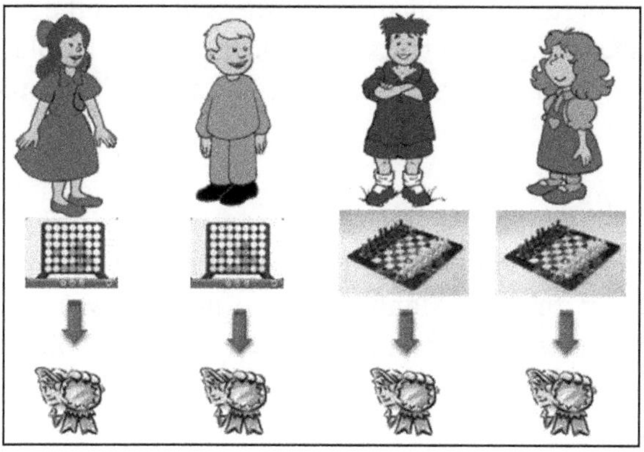

Figure 5.6. An example of Condition B – DE contexts.

(40) Sperimentatore: "Questi quattro bambini si chiamano Anna, Marco, Michele e Lisa. Ieri hanno partecipato ad alcune gare. Anna e Marco hanno giocato a Forza Quattro, mentre Michele e Lisa hanno giocato a scacchi. Siccome sono stati molto bravi, tutti e quattro hanno vinto una medaglia. Chiediamo a Cappuccetto Rosso se ha capito cos'è successo. Cappuccetto, cos'è successo?
Cappuccetto: "Ogni bambino che ha giocato a Forza Quattro o a scacchi ha vinto una medaglia".

('Experimenter: "These four children are Anna, Marco, Michele and Lisa. Yesterday they took part to some competitions. Anna and Marco played Connect Four, whereas Michele and Lisa played chess. Since they were all very skilled, all of them won a medal. Let's ask Little Red Riding Hood if she understood what happened in this story. Little Red Riding Hood, what happened?"
LRRH: "Every child who played Connect Four or chess won a medal'".)

In this condition, disjunction occurs in the restriction of the quantifier *every*, which, as observed above, is a downward entailing context, and it receives an inclusive interpretation, since the implicature does not arise. Consequently, the sentence must be considered correct, given that both children who played Connect Four and children who played chess won the medal. If the subject computes the implicature, assigning an exclusive interpretation to disjunction, she will reject the puppet's utterance, since she will reason that either the children who played Connect Four or the children who played chess, but not both, should have won the medal.

4.4.3. Results

All subjects included in the four groups gave the correct answer to the vast majority of the fillers and therefore nobody was excluded from the sample. Descriptive statistics are reported in Table 5.9, whereas the error rates shown by the four groups of participants are reported in Graph 5.4.

Table 5.9. Descriptive statistics of Exp. 4.

	Group	N	Mean Error Rate	Std. Deviation
Non-DE context	DC	18	0.47	0.36
	AMCC	18	0.10	0.24
	CA	18	0.00	0.00
	YC	18	0.71	0.35
DE context	DC	18	0.06	0.11
	AMCC	18	0.11	0.25
	CA	18	0.00	0.00
	YC	18	0.04	0.10

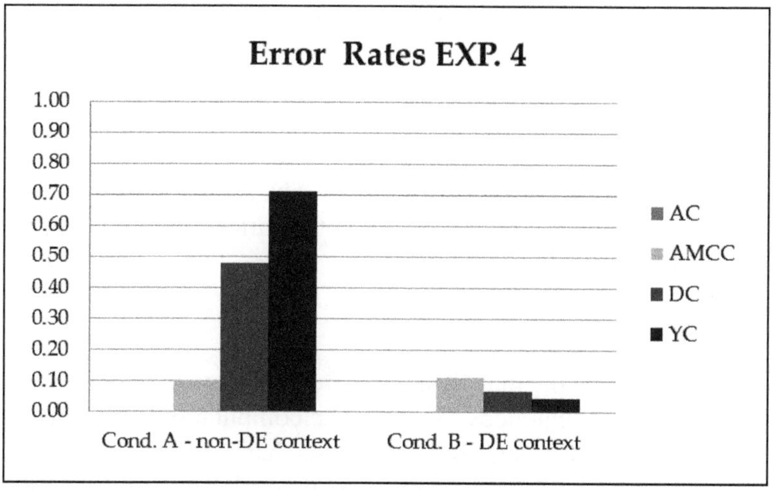

Graph 5.4. Mean Error Rates of the three groups in Exp. 4.

Graph 5.4 represents the error rates displayed by each group respectively in Condition A (non-DE context) and in Condition B (DE context). It is immediately evident that both dyslexics and younger children perform significantly worse than control children and adults in Condition A, whereas their error rates decrease radically in Condition B, where their performance is much more correct. A one-way ANOVA was conducted (α-level= 0.05), with 'Group' (DC; AMCC; YC; CA) selected as the dependent factor.

For what concerns Condition A "non-DE context 'Group' is highly significant, revealing that there are highly significant differences amongst the four groups of subjects and that the error rates are significantly affected by the group to which subjects belong (F (3, 68) = 24.429, $p < .001$, $\eta 2 = .52$). Levene's test for homogeneity of variances resulted significant: $p < .001$. Therefore, a subsequent post hoc comparison test for equal variance not assumed (Dunnett T3), with a α-level of 0.05 showed that DC's performance differs significantly from AMCC's ($p < .01$). and CA's one ($p < .001$). DC do not perform differently from YC ($p = .302$); AMCC's and CA's scores do not differ significantly, too ($p = .717$). There is also a statistically significant difference between YC and AMCC ($p < .001$).

Different results have been found for Condition B "DE context": 'Group' is not significant, showing that there are not significant differences amongst the four groups (F (3, 68)= 1.655, $p = .185$, $\eta 2 = .07$).

Summarizing, DC manifest a great difficulty to interpret disjunction in DE-context, where the computation of SIs is required, whereas they behave adultlike in non DE-context. The same tendency is exhibited by YC, while AMCC and CA do not manifest difficulties in either of the two conditions.

4.4.4. Discussion

Results indicate again that dyslexics are remarkably impaired in the comprehension of sentences requiring the computation of scalar implicatures. They perform significantly worse than age-matched typically developing children, who display an adultlike behaviour, but not dissimilarly from preschool children, five years younger than them.

In the second condition, instead, where the disjunction operator *or* occurs in a downward entailing context and the implicature does not arise, all groups of subjects manifest a correct performance.

These results show that the difficulties exhibited by dyslexics and younger children in Condition A, as well as in Experiments 1, 2 and 3, are actually due to the processing load associated to the computation of implicatures. This is consistent with the Pragmatic Approach and incompatible with the Structural Approach, which predicts that processing is even heavier in DE contexts, since the implicature, computed by default, must be deleted, involving a further operation. Finally, the results of Experiment 4 confirm that dyslexics manifest remarkable difficulties due to their working memory limitations, similarly to younger children, whose working memory has just started to develop.

4.5. Experiment 5: A Felicity Judgment Task

In the previous experiments, results emphasized a general inability in dyslexics and young children to interpret scalar expressions in contexts that require the computation of a scalar implicature. Given that a number of studies have shown that dyslexic children experience working memory impairments and that younger children's WM is not yet fully developed, I propose that their difficulties with the computation of scalar implicatures arise from a processing limitation. The goal of this last experiment was to test this hypothesis, by assessing the interpretation of the disjunction operator *or* in sentences that involve the computation of a scalar implicature through the use of a different experimental technique, with the purpose of facilitating the subject's task. The Felicity Judgment Task, in fact, involves the explicit presentation of two alternative descriptions of the context under consideration, reducing the subject's job to the mere choice of the more appropriate one and hence radically decreasing the processing load required to perform the test.

4.5.1. Participants

The experiment was performed on the same 72 subjects who took part in Experiment 1 and 4, as reported below for convenience.

Table 5.10. Group data of the subjects who took part in Exp. 5.

Group	**Number**	**Mean Age (SD)**
DC	18	9;9 (1;5)
AMCC	18	9;8 (0;10)
CA	18	26;7 (13;8)
YC	18	5;4 (0;8)

4.5.2. Design and Procedure

A felicity judgment task was administered. The subject was shown some pictures on a computer screen portraying a short story that always involved five characters performing some actions. Then she was presented with two puppets, Santa Claus and Befana, who had the task to explain what happened in the story. The participant was told that only one of the puppets uttered an appropriate sentence and that her task was to establish which puppet best described what happened in each short story.

The task involved three experimental items intertwined with three fillers. In the experimental items, the subjects could choose between (i) a sentence containing the disjunction operator *or* in a context where conjunction would have been more appropriate and (ii) a sentence constructed with its stronger alternative *and.* An example of the task is reported below:

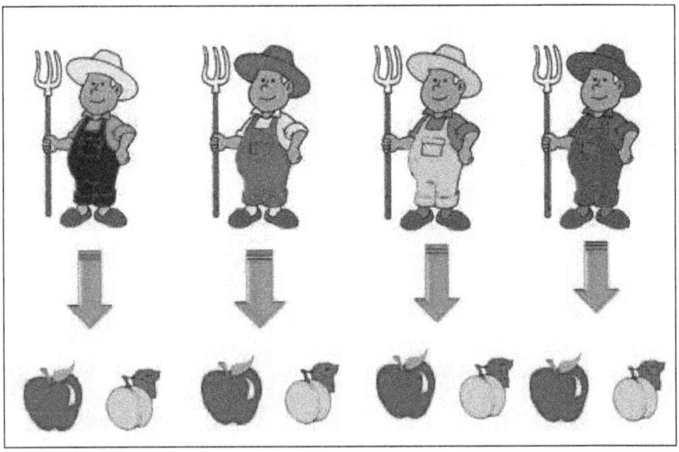

Figure 5.7. An example of Exp. 5.

(41) Sperimentatore: "Questi quattro contadini stanno coltivando della frutta nel loro orto. Vediamo un po'cosa hanno raccolto il mese scorso. Il primo contadino ha raccolto delle mele e delle pesche, anche il secondo ha raccolto delle mele e delle pesche, anche il terzo e anche il quarto hanno raccolto delle mele e delle pesche. Chiediamo a Babbo Natale e alla Befana cosa è successo secondo loro".

Babbo Natale: "Ogni contadino ha raccolto mele o pesche"
Befana: "Ogni contadino ha raccolto mele e pesche"

('Experimenter: "These four farmers are growing some fruit in their farms. Let's see what they harvested last month. The first farmer harvested apples and peaches, the second harvested apples and peaches, too and also the third and the fourth farmer harvested apples and peaches. Let's ask Santa Claus and Befana what happened in the story".
Santa Claus: "Every farmer harvested apples or peaches".
Befana: "Every farmer harvested apples and peaches"'.)

Notice that in this case only Befana said the truth, since all farmers harvested both apples and peaches. The explicit presentation of the two alternative descriptions of the sentences should facilitate the subject's ability to perform the task: therefore, a lower error rate is expected for both preschool children and dyslexics, in accordance with the hypothesis claiming that their difficulties arise from processing limitations. On the contrary, if they completely lack pragmatic knowledge, they should not find any difference between the two sentences uttered by the puppet.

4.5.3. Results

Although adults and age-matched typically developing children did not meet difficulties choosing the appropriate description of the story, two dyslexic children and three younger children were not able to perform the task and were therefore excluded from the sample. Descriptive statistics are reported in Table 5.11, whereas the error rates shown by the four groups of participants are reported in Graph. 5.5.

Table 5.11. Descriptive statistics of Exp. 5.

	Group	N	Mean Error Rate	Std. Deviation
Felicity Judgment Task	DC	16	0.12	0.20
	AMCC	18	0.01	0.07
	CA	18	0.00	0.00
	YC	15	0.15	0.21

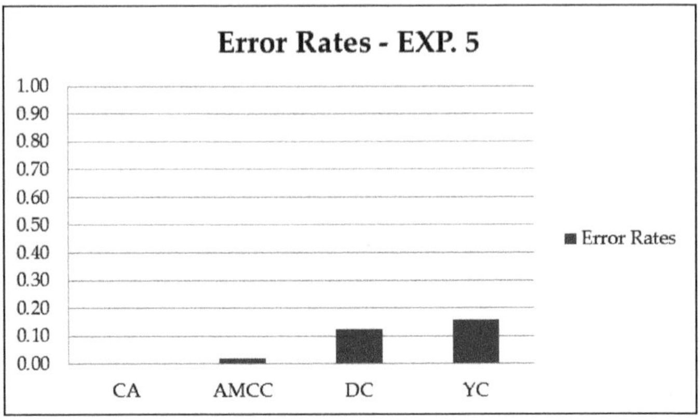

Graph 5.5. Mean Error Rates of the three groups in Exp. 5.

As the graph displays, dyslexic children and younger children manifest a very low error rate, choosing the appropriate description of the stories in the vast majority of the cases. Adults' and age-matched control children performed correctly, too.

A one-way ANOVA was conducted (α-level= 0.05), with 'Group' (DC; AMCC; CA; YC) selected as the dependent factor. 'Group' is significant, revealing that there are significant differences amongst the groups (F (3, 68) = 4.447, $p < .01$, $\eta 2 = 0.17$). Levene's test for homogeneity of variances resulted significant: $p < .001$. However, a subsequent post hoc comparison test for equal variance not assumed (Dunnett T3) resulted non significant, showing that there are not significant differences amongst the four groups. Specifically, no differences were reported between DC and AMCC (p = .321), between DC and CA (p = .149), DC and YC (p = .999), AMCC and YC (p = .160), AMCC and CA (p = .890), CA and YC (p = .074).

Summarizing, dyslexic children and preschool children perform adultlike, as well as age-matched control children. This confirms that they are greatly facilitated by the explicit presentation of the two alternatives, indicating therefore that the difficulties met in the previous experiments are not due to a lack of pragmatic knowledge but rather to a processing limitation that affects their ability to construct, maintain in memory and compare the alternative sentences at the same time.

4.5.4. Discussion

The results of this last experiment suggest that dyslexics' and preschool children's difficulties with the computation of scalar implicatures are actually due to the processing load requested to accomplish the task. The Felicity Judgment Task, in fact, has been used with the aim of reducing the processing costs associated with the computation of implicatures, as predicted by the hypothesis that implicatures involve Reference Set Computation. In this kind of task, indeed, the subject is not required to construct and contemporarily maintain in memory the two alternative sentences, containing respectively the weaker and the stronger scalar terms, since they are explicitly presented. Therefore, all what the subject has to do is to choose the most appropriate one between the two given sentences.

In line with our predictions, dyslexics and younger children derive a significant benefit from this kind of help, as indicated by the absence of significant differences amongst the four groups of participants. Finally, these results offer a further argument in favour both of the Pragmatic Approach, claiming that the computation of implicatures is costly, and of the Phonological and Executive Working Memory Deficit Hypothesis, arguing that dyslexics' processing resources are more limited, hampering the execution of particularly demanding tasks.

5. General discussion

The results of the experiments administered in this protocol showed that dyslexic children are impaired in their ability to compute scalar implicatures, performing much worse than age-matched typically developing children, who displayed instead an adultlike and almost always accurate behavior. These findings are consistent with the predictions made by the Phonological and Executive Working Memory Deficit Hypothesis, according to which dyslexics are impaired in those complex operations that impose high processing costs, like the computation of implicatures. Dyslexic children show a very poor performance in the statement evaluation task and in all three truth value judgment tasks, displaying a behavior similar to that shown by younger children, whereas age-matched control children perform adultlike.

In Experiment 1, a statement evaluation task, subjects were asked to evaluate pragmatically infelicitous sentences containing the disjunction operator *or*, such as "People have arms or legs", or the quantifier *some*, such as "Some birds have wings". Results showed that both dyslexics and preschool children tend to accept these infelicitous statements in the majority of the cases, far more often that control children and adults. In particular, they interpret scalar expressions logically rather than pragmatically, treating the quantifier *some* as compatible with the quantifier *all* and the disjunction operator *or* as compatible with the conjunction operator *and*. This marked tendency to give scalar terms a logical interpretation indicates that they are avoiding to compute implicatures, suggesting that this task is too difficult for them and exceeds their actual capacities. Conversely, age-matched typically developing children manifest an adultlike behavior, displaying a significantly lower error rate.

The interpretation of quantifiers was further tested in Experiment 2, a truth value judgment task, where subjects were asked to judge utterances containing the quantifiers *some* and *most* in pragmatically infelicitous contexts where *all* characters performed the same action. For this reason, subjects were forced to compute scalar implicatures by the context, given that a logical interpretation of a sentence like "Some children received the candies" is not appropriate in a scenario in which *all* children received the candies. Results confirmed that also in this kind of experiment dyslexics underperform in comparison to controls, failing thus to draw scalar inferences, whereas their behavior is similar to that shown by first-class children, three years younger than them.

The same tendency was found in Experiment 3, a truth value judgment task testing the interpretation of the frequency adverbs *sometimes* and *often* in pragmatically infelicitous contexts where it would have been more appropriate to use the adverb *always*. Again, results are very clear: dyslexics and first-class children are remarkably more impaired than age-matched control children, accepting significantly more often utterances such as "Sometimes Luca washed his face" in a context in which Luca washed his face *every day*.

The interpretation of disjunction was examined in Experiment 4, a truth value judgment task, where subjects had to interpret disjunction in two different conditions. In Condition A the disjunction operator *or* occurred in a non-downward entailing context, where scalar implicatures have to be computed, and the subject was asked to judge sentences such as "Every child ate cake or pizza" in a scenario where all children ate both cake *and* pizza. In Condition B, instead, disjunction occurred in a downward entailing context, where scalar inferences do not arise, and the subject had to provide a truth value judgment for utterances such as "Every child who played Connect Four or chess won a medal", in a scenario where both children who played Connect Four *and* children who played chess won a medal.

Again, results are very interesting: both dyslexic children and preschool children display a remarkably poor performance in non-DE contexts, where the implicatures should have been computed, whereas they exhibit an adultlike behavior in Condition B, when disjunction occurred in downward entailing environments and scalar inferences did not arise. On the contrary, age-matched typically developing children do not experience any difficulty, performing as adults in both conditions.

These results indicate that dyslexic children's and younger children's problems do not arise from a general inability to interpret the disjunction operator *or*, given that their performance is accurate in DE contexts, but rather from a processing limitation linked to the computation of the scalar implicature.

Summarizing, dyslexics exhibit remarkable deficits in the interpretation of the quantifiers *some* and *most*, the frequency adverbs *sometimes* and *often* and the disjunction operator *or* in contexts in which the computation of a scalar implicature is required. Interestingly they perform as younger children, while age-matched children do not experience problems, computing the implicatures in all contexts without difficulties.

These results are consistent both with the Pragmatic Approach illustrated above and with the Phonological and Executive Working Memory Deficit Hypothesis, predicting higher error rates for those subjects whose processing resources are more limited. To interpret these outcomes, in fact, I adopt Reinhart's framework, according to which the computation of scalar implicatures imposes a great burden on Working Memory, since it involves a Reference-Set Computation (i.e. the construction and comparison of two alternative descriptions of the sentences), which is an operation remarkably demanding in terms of processing resources.

As predicted by this account, younger children experience significantly more difficulties than older children, because their working memory is not yet fully developed. Moreover, since dyslexics' performance resembles that of younger children in all four experiments, it is reasonable to argue that their difficulties arise precisely from a processing limitation, consistently with the Phonological and Executive Working Memory Deficit Hypothesis.

To test even more directly this hypothesis, the subjects' competence has been further examined in Experiment 5, assessing the interpretation of disjunction with a different methodology, the felicity judgment task. Since this technique involves the explicit presentation of the two alternative descriptions of the target sentence, the processing load required to execute the task is significantly reduced. The subject, in fact, does not need to construct the two different representations of the target sentence, which are explicitly presented, but she has simply to choose the most appropriate one amongst them.

Again, results are interesting: consistently with the Phonological and Executive Working Memory Deficit Hypothesis, dyslexic children's and preschool children's error rates are significantly lower in this experiment. Moreover, there are not statistically significant differences between their performance and the performance shown by age-matched typically developing children. This finding confirms that the difficulties exhibited by dyslexics and younger children in previous experiments were indeed caused by the excessive computational demands of the tasks, which surpassed their available WM resources. Once the computational load is reduced, as in the case of a felicity judgment task, both dyslexics and younger children can achieve an accurate performance.

To conclude, then, all five experiments administered to test scalar implicatures' computation provided interesting data revealing that dyslexic children are significantly more impaired than age-matched typically developing children, whereas their behavior is similar to that proper of younger children, three and five years younger than them. Arguably, their poor performance is due to a processing limitation, providing further support to the Phonological and Executive Working Memory Deficit Hypothesis.

6. Summary and Conclusions

In this Chapter I have reported the results of five experiments testing the interpretation of sentences that require the computation of a scalar implicature and providing further support to the Phonological and Executive Working Memory Deficit Hypothesis, according to which dyslexic individuals suffer from an impairment affecting their phonological memory and executive functions. As extensively discussed in Chapter 4, this deficit hampers their ability to perform complex operations whose processing demands exceed their actual Working Memory capacities.

Throughout this chapter we have observed that computing a scalar implicature is indeed an expensive task, since it requires the subject to perform a Reference-Set Computation, constructing and comparing the two distinct representations of the target sentence. This kind of computation is arguably too expensive for dyslexic children and younger children, whose processing resources are not up to the task.

Consistently, results clearly showed that dyslexic children's pragmatic competence is impaired, since they exhibit a very poor performance in comparison to age-matched typically developing children and adults in the first four experiments, performing similarly to younger children. Conversely, they show a more accurate behavior in Experiment 5, where a different methodology was adopted to reduce the computational load of the task, further confirming that their difficulties are determined by a processing deficit. To interpret these results, hence, I assume that the computation of scalar implicatures imposes high processing costs and I propose that dyslexic children's difficulties arise from a working memory impairment. Similarly, I suggest that younger children's poor performance is related to the fact that their working memory is not yet completely developed.

Summarizing, the results reported in this chapter are consistent with the Phonological and Executive Working Memory Deficit Hypothesis, demonstrating that dyslexics experience remarkable difficulties in those tasks that are quite demanding in terms of processing resources, such as the computation of scalar implicatures.

Chapter 6

The Interpretation of Negation in Developmental Dyslexia

1. Introduction

In this chapter I will present the results of an experimental protocol administered on a group of dyslexic children and on a group of age-matched typically developing children to test their interpretation of negative sentences. The protocol was composed of two distinct experiments testing respectively the interpretation of active negative sentences (Exp. 1) and the interpretation of passive negative sentences.

As it will become evident throughout this discussion, negation is an intriguing topic of research, since despite its apparent simplicity – it is just one of the connectives of propositional logic – it seems to impose a significant burden on Working Memory, demanding more processing resources than one should expect from a connective. Before presenting and discussing the results of my experimental protocol, I will review the recent literature on negation, focusing especially on the processing costs imposed by the interpretation of negative sentences.

I will argue that the processing difficulty associated with negation cannot be ascribed to structural, but rather to pragmatic factors. Negative sentences, in fact, are generally used in supportive contexts with the precise communicative intention to negate a previously asserted or implied affirmation. This intuition was already grasped by Wason (1965), who argued that a negative sentence can be uttered felicitously only in "contexts of plausible denial", that is, in those contexts in which its affirmative counterpart can be uttered felicitously.

A similar intuition underpins the hypothesis recently put forward by Kaup, Zwaan and Lüdtke (2007), known as the "Two Step Simulation Hypothesis". According to this proposal, the processing of a negative sentence involves the mental simulation of an expected state of affairs (i.e. the affirmative counterpart of the negative sentence), which must be successively deleted and replaced by the simulation of the actual state of affairs. It is precisely this step that requires high processing resources, rendering negation more difficult to process than affirmation.

It can be interesting, therefore, to verify how dyslexics perform in comparison to age-matched typically developing children in tests involving the interpretation of negation in order to verify the predictions of the Phonological and Executive Working Memory Deficit Hypothesis.

2. The semantics of negation

Negation is a linguistic tool highly specific and peculiar of human language, which is employed to accomplish different tasks such as denying, contradicting, refusing concepts, correcting wrongly made inferences, but also lying and speaking ironically. For its fundamental role in human language, negation has been extensively studied throughout the centuries. It has been a matter of research for philosophers as Plato and Aristotle and it has been dealt with in classical logic. In the late 1800s and in 1900s research on negation has been linked to the study of presupposition and it has gained an increasing attention that persists nowadays.

2.1. Negation in classical logic

The first studies on negation and opposition can be traced back to Plato, who identifies negation, the not-proposition or not-*p*, with the concept of otherness, that is, what is different from *p*. In fact, it is not always the case that negation must be read as opposition or contrariety: as Plato's spokesman, the Stranger, observes, when we argue that something is "not great", we are not assuming that it is small, but simply that it is different from being great.

With Aristotle, the study of negation moves from the domain of ontology to that of logic and language. Aristotle offers two fundamental contributions to the research on negation: first, he recognizes that there are distinct types of oppositions, distinguishing the notion of *contrariety* from the notion of *contradiction*; secondly, he formulates the two principal laws about negation, namely, the Law of Contradiction and the Law of the Excluded Middle. Aristotle's theory of negation, indeed, considers four distinct types of opposition: (i) correlation (e.g. *double* vs. *half*), (ii) contrariety (e.g. *good* vs. *bad*), (iii) privation (e.g. *blind* vs. *sighted*) and (iv) contradiction (e.g. *he sits* vs. *he does not sit*). Contradiction, which concerns the actual opposition between affirmative and negative sentences, can be distinguished from the other classes of oppositions for two main reasons: first, it can be applied only to propositions and not to single terms. Secondly, only in contradictory opposition it is necessary that one member be true and the other be false.

The notions of contrariety and contradiction are dealt with in first-order logic and in the square of oppositions, as reported below.

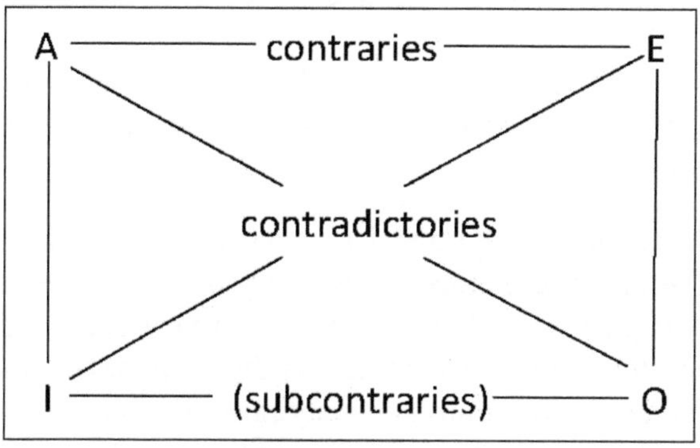

Figure 6.1. Aristotle's Square of Opposition.

In the square of oppositions the capital letters "A", "E", "I" and "O" represent the vowels of the Latin verbs *affirmo*, ('I affirm') and ***nego*** ('I deny'); the horizontal axis defines a quality distinction between affirmation and negation, whereas the vertical axis represent a quantity distinction between universals and particulars, as summarized in (1).

(1) **A** (∀) universal affirmative: e.g., "Every student solved the problem".

E (¬∃) universal negative: e.g., "No student solved the problem".
I (∃) particular affirmative: e.g., "Some students solved the problem".
O (¬∀) particular negative: e.g., "Not every student solved the problem".

Therefore, four kind of oppositions are possible:

(i) A/I: the universal affirmative ("Every student solved the problem") versus the particular affirmative ("Some students solved the problem").
(ii) A/E: the universal affirmative ("Every student solved the problem") versus the universal negative ("No student solved the problem").
(iii) E/O: the universal negative ("No student solved the problem") versus the particular negative ("Not every student solved the problem").
(iv) I/O: the particular affirmative ("Some students solved the problem") versus the particular negative ("Not every student solved the problem").

Aristotle identifies the A/O and I/E pairs as contradictories, since in any state of affairs one member must necessarily be true and the other false. The A/E pair instead, represents a contrary opposition: A and E are namely mutually inconsistent, that is they cannot be simultaneously true, though they can be simultaneously false. For instance, A and E are both false in a context where only some of the students solved the problems. Finally, a further subtle distinction should be made between the A/E pair and the I/O pair: Aristotle, indeed, argues that I and O are "only verbally opposed", observing that propositions as "Some students solved the problem" and "Not every student solved the problems" are mutually consistent, that is they can both be true at the same time, unlike A and E. Aristotle's logic of opposition is based on two fundamental principles, considered basic and indemonstrable: (i) the Law of Contradiction and (ii) the Law of the Excluded Middle. The Law of Contradiction states that it is impossible for one property to be asserted and negated at the same time for the same object and in the same respect. Aristotle argues that this is the most certain principle of all and that it applies to both contrary and contradictory opposition. What distinguishes contraries and contradictories, instead, is the second indemonstrable principle, the Law of the Excluded Middle, which states that for any proposition *p*, either *p* is true, or its negation $\neg p$ is. This principle applies only to contradictories, since as Aristotle observes, "nothing can exist between two contradictories, but something may exist between contraries". Two contraries, as *hot* and *cold*, in fact, cannot be both true, but they can certainly be both false: nothing can be both hot and cold at the same time, but something can be neither hot nor cold.

Conversely, two contradictories such as *alive* and *dead* cannot be both false: if the one is false, the other must be true, and vice versa. Contradictories, then, are mutually exhaustive as well as mutually inconsistent, since one member of the pair must be true and the other false, as schematized below.

Table 6.1. Mutual Exhaustiveness of contradictories.

p **(Socrates is ill)**	**¬p** **(Socrates is not ill)**
T	**F**
F	T

Moreover, an important clarification should be made: these laws apply only when the entity that corresponds to the subject of predication in the proposition exists. Things radically change, instead, whenever the subject of the sentence is an empty (non-denoting) entity. Consider the examples in (2).

(2) a. Socrates is ill.
b. Socrates is well.
c. Socrates is not ill.

Aristotle argues that the two affirmative sentences (2a) and (2b) will be one true and the other false, if Socrates exists, whereas they will be both false, if Socrates does not exist. With respect to the negative sentence in (2c), instead, he points out that the proposition will be either true or false, if Socrates exists, whereas it will be true, if Socrates does not exist. Aristotle motivates this distinction between affirmation and negation arguing that if Socrates does not exists, it is false to say that he is ill, while it is true to say that he is not ill. Specifically, he points out that denying what is predicated or the predicate itself of an empty non-existing entity results in a true statement, because a predicate denial such as *A is not B* is true if and only if the corresponding affirmative proposition, *A is B*, is false. In other words, since "Socrates is ill" is false, whenever Socrates does not exists, the negative sentence "Socrates is not ill" must be true. The question of which truth value should be assigned to the predications of nonexistent objects has been matter of an intense debate which has been revived in the last centuries.

2.2. *Negation and presuppositions*

In the previous paragraph we have observed that denying the predicate of an empty entity is considered true in Aristotelian logic. This position has been both criticized and vindicated first in the philosophical and then in the linguistic literature. The debate has been redrawing attention starting from Frege (1892), who develops the notion of *presupposition*. Specifically, he argues that both the affirmative and the negative sentences in (3) convey a presupposition of existence, that is the presupposition that Kepler has a referent or, in other words, that Kepler existed.

(3) a. Kepler died in misery.
b. Kepler did not die in misery.

Specifically, Frege claims that every sentence with a singularly referring subject, regardless of whether it is affirmative or negative, presupposes the existence of a referent for that subject. Whenever this presupposition fails, then, there is a truth value gap: the sentence cannot be assigned a truth value and consequently it cannot be used to make an assertion. This solution is rejected by Russell (1905), who goes back to Aristotle's original position, arguing that by the Law of the Excluded Middle a proposition must be necessarily either true or false. To solve the problem posed by sentences with non-referring entities, he proposes that negative sentences are ambiguous, depending on the scope of negation. He notes, indeed, that it is possible to distinguish two types of negation (internal and external), giving rise to different truth values.

Consider, for instance, the sentences in (4).

(4) a. The king of France is bald.
b. The king of France is not bald.

In Russell's framework, the affirmative sentence in (4a) must be judged false since the subject is a non-referring entity: it is, in fact, false that there is a unique entity with the property of being the King of France and of being bald. (4a) can be represented as an existentially quantified conjunction, as reported in (5a) below.

(5) a. $\exists X\ (Kx \wedge \forall y\ (Ky \rightarrow y = x) \wedge Bx)$
b. $\exists X\ (Kx \wedge \forall y\ (Ky \rightarrow y = x) \wedge \neg Bx)$
c. $\neg \exists X\ (Kx \wedge \forall y\ (Ky \rightarrow y = x) \wedge Bx)$

The negative sentence in (4b), instead, is considered ambiguous since it gives rise to an external and an internal reading, depending on the scope of the negation operator *not*. These two different readings are represented with distinct logical forms and they give rise to different truth values. The two representations are reported below. In (5b) the negation is internal and it falls within the scope of the definite description "the king of France"; we can interpret this proposition as arguing that there is a king of France and that he is not bald. Given that there is no king of France, the sentence is false. In (5c), instead, negation is external and it has wide scope over the definite description. In this case, the proposition means that there is no unique individual that has both the property of being the king of France and the property of being bald. Since there is no one satisfying the property of being king of France, one of the two conjuncts is false, to the effect that the sentence (which amounts to negating a conjunction) is to be judged true.[1] In Russell's approach,

1 It can be interesting to note that in this approach negation can be also used as a test in order to check whether the grammatical subject of a sentence is referential or not. Consider the sentences below:

(6) a. It is not the case that Eric is bald. $\rightarrow$ Eric is not bald.
b. It is not the case that the King of France is bald. $\nrightarrow$ The King of France is not bald.

Observe that only when the grammatical subject of the sentence is referential, as in (6a), negating the sentence coincides with negating its predicate. On the contrary, if the subject is not referential, as in (6b), negating the sentence and negating

hence, (5a) and (5c) are contradictories and the Law of the Excluded Middle is satisfied, since the former is false and the latter is true.

Russell's proposal of considering negation as ambiguous depending on the scope of the negation operator is criticized by Strawson who argues, as Frege, that a negative sentence with a non-denoting subject like (4b) cannot be attributed a truth-value. In Strawson's account, the question of the truth value of the sentence fails to arise, given that the presupposition of existence is not satisfied; to say it with Horn (1989), in Strawson's proposal any statement about a non-existent entity is not false, "but rather immune to concerns of truth and falsity" (109).

The feeling that classical logic is inadequate to account for sentences with non-denoting entities has opened the way to Multivalued Logic, which differentiates from classic bivalued logic since it postulates the existence of more than two truth-values. The impossibility of evaluating sentences such as (4b) has been interpreted as a "truth conditional black-hole", equivalent to "the formal design of assigning a third truth value" (Horn, ibid). In the three-valued logic proposed by Lukasiewicz (1930; 1957), for instance, the third truth value "unknown" is added to the classic truth values "true" and "false", which is generally dubbed N, for "neuter" (or Nonsense, or Neither true nor false). As a consequence, sentences with empty reference are judged "unknown"; furthermore, "true" and "false" are not seen as contradictories anymore, as in classical bivalent logic, but rather as contraries, since it is no more the case that a proposition must be necessarily either true or false (Lukasiewicz 1930; 1957).

Within Multivalued Logic, then, an affirmative sentence with a non-denoting subject gets the "unknown" (N) value, whereas negative sentences are seen as ambiguous between internal negation and external negation. Sentences with an internal negation are judged "unknown", as affirmatives, whereas sentences with an external negation are considered true, as schematized below. For this reason, internal negation is defined presupposition-preserving, whereas external negation is presupposition-canceling.

---

its predicate yield different interpretations. The same observation can be extended to quantifiers, as shown by the contrast below:

c. It is not the case that every man is bald. → Every man is not bald.

As in (6b), also in this case negating the whole sentence does not coincide with negating its predicate.

Table 6.2. Negation in Multivalued Logic.

p **Affirmative Sentence**	¬p **Internal Negation**	−p **External Negation**
T	F	F
F	T	T
N	N	T

However, not even this theory is free of complications. Strawson (1964), for instance, observes that truth-value gaps arise only when empty singular terms have a referential position in the sentence, i.e. when they are the subject or the topic of the utterance. Consider, for instance, the sentences in (7) and (8):

(7) a. The king of France visited the exhibition.
b. The king of France didn't visit the exhibition.

(8) a. The exhibition was visited by the king of France.
b. The exhibition wasn't visited by the king of France.

According to Multivalued Logic, an "unknown" value should be assigned to the couple of sentences in (7), given that both affirmative and negative sentences with an internal negation are supposed to be neither true nor false when the subject is a non-referring entity. Nevertheless, we are perfectly able to evaluate the sentences in (8), judging (8a) false and (8b) true. Strawson explains this fact arguing that the presupposition of existence stating that "There is a king of France" does not arise, since the definite description "The king of France" is neither the subject nor the topic of the sentence, which is instead about the exhibition. A different perspective is adopted by Horn (1996), who draws the distinction between truth and verification, considering sentences like (9).

(9) The king of France is standing next to me.

In Horn's approach, the assertion that the king of France is not standing next to me can be easily falsified, given that whoever is standing next to me, if there is someone, he does not have the property of being the king of France, regardless of whether France has or not a king. Conversely, the truth value of sentence (4a), stating that that the king of France is bald, cannot be determined straightforwardly, but rather only implicitly, arguing that France is not a monarchy. Significantly, this approach seems to suggest that there is a strict relationship between a presupposition and its context of utterance, proposing that presuppositions are a matter of pragmatics, instead of semantics. This position is supported also by scholars as Karttunen (1974) and Stalnaker (1974; 1978), who emphasize the importance of the discourse context, arguing that a proposition is presupposed if it is non-controversially true in every world within the working context set. According to the pragmatic approach, presuppositions are "restrictions on the common ground, rather than conditions on truth and falsity" (Horn 1996: 307). Consequently, when presuppositions fail, as in the case of the non-existing king of France, sentences are simply considered infelicitous or inappropriate and it does not make sense to assign them a truth value.

However, when a presupposition is not part of the common ground, it can be accommodated, as proposed by Lewis (1979), who formulates a rule for the accommodation of presuppositions.

(10) Lewis' rule of accommodation for presuppositions
If at time *t* something is said that requires presupposition *P* to be acceptable, and if *P* is not presupposed just before *t*, then – *ceteris paribus* and within certain limits – presupposition *P* comes into existence at *t* (Lewis, 1979).

To understand how accommodation works, consider the couple of sentences in (11).

(11) a. Eric doesn't smoke anymore.
b. Eric used to smoke.

Sentence (11a) carries the presupposition reported in (11b). Even in the case that the hearer didn't know that Eric used to smoke, he is forced to accommodate the presupposition in (11b) by adding it to the common ground.

2.3. *Markedness of negation*

As noted by Horn (1989), the symmetry displayed by affirmation and negation in logic is not reflected by a comparable symmetry in language structure and use. Consider, for instance, the sentences below:

(12) Lisa thinks that Eric solved the problem.
(13) Lisa doesn't think that Eric didn't solve the problem.

In first order logic, sentences (12) and (13) should be equivalent, since they share the same truth-conditions: if (12) is true, (13) must be true as well, and vice versa. However, it seems that the negative sentence in (13) entails a different communicative effect which is not present in its affirmative counterpart; moreover, it appears that (13) requires a higher cognitive effort to be processed. Observing the semantic asymmetry shown by sentences such as (12) and (13), researchers generally agree considering negation the marked form respect to affirmation. Accordingly, speakers generally use the positive form to convey a piece of information, whereas they resort to the negative form to express some additional communicative effect.

Beyond this semantic markedness, negation is also formally marked, since it always requires the presence of a specific operator, differently from affirmation, which does not require a special marking. This generalization is universally valid for human languages: as Greenberg (1966) notes, negative sentences always receive an overt expression, whereas affirmative sentences are formally less complex and they are generally realized with a zero expression. Moreover, Greenberg observes that this pattern occurs also in mathematics: negative numbers, in fact, must bear a formal overt mark (e.g. "-3"), while positive numbers may lack it (e.g. "3, +3"). As DeSwart (2009) notes, negation is marked in the sense that it involves special grammatical means, leading to greater syntactical and morphological complexity.

Another factor contributing to the markedness of negation is the fact that negative sentences are generally less informative than their affirmative counterparts, as stated in the Principle of Negative Uninformativeness proposed by Leech (1981). Consider, for instance, the sentences below:

(14) China is the most populous country in the world.
(15) India is not the most populous country in the world.

Even though both sentences are true, (15) is far less informative than (14): assuming that there are 194 countries in the world, in fact, (15) can be seen as 193 times less informative than (14). As pointed out by

Leech, a negative sentence like (15) must be uttered in a specific context to be appropriate, as in the conversational exchange reported in (16):

(16) Eric: "India is the most populous country in the world."
Lisa: "No, you're wrong! India is not the most populous country in the world. China is the most populous country in the world!"

Otherwise, if (15) is uttered out of the blue, it is perceived as inappropriate, since it infringes the Maxim of Quantity making part of the Conversational Maxims theorized by Grice (1975) and asserting "Make your contribution as informative as required" (see Chapter 5). A speaker trying to be cooperative, would in fact utter (14) instead of the less informative (15), unless she has a particular communicative intent, as in (16). However, note that it is not always true that negative sentences are less informative than their affirmative counterparts. Take, for instance, the couple of sentences below:

(17) The radio is on.
(18) The radio is not off.

Although (17) and (18) convey precisely the same information, the decontextualized occurrence of (18) seems intuitively harder to interpret than (17). But what precisely determines the higher processing cost that seems to be associated with negation? This question will be handled with in the following paragraph, where the results of experimental studies and the theories elaborated to account for them will be exposed.

3. Processing of negation

The processing of negation has been the matter of a considerable amount of research in the 1960s and 1970s. In most of the studies conducted, participants were asked to verify affirmative and negative sentences either against their background knowledge (sentence-verification tasks), or against a picture (picture-verification task). From the results it clearly emerged that negative sentences were more difficult to process than their affirmative counterparts, as shown by higher error rates or longer reaction times.

Amongst the various hypotheses elaborated to account for these data, the most convincing account is the pragmatic one, which focuses on the importance of the context of utterance, claiming that negative sentences are more difficult when they occur in an infelicitous context. Afterwards, the processing of negation has gained increasing interest in the late 1990s, with a number of experimental studies testing in particular the accessibility of the concepts mentioned in negated phrases. Results have shown that negation reduces the accessibility of information that occurs within its scope.

In line with the pragmatic hypothesis, a further approach to the processing of negation has been recently proposed, known as the "Two-Step Simulation Hypothesis" (Kaup et al. 2007). According to this proposal, a negative sentence always requires the presence of its affirmative counterpart, which gets negated. The affirmative counterpart can be either already present in the discourse context, as in the examples discussed in the previous section, or it must be recovered or constructed by the comprehender. In other words, when processing a negative sentence, the comprehender is forced to retrieve or create a representation of its affirmative counterpart. Therefore, she must construct two mental simulations, the one for the actual state of affairs and the other for the expected state of affairs, and compare them. An operation that is accordingly very expensive in terms of processing resources.

In the following sections I will discuss the earlier experimental protocols conducted to test negation and I will present the pragmatic hypothesis. Afterwards I will report the results of the most recent studies, considering also neurological fMRI-studies, and I will illustrate in detail the Two-Step Simulation Hypothesis.

3.1. *The earlier experimental studies on negation: Wason (1961) and Carpenter and Just (1975)*

One of the earliest experimental protocols testing negation was administered by Wason (1959, 1961), obtaining interesting and quite surprising results. The experimental protocol comprised a sentence verification task, in which subjects were asked to provide a truth value judgment for sentences about their encyclopedic knowledge; the target sentences were divided in 4 groups:

(i) True affirmative sentences (e.g., "Twenty-four is an even number".).
(ii) False affirmative sentence (e.g., "Thirty-nine is an even number".).
(iii) True negative sentences (e.g., "Fifty-seven is not an even number".).
(iv) False negative sentences (e.g., "Ninety-two is not an even number".).

Both error rates and response times were considered. Results show a significant effect of negation, with negative sentences taking longer to process than their affirmative counterparts. The accuracy of responses was further analyzed, showing that true negative sentences are the most difficult ones, with the highest error rate. This result was quite surprising, since it was expected that false affirmatives were harder than true affirmatives and that false negatives were harder than true negatives. Instead, an asymmetry was found between affirmative and negative sentences, with the following ranking:

(19) true affirmatives > false affirmatives > false negatives > true negatives

The same results were reported by Carpenter and Just (1975), who administered a sentence-picture verification task. In this experiment subjects were asked to evaluate sentences against pictures and response times were measured. In this case, external negation has been tested. There were four experimental conditions:

(i) True affirmative sentences: subjects had to evaluate a sentence as "It is true that the dots are red" against a picture of red dots.
(ii) False affirmative sentences: subjects had to evaluate a sentence as "It is true that the dots are red" against a picture of black dots.
(iii) True negative sentences: subjects had to evaluate a sentence as "It is not true that the dots are red" against a picture of black dots.
(iv) False negative sentences: subjects had to evaluate a sentence as "It is not true that the dots are red" against a picture of red dots.

The results reported both an effect of negation, with negative sentences being more difficult than affirmative sentences, and an effect of truth. True affirmative sentences, in fact, were evaluated faster than false affirmatives and false negatives were evaluated faster than true negatives. As in the experiment administered by Wason (1961), true negative sentences appeared to be the hardest to process. Moreover, the fact that the two experiments yielded similar results indicates that internal and external negations are processed in the same way.

3.2. *First solutions: Wason's "context of plausible denial" and the pragmatic theory of negation*

Different proposals have been developed to explain the reason why negative statements were processed less accurately and more slowly than positive statements. A first tentative explanation is that negative sentences are more difficult because they are phonologically longer than positive sentences, as they contain an extra-syllable, i.e. the negation operator. However, this hypothesis has been filtered out by Clark and Chase (1972), who estimated that the time needed to process an extra-syllable was significantly lower than the time needed to process negation in comparison to affirmation. Moreover, negatives were harder even in those experiments in which length was controlled and both affirmative and negative sentences had the same number of syllables (Just and Carpenter 1971).

Another hypothesis focused on the higher syntactic complexity of negative statements, which were expected to involve a greater number of grammatical transformations. However, this hypothesis has not been confirmed directly and it has been considered implausible both for theoretical and empirical reasons (Partee 1970; Gough 1965).

A further approach considered the psychological dimension of negation, arguing that positively presented information is more valuable, whereas negative concepts have an unpleasant connotation, since they are generally associated with the concept of prohibition. Also this approach has been discarded.

The most persuading hypothesis about the processing of negation is the pragmatic one, claiming that negative sentences are particularly difficult to process when they are used in an unsupportive context. At the basis of this consideration there is Wason's (1965) proposal, known as the hypothesis of the "Context of plausible denial". Observing sentences like those reported below, Wason notes that (21) seems odder than (20).

(20) The whale is not a fish.
(21) The whale is not a bird.

Even though both statements are negative and share the same truth-value, (21) takes longer to be processed and seems less appropriate. Wason focuses precisely on this feeling of inappropriateness, noting that there is an association between the appropriateness of a negative sentence and the plausibility of its affirmative counterpart. In fact, it seems perfectly plausible to wonder whether a whale is a fish, whereas it would seem far more strange to wonder whether it is a bird.

According to Wason, (20) is pronounced in a supportive context, because there is an expectation to be denied (i.e. that the whale is a fish) or an exception to be noted (i.e. that the whale is a mammal). In this sense, negatives have the function to emphasize a fact that deviates from the expectations and therefore they depend on a prior state of affairs that has to be negated. It is unlikely that the sentence "It is not x" would be uttered unless there were good reasons to suppose that it might have been "x" or that someone thought it might" (Cornish and Wason 1970: 113). In this approach, then, the plausibility of a negative sentence is indissolubly connected to the presence of a prior statement that is to be denied. In other words, it is possible to say that negative statements presuppose the existence of an affirmative sentence that has to be denied.

A number of studies have provided results corroborating this hypothesis and showing that negation is processed more easily and more rapidly when it is used to negate a proposition previously introduced in the context and when its affirmative counterpart is plausible. Interestingly, this tendency has been shown also by two- three- and four- years old children, who appear to be aware of the pragmatic requirements of negative sentences (De Villiers and Flusberg 1975).

Summarizing, according to Wason the negative sentences tested in the experiment reviewed in the previous sections were more difficult to process than the affirmative sentences, since they were uttered in an unsupportive and infelicitous context.

It seems, then, that negative sentences *presuppose* the existence of a prior statement presenting a state of affairs that must be corrected. In those cases where there is no previous statement (e.g. "Eric didn't eat fish at the restaurant" uttered out of the blue), the presupposition is disregarded and the sentence turns to be infelicitous sounding inappropriate. Hence, to understand these sentences, comprehenders must accommodate the presupposition and reconstruct a supportive context on their own (e.g. "Eric was supposed to eat fish at the restaurant"). Similarly, the experiments by Wason (1959; 1961) and (Carpenter and Just 1975) presented sentences uttered out of the blue, without a supportive context: to comprehend them, hence, subjects were forced to construct their affirmative counterparts in order to accommodate the presupposition. Whence the longer response times.

Similarly, Givon (1978) argues that negative sentences require a particular pragmatic context within which they are processed to counter the presuppositions held by the listener. This view is shared also by Horn (1989), who claims that the prototypical use of negation is precisely to deny a previously asserted proposition.

Experimental data support this pragmatic hypothesis of negation. Glenberg et al. (1999), in particular, show that it is not always the case that negation is more difficult to process that affirmation. Indeed, they claim that negative sentences are as easy as their affirmative counterparts when they are presented in a supportive context. To test this hypothesis, they developed an experimental protocol measuring reading times of affirmative and negative statements presented in supporting and non-supporting contexts. An example of their experiment is reported below:

(22) Marcy needed a new couch for her family room.

a. Supportive context: She wasn't sure if a darkly colored couch would look the best or a lighter color. She finally picked one out and had it delivered to her home.

b. Non-supportive context: She wasn't sure what kind of material she wanted the couch to be made of. She finally picked one out and had it delivered to her home.
c. Target positive sentence: The couch was black. It looked very nice in her family room.
d. Target negative sentence: The couch wasn't black. That probably would have been too dark.

Results show that subjects processed negated sentences as easily as affirmative sentence when they occurred in a pragmatically supporting context, corroborating the pragmatic hypothesis of negation.

3.3. Carpenter and Just's Psycholinguistic Model of Sentence Verification

Leaving aside general discussions about the processing of negation, Carpenter and Just (1975) developed a model to explain the results obtained in their experiments which, as we have seen before, showed that false affirmatives take longer to verify than true affirmatives and that true negatives take longer than false negatives. To account for this asymmetry, they proposed a model of the verification process based on the notion of congruence. Their "Constituent Comparison Model" takes into consideration two kinds of *constituents*, whose congruence is to be checked:

(i) Inner proposition: it refers to what the sentence and the picture are about.
(ii) Polarity: it refers to the polarity of the picture, which is by definition always positive, and that of the sentence, which can be either affirmative or negative.

Following Gough (1965), Carpenter and Just noted that it is easier to compare two constituents when they are congruent. Consider first the "inner proposition" constituents: when there is a match between what is represented in a picture[2] (e.g. red dots) and what is stated in the sentence

2 Carpenter and Just argue that sentence and picture representations are represented in an abstract propositional format, so that they can be compared at an abstract level. Referring to the work by Chase and Clark (1972) and Clark and

(e.g. "It is true that the dots are red") the comparison process necessary to evaluate the sentence is facilitated. Conversely, when there is a mismatch (e.g. a picture of black dots and the statement "It is true that the dots are red") an extra time, called *falsification time*, is consumed. This extra-time is responsible for the longer latencies needed to evaluate false affirmatives in comparison to true affirmatives. Note that the same reasoning can be applied for negative sentences, where, however, the situation is upside down: the picture matches with the sentence in the false negative condition (e.g. "It is not true that the dots are red" against a picture of red dots), whereas there is a mismatch in the true negative condition (e.g. "It is not true that the dots are red" against a picture of black dots). The falsification time, then, determines the greater difficulty manifested in the processing of false affirmatives versus true affirmatives and of true negatives versus false negatives.

The same procedure applies when the congruence of the "polarity" constituents is checked: affirmative sentences, in fact, are predicted to be easier since there is a match between the polarity of the sentence and that of the picture. With negative sentences, instead, there is a mismatch, since the polarity of the sentence is negative.

To sum up, the number of mismatches entailed by each condition are reported below:

(i) True affirmative: sentence-picture match, polarity match (0 mismatches).
(ii) False affirmative: sentence-picture mismatch, polarity match (1 mismatch).
(iii) True negative: sentence-picture mismatch, polarity mismatch (2 mismatches).
(iv) False negative: sentence-picture match, polarity mismatch (1 mismatch).

As the reader may have noted, this proposal can account for the greatest processing difficulty required by true negatives, which involve two mismatches, but it cannot explain why false negatives are more difficult

Chase (1972), they claim in fact that there is a level of representation which is neither linguistic nor pictorial and which can represent information of both domains.

than false affirmatives, since they both entail only one mismatch. To solve this problem, Carpenter and Just are forced to introduce some stipulations:

(i) Inner propositions are to be compared obligatorily before polarity.
(ii) Whenever a mismatch is found, the entire process must be reinitialized.
(iii) When a mismatch is found, the two constituents are tagged so that when the process is reinitialized they will be treated as a match.
(iv) The mismatch that is found later in the comparison process, i.e. the polarity mismatch occurring with negative sentences, results in more recomparisons than a mismatch on earlier constituents, so that "the total latency is a function of both the number of mismatches and their locus in their respective representations" (Carpenter and Just 1975: 48)

Keeping in mind these assumptions, we can now verify how the Constituent Comparison Model works, following the flowchart predisposed by Just and Carpenter and reported below.

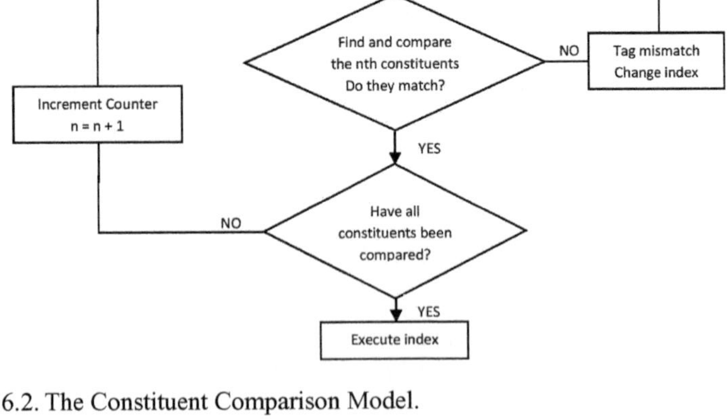

Figure 6.2. The Constituent Comparison Model.

Following these instructions, we can see how the model accounts for the processing required by each condition:

(i) True affirmative: sentence and pictures are represented in an abstract format, the response index is set to true. Since both the inner proposition and the polarity marker constituents match, the index can be executed "true", for a total of 2 comparisons.
(ii) False affirmative: since the inner proposition constituents mismatch, the constituents are tagged and the index is changed to false. The process must be reinitialized, the inner constituent are compared and they match. Since there is a "polarity" match, the index "false" can be executed, for a total of 3 comparisons.
(iii) False negative: there is an inner constituent match. However, since there is a polarity marker mismatch the index is changed to false and the entire process must be reinitialized with the inner constituent comparison and the polarity comparison. In the end, the index "false" is executed for a total of 4 comparisons.
(iv) True negative: there is an inner proposition constituent mismatch, which changes the response index to false. The process is reinitialized. There is a second mismatch regarding the polarity marker, the index is turned to true and the process is entirely restarted. Finally, the index "true" is executer for a total of 5 comparisons.

As we have shown, this model permits to account for the latencies found in the previous experiments. However, the major weakness of this model lies in its stipulative nature. Why, in fact, should it be necessary to restart entirely the process every time that there is a mismatch?

In the following section I will report the results of a number of experiments performed in the last decade and I will discuss a new hypothesis recently developed to account for the processing difficulty related to negation. Then, in the light of this new hypothesis, I will present an original model that I developed to explain the processing of negation in sentence-picture evaluation experiments.

3.4. *Negation and Accessibility*

In the previous section, we have seen that the first experimental studies performed on negation showed that negative sentences require higher processing costs to be interpreted in comparison to their affirmative counterparts. Moreover, we have argued, following Wason, Givon and Horn, that this difficulty may be due to the lack of an appropriate pragmatic context which can be used to reject the presupposition of the affirmative counterparts. More recent works on negation has focused, instead, on the accessibility of the concepts occurring under the scope of negation. MacDonald and Just (1989), in particular, developed an experiment protocol to test directly this issue. They asked participants to read sentences like (23) and, immediately after, they measured the accessibility of negated and non-negated concepts by means of a probe-recognition or a word-naming task.

(23) Almost every weekend, Mary bakes some bread but no cookies for the children.

Results were interesting, indicating that negated terms such as *cookies* were less accessible than non-negated terms, such as *bread*, as shown by longer recognition and naming latencies. To explain these results, MacDonald and Just argued that readers construct a propositional representation of the sentence in which the negation operator encapsulates the information occurring in its scope, reducing therefore its accessibility. Hence, negation is essentially seen as an accessibility reducing operator.

However, this view is challenged by Kaup et al. (1997), who demonstrated that it is not always the case that negated concepts are less accessible than non-negated concepts. In particular, they observed that another relevant variable determining the lower accessibility of negated terms is the presence of the entity in the described situation. In particular, they took into consideration two distinct kinds of sentences, involving respectively verbs of creation (e.g. to cook) and verbs of destruction (e.g. to destroy). To test the accessibility of creation passages they employed sentences similar to those proposed by MacDonald and Just, as in (23), whereas for destruction passages they used sentences such as (24):

(24) Elizabeth tidied up her drawers. She burned the old letters but not the photographs. Afterwards she cleaned up.

As in the experiment by MacDonald and Just, subjects had to read the target sentences and immediately after they were presented with a probe word, such as "bread" or "cookies" and "letters" or "photographs", and they were asked to decide whether that word was present in the text. Recognition times were then measured. Significantly, results showed that negated terms are less accessible than non-negated terms in creation passages, as demonstrated by MacDonald and Just; however, this tendency was not present in destruction passages. In this case, in fact, no accessibility difference was found between negated and non-negated concepts. The same results were replicated by Kaup (2001), opening the way to a radically new hypothesis about the processing of negation, proposed by Kaup, Lüdtke and Zwaan (2007) and known as the "Two-Step Simulation hypothesis".

3.5. *Kaup, Lüdtke and Zwaan (2007): The Two-Step Simulation Hypothesis*

The Two-Step Simulation Hypothesis rests upon the experiential view of language comprehension, claiming that comprehending a text involves the construction of a mental representation of the described state of affairs, the so-called *situation model* (also *mental model*; for a review, see Zwaan and Radvansky 1998). This hypothesis is supported by a large body of empirical evidence, suggesting that comprehenders mentally simulate the state of affair that is described in the utterances in a way that is similar to directly experiencing it. Neuroscience studies, indeed, have found a significant overlap between the mental subsystems involved in the representation of linguistically conveyed information and those used to perceive or enact the same situations (Pulvermüller 2002). Moreover, behavioral experiments have shown that nonlinguistic cognitive processes such as perception, action planning or imagery depend on the same mental subsystems involved in the creation of representations used for language comprehension (see Kaup et al. 2007 for a detailed review).

However, the existence of linguistic operators such as negation, poses a potential problem for this view, since they do not seem to have a direct equivalent in experience. Therefore, researchers tried to answer the question of how negative text information is represented.

First, it has been proposed that negated information is simply absent from the experiential representation of the state of affairs; however, this hypothesis has been discarded, considering examples as the following.

(25) Charles had been very lucky to get hold of tickets for a concert by the Berlin Philharmonic Orchestra for tonight. He was now sitting in the fifth row of the concert hall, from where he had a real good view of the stage. Finally, the musicians entered the hall. Charles knew that the concert would begin any minute now. Then, he suddenly realized that the conductor was not present (Kaup et al. 2007: 266).

In this case, the presence of the conductor is explicitly negated and thus the simulation of the situation should not contain a representation of the conductor. However, if it were the case, the comprehender would not be able to understand what the text is about or, more specifically, "whether the text specified the conductor as being absent, or whether there just had not been any information regarding the conductor" (ibid).

In other cases, however, the representation of a negated entity can be obtained representing its affirmative counterpart: when simulating a sentence like (26), for instance, the comprehender would represent a turned-on television.

(26) When she entered the room, Lisa noticed that the television was not off.

To solve this impasse, Kaup and colleagues resorted to an idea very similar to the pragmatic considerations about negation proposed by Wason, Givòn and Horn, who argue that negative statements are generally uttered to deny a corresponding positive presupposition attributed to the listener.

Kaup et al., indeed, observed that negation seems to be used to communicate to the listener a deviation from her expectations. For instance, (26) can be uttered felicitously only in a context in which the television should have been turned off, i.e. where its being turned off was presupposed. Intuitively, thus, it seems that negation invites to delete a previously built expected state of affairs (e.g. the television being turned off), replacing it with the representation of the actual state of affairs (e.g. the television being turned on). Comparing these two simulations allows the comprehender to determine what the sentence is about.

According to the Two-Step Simulation Hypothesis, then, the comprehension of negation involves (i) the retrieval (or the construction, e.g. in unsupportive contexts) of a simulation of the expected state of affairs, which corresponds to the state of affairs that is being negated in the sentence and (ii) the construction of a simulation of the actual state of affairs.

Two cases can be distinguished: when the negated state of affairs is already present in the discourse representation before encountering negation, the comprehender must simply correct the expectation by simulating the actual state of affairs. Conversely, when the negated state of affairs is not present in the discourse context, e.g. when the sentence is uttered out of the blue, the comprehender must construct a mental simulation of the expected state of affairs and then turn towards the representation of the actual state of affairs.

Importantly, then, this hypothesis permits also to explain why negation is more easily processed when it occurs in a felicitous, supporting context. Consider the following examples:

(27) a. Lisa finished late working. While she was driving home, she thought that her husband was preparing dinner. But when she arrived home, she realized that her husband was not there.
b. When she arrived home, Lisa realized that her husband was not there.

In (27a) the context informs the comprehender that Lisa's husband is expected to be at home preparing dinner. This information constitutes the simulation of the expected state of affairs: all the comprehender has to do to process the negative sentence "her husband was not at home", then, is to correct the expectation and to construct a mental simulation of the actual state of affairs, which deviates from the prior simulation, representing, for instance, an empty house.

Conversely, when (27b) is uttered out of context, an additional step is required: first, the comprehender has to create a mental simulation of the expected state of affairs, corresponding to the state of affairs that is being negated in the utterance (e.g. Lisa's husband at home). Secondly, she has to construct a mental simulation of the actual state of affairs. Consequently, the comprehension of a negative sentence uttered out of a non-supportive context is expected to be more difficult, since it requires to construct a simulation of the expected state of affairs, demanding higher processing resources.

Often, as Kaup and colleagues observed, it is not possible to infer precisely the actual state of affairs with respect to the dimension affected by negation. The utterance in (28), for instance, does not specify what Eric was doing at the moment.

(28) Eric was not preparing dinner.

In cases like this, the dimension of the negated property (i.e. what Eric is doing) remains unspecified. Only with complementary negation it is possible to infer the actual state of affairs with certainty; in (29), for instance, the comprehender can safely simulate a state of affairs in which Eric was sleeping.

(29) Eric was not awake.

To summarize, the Two-Steps Simulation Hypothesis claims that negation represents a deviation from a previous expectation and that it involves the comparison between the expected and the actual state of affairs.

To test this hypothesis, Kaup et al. (2007) conducted an experimental protocol that provided supporting results. Participants were presented with sentences with indefinite negation, such as (30), or definite negation, as (31):

(30) There was no eagle in the sky.
(31) The eagle was not in the sky.

Immediately after they were shown a picture and they were asked to indicate whether the depicted object had been mentioned in the target sentence. There were two experimental conditions: in both cases the object depicted in the picture presented after (30) or (31) was an eagle, and therefore the correct answer was always 'yes'. However, in the first condition the picture matched the shape of the object in the negated situation (e.g. an eagle with outstretched wings), whereas in another experiment condition there was a mismatch (e.g. an eagle with folded wings).

As predicted by the Two-Step Simulation Hypothesis, response times were faster when the picture matched the negated state of affairs. The same result was found in a further experiment testing sentences with definite negation as (31).

This result confirms that when processing a sentence like (31) subjects need to construct a mental simulation of an eagle flying in the sky, suggesting that the processing of a negative sentence and the processing of its affirmative counterpart trigger the same simulation. The only difference between the affirmative and the negative sentence lies in the fact that the latter also requires the subject to construct an additional simulation, causing its higher processing difficulty.

Moreover, in a further experiment, Kaup and colleagues show that the processing of a negative sentence triggers the simulation of the actual state of affairs as well, but only after the simulation of the expected state of affairs has been created. In this experiment, the authors tested negative sentences with contradictory predicates, as reported in (32), and prolonged the delay at which the picture was presented from 250 ms to 1500 ms.

(32) The umbrella was not open.

Results show that with a 750-ms delay response times were faster for affirmative sentences, but not for negative sentences, when the picture matched the actual state of affairs. Conversely, with a 1500-ms delay responses were faster when negative sentences, but not affirmative sentences, were followed by a picture that matched the actual state of affairs.

These data provide significant evidence that comprehending a sentence requires the simulation of the actual state of affairs, demonstrating also that the actual state of affairs is simulated only after the expected state of affairs has been represented. Note that this proposal can also account for the findings reported in the previous sections and showing a greater processing difficulty associated with negative sentences and, in particular, for the utterances presented without an appropriate supporting context. In this case, reaction times increase, since higher processing costs are required to construct the simulation of the expected state of affairs that is not provided by the context.

The Two-Step Simulation Hypothesis permits also to explain the reduced accessibility shown by negated concepts in creation but not in destruction passages (section 3.4). The target sentences are reported below for convenience:

(33) Almost every weekend, Mary bakes some bread but **no cookies** for the children.

(34) Elizabeth tidied up her drawers. She burned the old letters but **not the photographs**. Afterwards she cleaned up.

To comprehend (33) the subject has to construct a mental simulation of the expected state of affairs (e.g. Mary that bakes bread and cookies) and of the actual state of affairs (e.g. Mary that bakes only bread) and to compare them. The absence of the negated entity (e.g. cookies) in the actual situation leads to a lower response time in comparison to the non-negated entity (e.g. bread), indicating that the negated concept is less accessible.

Conversely, to comprehend (34) the subject simulates the expected state of affairs (e.g. Elizabeth's drawers where there are neither letters nor photographs) and the actual state of affairs (e.g. Elizabeth's drawers where there are only photographs). In this case there is no reduced accessibility since the entity mentioned under the scope of negation is present in the simulation of the actual state of affairs.

Finally, the Two-Step Simulation Hypothesis can account for the different latencies found in sentence-picture verification tasks, arguing that responses are faster when the picture matches the negated state of affairs.

In the following section, I will present a model of sentence-picture verification that permits to account for the experimental findings by Gough and Carpenter and Just in the light of the proposal made by the Two-Step Simulation Hypothesis.

3.6. *An original proposal to account for the processing of negation in sentence-picture verification tasks: The Model of Sentence-Picture Match Processing for Negative Sentences*

As agreed above, Carpenter and Just's model of verification has a too stipulative nature. In the light of what proposed by the Two-Step Simulation Hypothesis, I will propose a model that can account for the greater processing difficulties of (i) negative sentences in comparison to affirmative sentences, (ii) false affirmatives in comparison to true affirmatives and (iii) true negatives in comparison to false negatives.

In the model that I am proposing, the Model of Sentence-Picture Match Processing for Negative Sentences, it is possible to capture the greater processing difficulty imposed by negative sentences, referring to the Two-Steps Simulation Hypothesis. Since the sentences presented in the experimental protocols that we have considered are uttered out of a specific supporting context, I propose that subjects must create a mental simulation of the expected state of affairs and compare it to the simulation of the actual state of affairs. An operation which is remarkably demanding in terms of working memory resources and which is responsible for the fact that negative sentences are more difficult to interpret than their affirmative counterparts.

Moreover, in sentence-picture verification tasks subjects have to cope with an additional difficulty: they have to compare the representation of a sentence to that of a picture in order to decide if the sentence describes correctly what happens in the picture. I propose that the picture provided in the experiment can be used to create the mental simulation: if the picture does not provide the subject with a representation of what the sentence is about (e.g. "It is not true that the dots are black" against a picture of red dots), the subject has to correct this mismatch, creating a representation of the sentence which can be compared against the picture (e.g. a representation of black dots). When the picture and the sentence match, instead, the subject's task is facilitated. This difference can explain the longer latencies reported for false affirmatives in comparison to true affirmatives and for true negatives in comparison to false negatives. In fact, in the "false affirmative" condition as well as in the "true negative" condition there is a mismatch between the sentence and the picture that is responsible for their higher complexity.

According to the Model of Sentence-Picture Match Processing for Negative Sentences, three main steps are required to evaluate target sentences against pictures:

(i) Sentence-Polarity Processing: the subject has to process sentence polarity. If the polarity is positive, she can represent the actual state of affairs; if it is negative, instead, she has to simulate first the expected state of affairs and then the actual state of affairs. Arguably, then, negative sentences are predicted to be more difficult than affirmative sentences, since they require the construction of two different representations, in accordance with the Two-Step Simulation Hypothesis.

(ii) Simulation of the Asserted[3] State of Affairs: after polarity has been processed, the subject has to create the representation of the asserted state of affairs. When possible, the subject can resort to the picture to simulate the state of affairs. Otherwise, if the picture does not match with the event described in the target sentence, an additional step is required, since the subject needs to build the simulation by herself. Consequently, the prediction is that a greater effort is required when the subject cannot resort to the picture in order to represent the state of affairs.

(iii) Sentence-Picture Match Processing: in the final passage, the subject has to verify if the picture and the representation of the asserted state of affairs are mutually consistent. If they are, she can answer "true", otherwise, she will answer "false".

The model of verification for negative sentences that I am proposing is reported below.

3 I prefer to use the term "asserted" state of affairs instead of "actual" state of affair to avoid ambiguities between the state of affairs described by the sentence and the one depicted in the picture.

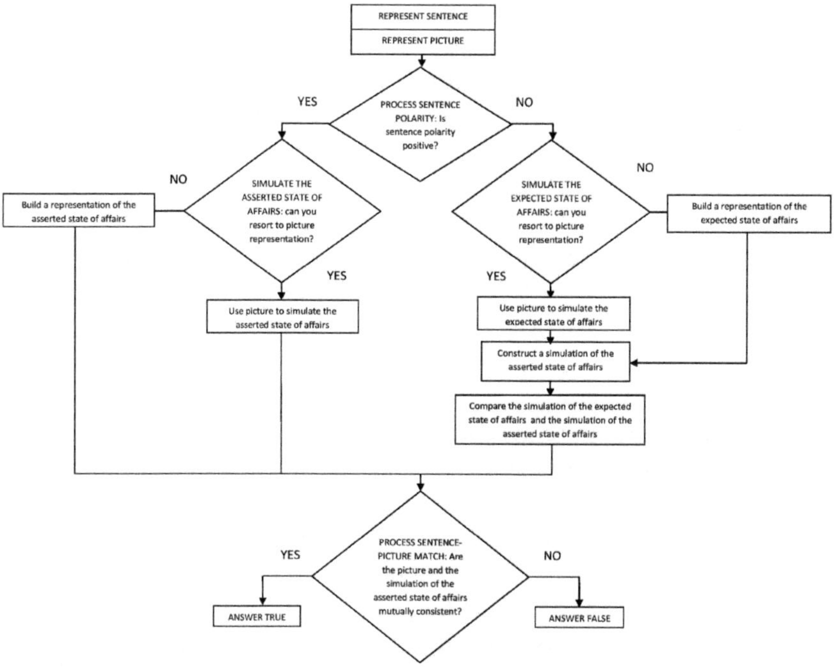

Figure 6.3. The Model of Sentence-Picture Match Processing for Negative Sentences.

Let us see how this model works, examining each condition. Suppose that the subject is presented with a picture depicting Cinderella who is combing her hair, like the one reported below, and afterwards with the target sentence.

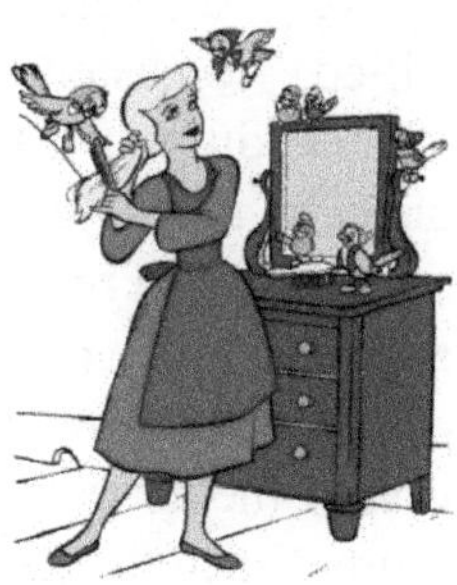

Figure 6.4. Cinderella combing her hair.

(i) True affirmative sentence: the target sentence is "**Cinderella is combing her hair**". According to the model, the subject has first to consider sentence polarity. Since it is positive, she can move to the second step, concerning the simulation of the asserted state of affairs. In this case, the picture provides the subject with a representation of what the sentence is about, namely Cinderella who is combing her hair. Therefore, the subject can use it as a source of help to simulate the asserted state of affairs. Finally, she has to compare the picture and the simulation: given that they are mutually consistent, she can answer "true".

(ii) False affirmative sentence: the target sentence is "**Cinderella is cleaning the house**". Again, sentence polarity is positive and the subject needs to represent the asserted state of affairs. In this case, however, the picture does not help the subject to build a representation of what the sentence is about and the subject must construct a mental representation of Cinderella cleaning the house. Arguably, this causes an extra-effort that may be taken as responsible for the longer latencies required by false affirmatives in comparison to true affirmatives. At last, the subject has to match the picture and the simulation of the asserted state of affairs: since they are not mutually consistent, she answers "false".

(iii) False negative sentence: the target sentence is "**Cinderella is not combing her hair**". In this case, polarity is negative and thus the subject has to simulate first the expected state of affairs (e.g. Cinderella who is combing her hair) and afterwards the asserted state of affairs (e.g. Cinderella who is doing something else, possibly unspecified), consistently with the Two-Step Simulation Hypothesis. This additional passage results in the higher processing load required by negative sentences in comparison to affirmative sentences. In order to represent the expected state of affairs, the subject can resort to the picture, since it actually offers a representation of what the sentence is about. Finally, she has to compare the simulation of the actual state of affairs with the representation in the picture. Since they are not mutually consistent, the sentence is judged false.

(iv) True negative sentence: the target sentence is "**Cinderella is not cleaning the house**". Also in this case, the polarity of the sentence is negative, requiring the simulation of both the expected state of affairs (e.g. Cinderella who is cleaning the house) and the asserted state of affairs (e.g. Cinderella who is doing something else, possibly unspecified). However, the subject cannot resort to the picture to create the two representations, but she has to mentally simulate them. Finally, since the simulation of the asserted state of affairs and picture representation are mutually consistent, the target sentence is judged true.

Summarizing, the greatest difficulty found in the processing of negative true sentences is due to two distinct factors: firstly, to the negative polarity of the sentence, requiring the subject to construct and compare two representations, and secondly to the impossibility for the subject to use the picture as a source of help in order to generate the simulation of the state of affairs at stake. This second factor is responsible for the longer latencies found with negative true sentences in comparison to negative false sentences.

In conclusion, this model of verification can account for the greater difficulty found with negative sentences in comparison to affirmative sentences, assuming that subjects are forced to simulate two representations when processing a negative sentence, both for the expected and the actual state of affairs. It can also account for the higher complexity of false affirmatives in comparison to true affirmatives and of true negatives in comparison to false negatives, arguing that false affirmatives and true negatives require the subject to create *ex novo* a representation of what the sentence is about, without using the picture representation as a source of help.

4. Experimental Protocol

In this section I will present and discuss the results of an experimental protocol that I administered to test how dyslexic children compute negative sentences in sentence-picture verification tasks in comparison to age-matched typically developing children. The experimental protocol comprised two different tasks, testing respectively the computation of negative sentence (Exp. 1) and the computation of negative passive sentences (Exp. 2).

As we will see throughout the discussion, dyslexic children manifested greater difficulties in comparison to control children in all tasks, as demonstrated by higher error rates and slower response times. To interpret these results, I adopt the framework outlined by Kaup et al. (2007), according to which negation conveys a deviation from expectancies. Specifically, negation invites the comprehender to retrieve, or, if necessary, to build a simulation of the expected state of affairs, which has the role to represent the affirmative counterpart of the negative sentence. Arguably, this operation is remarkably expensive in terms of processing resources. Therefore, assuming that dyslexic children display a working memory limitation, they are expected to underperform in comparison to control children.

4.1. Participants

The experiment was conducted on a group of dyslexic children and a group of age-matched typically developing control children.

The group of Dyslexic children (DC) included 17 children (11 males), all native speakers of Italian. At the moment of testing, the group mean age was 9 years and 8 months (SD = 0;11). All children have been chosen from those who had independently received a diagnosis of dyslexia, specifically by the "Servizio di Neuropsichiatria Infantile" in Rovereto (TN): in particular, dyslexic children were selected according to different factors: (i) absence of neurological diseases or genetic pathologies, (ii) absence of sensorial diseases, (iii) absence of psychopathological diseases, (iv) IQ > 80 (WISC – R) and (v) fluent and correct reading and writing abilities under 2 SD (Tressoldi et al. Battery, Prove MT).

The group of age-matched control children (AMCC) was composed by 17 primary school children (4 males), all native speakers of Italian. At the moment of testing, the group mean age was 9 years and 8 months (SD = 1;5). Children were selected from those who had no history of reading problems or language disorders. The main features of the two groups are reported in Table 6.3.

Table 6.3. Group data of the subjects who took part in Exp. 1.

Group	Number	Mean Age (SD)
DC	17	9;8 (1;5)
AMCC	17	9;8 (0;11)

4.2. *Design and Procedure*

4.2.1. *Experiment 1: The interpretation of negative sentences*

A sentence-picture verification task was administered. As in Carpenter and Just (1975), subjects were presented with a picture depicting a situation. The experimenter introduced them with a puppet, Little Red Riding Hood, who had the task to explain what was happening in the picture. The subject was told that Little Red Riding Hood was not always able to describe correctly what was happening in the story. Therefore, the subject's task was to decide if Little Red Riding Hood described the picture correctly or not by pressing a smiling face for the right answer and a crying face for the wrong answer.

The task involved 12 experimental items, intertwined with 6 fillers. There were four experimental conditions, an example of each is reported below:

(i) Condition A: True Negative Sentence with Internal Negation (NT). The subject had to compare a sentence such as ***"La gallina non sta facendo la spesa"*** **('The hen is not going shopping')** against the picture of the hen that is reading the newspaper.

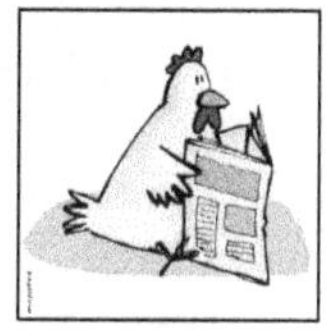

(ii) Condition B: False Negative Sentence with Internal Negation (NF). The subject had to compare the sentence ***"Il bambino non sta andando in bicicletta"*** **('The boy is not riding the bicycle')** against the picture of a boy who is riding the bicycle, as reported here.

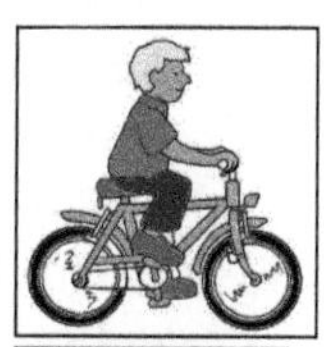

(iii) Condition C: True Negative Sentence with External Negation (ENT). The subject had to compare the sentence ***"Non è vero che Biancaneve sta litigando con un nano"*** **('It is not true that Snowhite is quarrelling with a dwarf')** against a picture depicting Snowhite who is dancing with a dwarf.

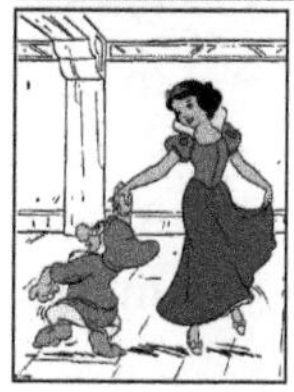

(iv) Condition D: False Negative Sentence with External Negation (ENF). The subject had to compare a sentence like ***"Non è vero che il toro sta rompendo una roccia"*** **('It is not true that the bull is breaking the rock')** against a picture depicting the bull which is indeed breaking the rock.

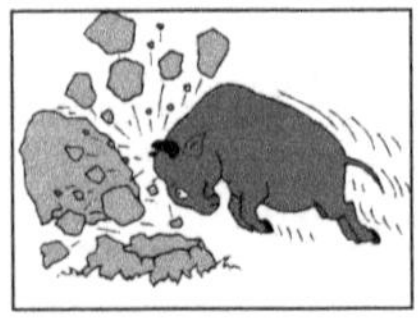

4.2.2. Experiment 2 – The interpretation of passive negative sentences

The experimental task was performed to test the computation of passive negative sentences. Both internal negation and external negation have been tested. As in Experiment 1, a sentence-picture verification task has been administered. The subject was shown a picture portraying two characters performing an action. For clarity, the experimenter described the picture telling the subject what exactly happened in the story. Then, he introduced the subject with a puppet, Little Red Riding Hood, who had the task to explain what was happening in the picture. The subject's task was to decide if Little Red Riding Hood described the picture correctly or not by pressing a smiling face for the right answer and a crying face for the wrong answer. The task involved 12 experimental items, intertwined with 6 fillers. Both sentences with internal negation and external negation were tested. There were four experimental conditions, with three experimental items for each condition:

(i) Condition A: True Negative Passive Sentence with Internal Negation (NPT). The subject had to compare a sentence such as ***"Trilli non è baciata da Peter Pan"*** **('Tinker Bell is not kissed by Peter Pan')** against the picture of Tinker Bell who kisses Peter Pan.

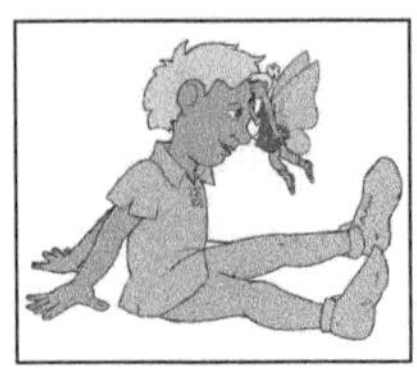

(ii) Condition B: False Negative Passive Sentence with Internal Negation (NPF). The subject had to compare the sentence ***"Gatto Silvestro non è colpito da Titti"*** **('Sylvester is not hit by Tweety')** against the picture of Tweety who is hitting Sylvester.

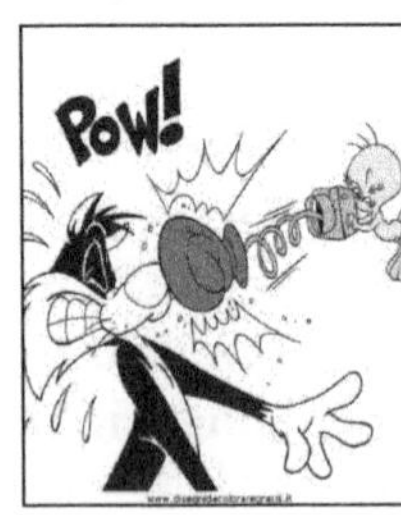

(iii) Condition C: True Negative Passive Sentence with External Negation (ENPT). The subject had to compare the sentence ***"Non è vero che il cerbiatto è seguito dal coniglio"* ('It is not true that the fawn is followed by the rabbit')** against a picture depicting the fawn following the rabbit.

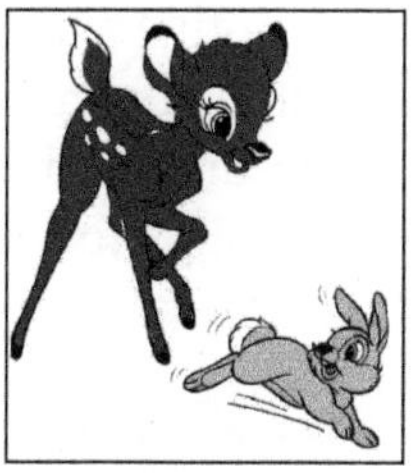

(iv) Condition D: False Negative Passive Sentence with External Negation (ENPF). The subject had to compare a sentence like ***"Non è vero che la bambina è pettinata dalla mamma"* ('It is not true that the girl is combed by her mother')** against a picture depicting the mother combing the girl's hair.

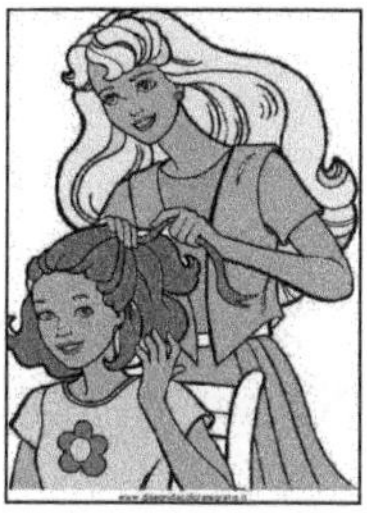

4.3. Results

4.3.1. Results of Experiment 1

All subjects were able to complete the test and to respond correctly to the vast majority of the fillers; therefore, nobody was excluded from the sample.

To exclude a yes-bias, the first measure collected is the overall number of "true" answers, as reported in Table 6.4. As shown by the data, neither DC nor AMCC manifested a tendency to provide "true" answer; conversely, both groups provided more "false" answers than "true" answers, arguably due to the greater difficulties of Condition NT and ENT.

Table 6.4. Number of true answers given by the children in Exp. 1.

Group	**True Answers**		
	Total Number	Out of	Mean (SD)
DC	88	204	.373
AMCC	101	204	.495

Descriptive statistics of the error rates displayed by the two groups of children are reported in Table 6.5, reporting the number of observations, the mean and the standard deviation of the error rates displayed by the two groups for each of the four experimental conditions. In Graph 6.1. the error rates displayed by the two groups of children are reported.

Table 6.5. Descriptive statistics of Exp. 1.

	Group	N	Mean	Std. Deviation
NT	DC	17	0.49	0.41
	AMCC	17	0.05	0.12
NF	DC	17	0.19	0.26
	AMCC	17	0.00	0.00
ENT	DC	17	0.39	0.33
	AMCC	17	0.05	0.12
ENF	DC	17	0.35	0.39
	AMCC	17	0.09	0.19

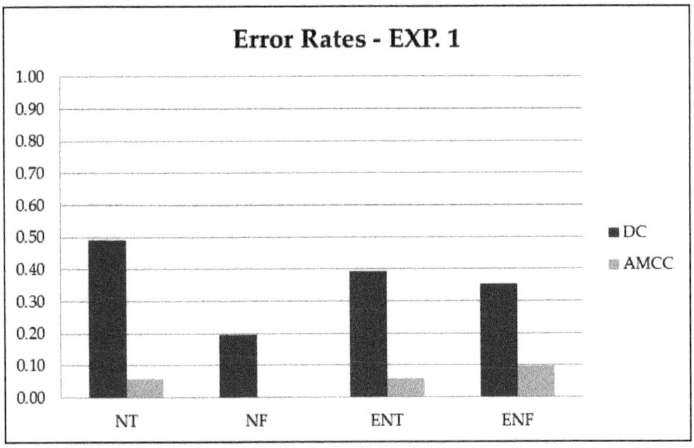

Graph. 6.1. Mean Error Rates of the two groups in Exp. 1.

Based on Graph 6.1, it is clear that dyslexics commit far more errors in comparison to control children. Specifically, it seems that NT is the most difficult condition for dyslexic children, followed by ENT (39,22%). The "false" conditions, instead, turns out to be easier, even though the error rate is still quite high.

A statistical analysis has been conducted on these data, to determine if there were statistically significant differences between the performances shown by the two groups of children. A 2 x 2 x 2 mixed design ANOVA was conducted. *Group* (DC; AMCC) was the between subject variable. *Type of negation* (internal; external) was the first within subject variable, considering subjects' performance in sentences constructed with internal negation and with external negation (comparing Conditions NT and NF to Conditions ENT and ENF). *Truth* was the second within subject variable, comparing true sentences to false sentences (Conditions NT and ENT to Condition NF and ENF).

There is a highly significant *Group* effect, $F(1, 32) = 16.910$, $p < .001$, partial $\eta^2 = .346$) indicating that dyslexic children perform significantly worse than control children. The *Type of Negation* variable is not significant, $F(1, 32) = 1.884$, $p = .179$, partial $\eta^2 = .056$, demonstrating that the form of negation (internal vs. external) does not affect the performance. Moreover, there is no significant *Type of Negation – Group interaction*, $F(1, 32) = .116$, $p = .736$, partial $\eta^2 = .004$, showing that the type of negation is significant neither for DC nor for AMCC.

The *Truth* variable, instead, is significant, $F(1, 32) = 5.308$, $p < .05$, partial $\eta^2 = .142$, even though the significant *Truth – Group* interaction, $F(1, 32) = 4.232$, $p < .05$, partial $\eta^2 = .117$, indicates that this variable is significant only for DC. This effect indicates that true sentences are more difficult to process than false sentences only for dyslexic children.

In sum, data show clearly that dyslexic children perform more poorly than age-matched typically developing children when asked to interpret negative sentences, displaying a significantly higher error rate. These results are consistent with the Two-Step Simulation Hypothesis, assuming that negation generally expresses a deviation from a prior expectation. In this perspective, what renders negative sentences more difficult to process in comparison to affirmative sentences is the need to retrieve or build a simulation for the expected state of affairs and a simulation for the asserted state of affairs. In this experiment, the task is further complicated by the request to verify the target sentence against a picture. As predicted by the Model of Sentence-Picture Match Processing for Negation outlined above, negative true sentences are more difficult to process than false sentences, as shown by a significantly higher error rate. This is due to the fact that in the "true" conditions (NT and ENT) the picture does not provide the comprehender with a representation of the event described in the sentence. Therefore, the subject must create *ex-novo* a mental representation of the sentence to be compared against the picture. This operation is arguably expensive in terms of processing resources and it contributes to make negative true sentences more difficult to interpret than negative false sentences. However, the statistical analysis has also revealed that this operation has a visible cost only for dyslexic children: we can argue that the absence of this effect for control children is due to their more efficient working memory, which allows them to accomplish the task effortlessly. On the contrary, dyslexic children poor working memory is not able to cope with the tasks, resulting in higher error rates.

Finally, results show that performance is not affected by the type of negation, i.e. whether it is internal or external. This result is consistent with the Two-Step Simulation Hypothesis, since it claims that negation is generally more difficult than affirmation for pragmatic and not for structural reasons.

4.3.2. Results of Experiment 2

All subjects were able to complete the test and to respond correctly to the vast majority of the fillers; therefore, nobody was excluded from the sample. To exclude a yes-bias, the first measure collected is the overall number of "true" answers, as reported in Table 6.7. As shown by the data, neither DC nor AMCC manifested a tendency to give true answer; conversely, both groups gave more "false" answers than "true" answers, arguably due to the greater difficulties of Condition NT and ENT.

Table 6.6. Number of true answers given by the children in Exp. 1.

Group	**True Answers**		
	Total Number	Out of	Mean (SD)
DC	76	204	.372
AMCC	89	204	.436

Descriptive statistics for the error rates reported by the two groups are displayed in Table 6.7, reporting the number of observations, the mean and the standard deviation of the error rates displayed by the two groups for each of the four experimental conditions. The error rates shown by the two groups of children are reported in Graph 6.2.

Table 6.7. Descriptive statistics of Exp. 1.

	Group	N	Mean	Std. Deviation
NPT	DC	17	0.48	0.41
	AMCC	17	0.11	0.12
NPF	DC	17	0.11	0.26
	AMCC	17	0.00	0.00
ENPT	DC	17	0.45	0.38
	AMCC	17	0.20	0.29
ENPF	DC	17	0.24	0.34
	AMCC	17	0.09	0.20

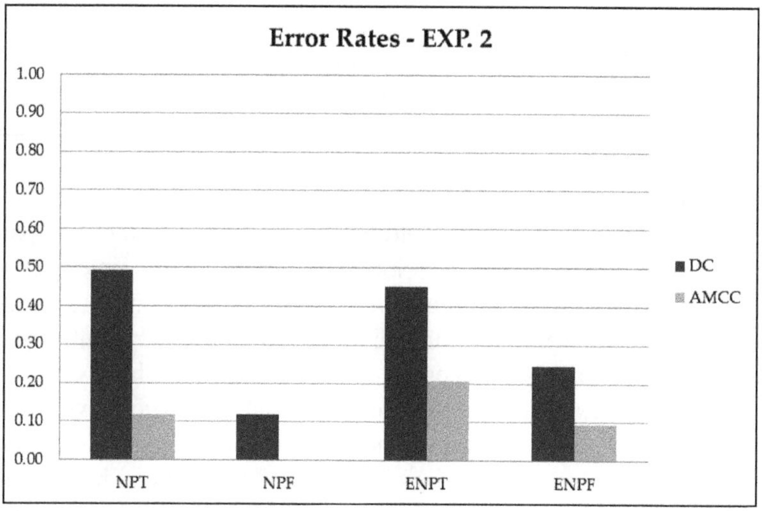

Graph. 6.2. Mean Error Rates of the two groups in Exp. 2.

As in Exp. 1, it is clear that dyslexic commit more errors in comparison to control children. Specifically, it seems that NPT is the most difficult condition for dyslexic children ENPT, whereas the "false" conditions turns out to be easier, even though the error rates are higher with respect to those shown by their peers.

A statistical analysis has been conducted on these data, to determine if there were statistically significant differences between the performances shown by the two groups of children. A 2 x 2 x 2 mixed design ANOVA was conducted. *Group* (DC; AMCC) was the between-subject variable. *Type of negation* (internal; external) was the first within subject variable, in order to check if the type of negation affected performance (comparing Conditions NPT and NPF with Conditions ENPT and ENPF). *Truth* was the second within subject variable, comparing true sentences with false sentences (Conditions NPT and ENPT with Conditions NPF and ENPF). There is a highly significant *Group* effect, $F(1, 32) = 19.761$, $p < .001$, partial $\eta^2 = .382$ indicating that dyslexic children perform significantly worse than control children. As in Experiment 1, the *Type of Negation* variable is not significant, $F(1, 32) = 2.721$, $p = .109$, partial $\eta^2 = .078$, demonstrating that the form of negation (internal vs. internal) has no influence on the performance. Moreover, there is no significant *Type of Negation – Group interaction*, $F(1, 32) = .318$, $p = .577$, partial $\eta^2 = .010$ showing that the type of negation is not significant either for DC or for AMCC. The *Truth* variable, instead, is significant, $F(1,32)=11.117$, $p<.01$. Furthermore, in this case there is a non-significant *Truth – Group* interaction, $F(1, 32) = 2.206$, $p = .147$ partial $\eta^2 = .064$, indicating that this variable is significant for both groups.

Summarizing, dyslexic children are significantly more impaired than age-matched typically developing children in the interpretation of negative passive sentences, as confirmed by higher error rates in all conditions. The interpretation of true sentences is more difficult than the interpretation of false sentences, as shown by the very high error rates exhibited by dyslexics and by the statistical analysis, which revealed that the *Truth* variable affects not only the performance of dyslexic children, as in Exp. 1, but also that of control children. This fact can be explained by acknowledging the higher complexity of the sentences used in Exp. 2, which also involve the processing of the passive construction. Arguably, then, we can claim that the greater processing difficulty associated with true sentences is determined by the higher amount of working memory resources required for the interpretation of passive sentences.

Finally, results show that also in this case the type of negative construction (internal vs. external) does not influence performance.

4.4. General Discussion

This experimental protocol was designed to test how dyslexic children interpret negative sentences in comparison to age-matched typically developing children. The protocol comprised two different experiments, testing respectively the computation of negative sentences (Exp. 1) and the computation of negative passive sentences (Exp. 2). The method used in both experiments was a sentence-picture verification task, in which subjects were asked to evaluate the sentences uttered by a puppet that had the task to describe what was represented in a picture.

In Exp. 1, in particular, dyslexics displayed a poorer performance in comparison to controls in all conditions, namely when asked to interpret true and false sentences with internal negation (Condition A and B), and true and false sentences with external negation (Conditions C and D). True sentences were significantly more difficult than false sentences for dyslexic children, whereas the type of negation (internal vs. external negation) did not affect the performance.

Similar results have been obtained in Exp. 2, which tested the interpretation of negative passive sentences. Also in this case dyslexics significantly manifested more difficulties than controls in all conditions, i.e. in true and false passive sentences with internal negation (Conditions A and B) and external negation (Conditions C and D), as shown by higher error rates. In this experiment, the truth of the target sentences affected the performance of both groups of subjects, whereas the type of negation had no impact. This fact can be considered as a consequence of the higher complexity of the task due to the presence of a passive construction.

In order to interpret these results, I adopt the framework of the Two-Step Simulation Hypothesis developed by Kaup, Zwaan and Lüdtke, claiming that negation is implicitly encoded in the sequencing of two distinct mental simulations, namely the simulation of the expected state of affairs, representing the affirmative counterpart of the negative sentence, and the simulation of the actual state of affairs, representing the negative sentence. This operation is arguably costly and imposes a great burden of Working Memory.

To explain the greatest difficulty reported in "true" conditions in comparison to "false" conditions, I refer to the Model of Sentence-Picture Match Processing for Negative Sentences. According to this model, when the picture does not provide the subject with a representation of what the sentence is about, she has to correct this mismatch, creating a representation of the sentence that can be compared against the picture. This is the case for negative true sentences, which were indeed more difficult to interpret, as indicated by higher error rates. Conversely, when the picture and the sentence matched, as in the "false" conditions, the subject's task was facilitated.

To sum up, the results of this experimental protocol show that dyslexic children are significantly more impaired than age-matched typically developing children when they are asked to interpret negative sentences. Their difficulty is due the fact that negative sentences are remarkably demanding in terms of processing resources and that their working memory is not efficient enough to cope with this task, as predicted by the Phonological and Executive Working Memory Deficit Hypothesis.

5. Summary and Conclusions

In this chapter I have provided further support to the Phonological and Executive Working Memory Deficit Hypothesis, showing that dyslexic children are remarkably more impaired than age-matched typically developing children in the interpretation of negation.

Throughout the discussion, in fact, we have observed that the interpretation of negative sentences constitutes a demanding task in terms of processing resources, as predicted by the Two-Step Simulation Hypothesis proposed by Kaup and colleagues (2007). According to this hypothesis, a negative sentence always requires the presence of its affirmative counterpart, which is then negated; this affirmative proposition can either be already present in the discourse contexts, or it must be constructed by the comprehender. Therefore, whenever she has to interpret a negative sentence, the comprehender is forced to retrieve or create its affirmative counterpart: she must construct two mental simulations, the one for the actual state of affairs and the other for the expected state of affairs, and compare them. As we have observed, this operation is very expensive in terms of memory and processing resources.

Adopting this perspective, the experimental protocol that I have presented in this section aimed at verifying how dyslexics performed in this kind of task with respect to controls, remembering that the Phonological and Executive Working Memory Deficit Hypothesis presented in Chapter 4 predicts that dyslexics underperform in demanding tasks due to their limited WM capacity. Consistently with this hypothesis, results confirmed that dyslexics actually performed worse than controls.

Chapter 7

The Interpretation of Pronominal Expressions in Developmental Dyslexia

1. Introduction

In this chapter I will present and discuss the results of an experimental protocol that I developed and administered to test how dyslexic children interpret anaphoric referential expressions. For what concerns the retrieval of the correct antecedent of a referential expression I adopt the framework of Accessibility Theory (Ariel 1991), according to which anaphoric expressions are accessibility markers ordered in a precise hierarchy. Their position in the scale informs the hearer about the accessibility degree of the referent, guiding her in the selection of the appropriate antecedent.

I will concentrate the discussion on the differences between zero pronouns, i.e. pronouns which are not phonetically realized and which are commonly used in *pro-drop* languages like Italian, and overt pronouns, which instead are pronounced. Specifically, zero pronouns occupy the highest position in Ariel's Accessibility Marking Scale, whereas phonetically realized pronouns are lower in the hierarchy. Capitalizing on Ariel's theory, I will propose an original hypothesis about the processing costs required for the interpretation of both types of pronouns. I will argue that the interpretation of anaphoric expressions is always demanding in terms of processing resources, but that the assignment of reference to realized pronouns is even more complex, since it involves the computation of an implicature. Given that, as discussed in Chapter 5, calculating an implicature imposes a great burden on Working Memory, I propose that the interpretation of overt pronouns is more difficult than the computation of zero pronouns.

As a consequence, testing anaphora resolution in dyslexic children provides substantial support to the hypothesis that they suffer from

WM deficiencies. To address this topic, I developed an experimental protocol with the aim of determining how dyslexics interpret zero pronouns and phonetically realized pronouns in comparison to age-matched typically developing children, control adults and two groups of younger children, the first attending the first class of the primary school and the second composed by preschoolers. The experimental protocol comprised a truth value judgment task with four conditions, testing the comprehension of zero pronouns and realized pronouns in both true and false sentences. In line with the predictions, results show that dyslexic children dramatically underperformed in comparison to age-matched controls, who instead exhibited an adult behavior, and even in comparison to first-class children, two years younger than them. Interestingly, instead, dyslexics' performance was similar to that shown by preschool children, more than 4 years younger than them. These data provide thus further and strong support in favor of the Phonological and Executive Working Memory Deficit Hypothesis.

2. The interpretation of referential expressions in the Accessibility Theory

As already stated in Chapter 1, anaphors, pronouns and referential expressions are expressions used to identify an individual or an object in a certain domain of interpretation. Imagine a situation in which a professor wants to tell his colleagues that a student wearing a red dress, Lisa, managed to solve a difficult problem. The professor can choose between different kinds of utterances to convey this information, opting, for instance, for one of the sentences below:

(1) She solved the problem.
(2) Lisa solved the problem.
(3) The student solved the problem.
(4) A student solved the problem.
(5) The student with the red dress solved the problem.

As the reader may have noted, all of these sentences could well suit the professor's communicative intention, but they would not be appropriate in every context. If, for instance, his colleagues do not know Lisa and are looking at a group of students in which the girl with the red dress can be easily identified, he can utter (5). If, instead, they already know the name of the student, he can choose (2). Or, again, if they were just talking about that student, he can simply utter (1).

However, what precisely guides the speaker to choose one expression instead of the other? A similar question arises regarding the interpretation of pronouns and referential expressions, which have to be assigned a correct antecedent in order to receive an interpretation. Consider the couple of sentences below:

(6) Frank explained the theory and then he left.
(7) Frank explained the theory and then x left, where x = Frank.

The sentence in (6) receives the interpretation in (7), where the pronoun *he* is interpreted as a variable that is assigned the same value as the subject of the sentence, i.e. Frank, which is its antecedent.[1] However, the situation can be made more complex by the presence of more than one possible antecedent for the referential expression. Take for instance the Italian sentence in (8):

(8) Il professore$_i$ ha spiegato la teoria allo studente$_j$ ed Ø$_{i,*j}$ è uscito dall'aula.
'The professor explained the theory to the student and Ø left the classroom.'

In (8), there are two possible antecedents for the zero pronoun represented as "Ø", i.e. *il professore* and *lo studente*. Nevertheless, Italian speakers can identify without difficulties *il professore* as the correct antecedent of the zero pronoun Ø.

But what precisely governs this reference assignment under anaphora resolution? And what allows the addressee to retrieve the correct antecedent of a pronoun or a referential expression? An answer to these questions is provided by the Accessibility Theory developed

1 Technically, this operation is dubbed *accidental coreference*, since the pronoun is assigned the same reference as the antecedent.

by Ariel (1991), which permits to explain how reference assignment works, aiming to capture the ways in which the human mind is able to select the most appropriate antecedent for a referential expression.

The concept of accessibility plays an important role in the relation established between anaphoric expressions and their antecedents. In an anaphoric relation, indeed, the anaphoric term refers back to an entity that has already been introduced in the discourse or activated by an antecedent. This entity is said to be *accessible* for the anaphoric expression. According to the Accessibility Theory, some entities are more readily retrievable than others in the participant's memory and the speaker can select, within a set of anaphoric expressions, the most appropriate one, in order to help the hearer to access the referent. In other words, we can imagine that each anaphoric expression is provided with a label that informs the hearer about how salient its antecedent must be in discourse. In the Accessibility Theory framework, then, referential expressions are seen as accessibility markers that are ordered in a precise hierarchy from a maximum to a minimum degree. The position of an anaphoric expression in the scale provides the addressee with appropriate instructions to retrieve its antecedent by indicating how accessible it is in the discourse. Different factors contribute to determine the accessibility degree of an antecedent: salience, distance, competition and unity. Let us briefly consider these concepts:

(i) Saliency: entities are said to be salient in the discourse if they are mental representations of the participants of the conversation, or if they are discourse or sentence topics. The more an entity is salient in the discourse, the higher its accessibility degree will be.
(ii) Distance: it concerns the distance between the anaphoric expression and its antecedent. Distance is determined by the number of DPs that occur between the referential expression and its antecedents. Shorter the distance, more accessible the antecedent.
(iii) Competition: it regards the number of other possible antecedent candidates for an anaphoric expression. If there are more than one possible antecedents, the competition becomes heavier and it is therefore more difficult to access the correct antecedent.
(iv) Unity: it informs us about how related the unit in which the antecedent occurs is to the unit in which the anaphoric expression finds

itself (i.e. it concerns the fact that the antecedent occurs in the same frame, world, point of view or segment of the paragraph).

These factors interact with each other contributing to determine the degree of accessibility of an antecedent. A detailed version of Ariel's Accessibility Hierarchy (see Ariel 1994), starting with the highest accessibility marker and ending with the lowest, is reported in (9).

(9) *Accessibility Marking Scale*
Zero pronouns (Ø)
Reflexives
Agreement markers
Cliticized pronouns
Unstressed pronouns
Stressed pronouns
Stressed pronouns + gesture
Proximal demonstrative (+NP)
Distal demonstrative (+NP)
Proximal demonstrative (+NP) + modifier
Distal demonstrative (+NP)+ modifier
First name
Last name
Short definite description
Long definite description
Full name
Full name + modifier

Ariel argues that the scale in (9) is essentially universal, since natural languages tend to encode the degree of accessibility relying on three principles: informativity, rigidity and attenuation.

(i) Informativity: the degree of informativity of a marker depends on the lexical information it provides. If a form is more informative than another, it is more likely that it will code a lower accessibility. Semantically lighter markers (as pronouns) signal higher accessibility. For instance, the long definite description *the girl with the red dress* is more informative than the pronoun *she*, and, hence, it is a lower accessibility marker. For this reason, if the speaker wants to refer to a non salient antecedent, she will use a lower but more informative accessibility marker.

(ii) Rigidity: the degree of rigidity determines how uniquely referring an expression is. If a form is rigid (i.e. it refers unambiguously to an individual or an object, as proper names do), it marks lower accessibility. For example, the proper name *Noam Chomsky* is more rigid and unambiguous than the definite description *the linguist*, and, hence, it is a lower accessibility marker.

(iii) Attenuation: the degree of attenuation depends on the phonological size of a form and on the presence or absence of the stress. Less attenuated forms are used for lower accessibility retrievals. A stressed pronoun is less attenuated then an unstressed one, and, hence, it conveys lower accessibility.

2.1. How the Accessibility Theory works

As we have observed above, the Accessibility Theory offers an account of reference assignment under anaphora resolution centered on the notion of accessibility. In this framework, the speaker can rely on the Accessibility Marking Scale to select the more appropriate expression to refer to a certain entity, according to its salience in the discourse, to the presence of other competitors, to the distance occurring between the NP and its antecedent and to the occurrence of the antecedent in the same unity of the anaphoric expression. If an expression is highly salient in the discourse, for instance, the speaker is guided to choose an expression conveying high accessibility, such a zero pronoun or a phonetically realized pronoun, instead of a lower accessibility marker, such as a long definite description. The hearer will exploit the Accessibility Marking Scale also to retrieve the correct antecedent of a referential expression: if the speaker opted for a high accessibility marker, the antecedent will be highly accessible in the discourse and, vice versa, if she used a lower accessibility marker, the hearer can infer that the antecedent is not very accessible in the discourse.

To better understand how Accessibility Theory works, let us consider how it permits to account for reference assignment in a sentence like (8), reported below for convenience.

(8) Il professore$_i$ ha spiegato la teoria allo studente$_j$ ed Ø$_{i,*j}$ è uscito dall'aula.
'The professor explained the theory to the student and Ø left the classroom.'

In this case, the speaker chose to use a zero pronoun, which occupies the highest position in the Accessibility Marking Scale. This permits the hearer to infer that the antecedent of the zero pronoun will be the most accessible one in the sentence, i.e. the topic of the sentence. Since in this case the topic of the sentences coincides with its grammatical subject, the hearer retrieves *il professore* as the appropriate antecedent of the zero pronoun. Therefore, the zero pronoun in (8) is interpreted as referring to *il professore*. Replacing the zero pronoun with a phonetically realized pronoun, instead, would give the sentence a radically different interpretation, as shown in (10):

(10) Il professore$_i$ ha spiegato la teoria allo studente$_j$ e poi lui$_{j,*i}$ è uscito dall'aula.
'The professor explained the theory to the student and then he left'.

According to the hierarchy in (9), the phonetically realized pronoun *he* occupies a lower position in the scale in comparison to the zero pronoun, and, hence, it provides us with the information that the appropriate antecedent is not the most salient expression in the discourse, i.e. the subject, but a less salient one. For this reason, the addressee selects *lo studente* as the referent of the pronoun *lui*. As we will discuss in the following section, this reasoning can be seen as the results of an inferential process involving the computation of an implicature (see Chapter 5).

To sum up, the Accessibility Theory claims that a high accessibility marker, such as a zero pronoun, informs the addressee that the antecedent is highly accessible in the discourse, while a low accessibility marker encodes the information that the antecedent is not highly salient in the discourse. Hence, the hierarchy helps the addressee reduce the number of possible candidates to the minimum, excluding incorrect and improper reference assignments.

Before we discuss the processing costs associated with the application of the Accessibility Theory, I will discuss the difference between zero pronouns and phonetically realized pronouns predicted by the theory.

2.2. *Processing costs of Accessibility Theory*

In the previous section we have observed that according to the Accessibility Theory referential expressions are accessibility markers ordered in a hierarchy and that their position in the Accessibility Marking Scale provides the addressee with the information necessary to retrieve the appropriate antecedent of an anaphoric expression. We have already noted that the kind of reasoning made by the hearer can be compared to that underpinning the computation of an implicature. The hearer, indeed, has to assume that the speaker wishes to stick to the Cooperation Principle, trying to be cooperative, and obeying, in the case of referent assignment, to the Accessibility Theory.

Moreover, as we will see in the following sections, I propose that the computation of an implicature is explicitly required to discriminate between zero pronouns and phonologically realized pronouns. In the next paragraph, I will concentrate precisely on the difference between zero pronouns and phonetically realized pronouns, focusing in particular on the processing costs they impose on the general computation of the sentence's meaning.

2.3. *The interpretation of zero pronouns and phonetically realized pronouns*

As established by the Accessibility Marking Scale in (9), zero pronouns (*zeros* henceforth) and phonetically realized pronouns (*pronouns* henceforth) are both high accessibility markers, even though not at the same degree. Pronouns, namely, are more rigid and fully articulated than zeros. The Italian pronoun *lui* ('he'), for instance, is more rigid (in the sense defined above) than Ø since it informs that its referent is male. The zero, instead, is less informative, more ambiguous and more attenuated (again in the sense defined above).

For this reason, zeros occupy the highest position in the hierarchy in (9), followed by pronouns, which mark a lower accessibility. Evidence in favor of this hierarchy is provided by the generalized preference manifested by those speakers whose mother tongue admits the use of zero pronouns, as Italian, for interpreting zero forms as referring to very salient antecedents in cases where both zeros and pronouns are grammatical. Consider, for instance, the sentences in (11) and (12):

(11) Questo è Gianni: Anna dice che è veramente un bravo linguista.
'This is John: Ann says that Ø is really a good linguist'.

(12) Questo è Gianni: Anna dice che lui è veramente un bravo linguista.
'This is John: Ann says that he is really a good linguist'.

Although both utterances are grammatically correct, the former is considered more appropriate and is actually preferred by speakers. Interestingly, people hearing a sentence containing a phonetically realized pronoun referring to the topic of the sentence, as (12), tend to attribute a slight contrastive meaning to the pronoun, inferring for instance that the speaker intended to say that John, *and not someone else*, is a good linguist. This tendency was already noted by Chomsky (1981), who tried to account for it by formulating the Avoid Pronoun Principle, reported in (13):

(13) Avoid Pronoun Principle
Lexical pronouns are blocked by empty pronouns if possible.

Even though it captures the general preference for sentences like (11) in *pro-drop* languages, this principle has been considered too vague. The reader may have noticed, indeed, that it leaves some questions open, since it cannot explain why in some cases speakers show preferences for realized pronouns, instead of zeros, in languages like Hebrew (Ariel 1991). Conversely, the Accessibility Theory is able to explain this phenomenon, arguing that once the accessibility of a given antecedent is perceived as relatively low, speakers tend to use a relatively lower accessibility marker, resorting to the pronoun.

3. Processing costs of zero pronouns' and phonetically realized pronouns' resolution: A proposal

In this section, I will present an original proposal about the distinct processing costs required in the interpretation of zero pronouns and full pronouns, arguing that the resolution of overt pronouns is more complex, since it involves a finer reasoning and the computation of an implicature.

Let us concentrate on Italian: as is well-known, Italian is a *pro-drop* language which allows the omission of the subject-pronoun. The zero pronoun, hence, can be used uniquely to refer to the subject of a sentence, whereas the realized pronoun is generally introduced to inform the addressee that a topic shift has occurred. Thus, when the addressee finds a zero pronoun, she has to retrieve the sentence topic, which generally coincides with the subject of the sentence, and to identify it as the appropriate antecedent.

We can formalize this procedure as indicated in (14):

(14) *Rule of Referent Assignment to the Zero Pronoun*
Select the topic of the sentence as the correct antecedent of a zero pronoun.

To understand how this rule works, consider sentence (15).

(15) Paperina ha ballato con Minnie e poi Ø ha preparato la cena.
'Daisy Duck danced with Minnie and then Ø prepared dinner.'

Applying the rule outlined above to the resolution of the zero pronoun in (15), we obtain that its appropriate antecedent is the sentence topic, i.e. Daisy Duck. Its competitor Minnie, instead, cannot be considered coreferential with the zero form, since it is the non-topic element.

However, this rule is of no help in presence of a realized pronoun whose resolution requires a more complex reasoning. The full pronoun can be seen, as shown above, as a variable which could be used both to refer to the topic and to the non-topic expression of a sentence. For this reason, while interpreting sentences as the one in (16), the addressee has to cope with an ambiguous sentence.

(16) Minnie ha ballato con Paperina e poi lei ha preparato la cena.
'Minnie danced with Daisy Duck and then she prepared dinner'.

To disambiguate the full pronoun *lei* ('she'), the addressee has to perform a more subtle reasoning, considering that if the topic had been the appropriate referent, the speaker would have used a zero pronoun, and concluding therefore that the topic cannot be the correct antecedent. Clearly, this reasoning involves the computation of a scalar implicature. We can assume, indeed, that the use of the phonetically realized pronoun to refer to a maximally accessible antecedent, such as a subject, is excluded by a conversational implicature. If the speaker had wanted to convey reference to a highly accessible antecedent, she would have used a zero pronoun, which selects the topic (i.e. the subject) as its appropriate antecedent, as established by the rule of Reference Assignment to the Zero Pronoun. The resulting implicature can be formalized as follows in (17):

(17) *Implicature for realized pronouns resolution*
If the topic had been the appropriate antecedent, the speaker would have used the zero pronoun to refer to it. Hence, select the non-topic expression as the correct antecedent of a phonetically realized pronoun.

Turning back to sentence (16), the addressee observes that if the speaker had wished to refer to the sentence-topic, i.e. Minnie, she would have used the zero pronoun. She is then forced to conclude that Daisy Duck is the appropriate referent to be chosen.

To see how the actual resolution of zeros and pronouns works, let us consider again the sentences reported in (18) and (19) for convenience:

(18) Lisa ha chiacchierato con Anna e poi Ø è tornata a casa.
'Lisa chatted with Anna and then Ø went home'.
(19) Lisa ha chiacchierato con Anna e poi lei è tornata a casa.
'Lisa chatted with Anna and then she went home'.

The second conjunct of (18) contains a zero pronoun; to retrieve its antecedent, the addressee has to apply the Rule of Referent Assignment to the Zero Pronoun formulated in (14) and to select the topic of the sentence, i.e. Lisa, as the appropriate referent of the zero. In (19), instead, she has to interpret a phonetically realized pronoun and therefore she is forced to compute the implicature as reported in (17), establishing that if the topic had been the appropriate antecedent, the speaker would have used the zero pronoun to refer to it. Her choice to use the phonetically realized pronoun permits to infer that the correct antecedent is not the topic, but a less salient expression in the sentence, in this case Anna.

Summarizing, the resolution of both types of pronouns seems to require a complex processing. However, in the light of the discussion about implicature computation in Chapter 5 (to which the reader is refereed), it should be clear that the processing costs required by the resolution of the zero and the overt pronoun are quite different. As we have observed, in fact, the computation of an implicature is very expensive in terms of processing resources, since it involves a reference-set computation (Reinhart 1999, 2006). According to Reinhart, indeed, the procedure of deriving an implicature requires the construction of an alternative sentence, which has then to be compared with the speaker's utterance. In order to interpret a sentence like (19), for instance, the addressee has to go through a number of steps: first, she has to construct an alternative sentence with the zero pronoun in place of the realized pronoun, as in (20). She has then to apply the Rule for Referent Assignment to the Zero Pronoun in (14), assuming that the topic of the sentence, i.e. Lisa, is the correct antecedent of the zero pronoun. However, since the speaker chose to use the phonetically realized pronoun, the addressee has to compute the implicature in (21), inferring that the alternative sentence in (20) is false and that, as a consequence, the correct antecedent of the pronoun is *Anna*.

(20) ALT: Lisa ha chiacchierato con Anna e poi è tornata a casa.
'Lisa chatted with Anna and then Ø went home'

(21) IMPL: Lisa ha chiacchierato con Anna e poi Anna, *e non Lisa*, è tornata a casa.
'Lisa chatted with Anna and then Anna, *and not Lisa*, went home'

Undoubtedly, the kind of reasoning required for the resolution of a phonetically realized pronoun is more complex and more demanding in terms of processing resources than that required for the interpretation of the zero pronoun. For this reason, it would be very interesting to analyze how dyslexic children can cope with the interpretation of this kind of sentences in comparison to age-matched typically developing children. If our starting hypothesis claiming that dyslexics suffer from an impairment affecting their working memory and processing resources is correct, greater difficulties are expected in tasks that are particularly demanding in terms of processing costs. This hypothesis has been addressed in the experimental protocol that will be presented in the following sections.

4. Experimental Protocol

In this section I will present and discuss the results of an experimental protocol, a truth value judgment task, performed to verify how dyslexic children interpret sentences containing a zero pronoun or a phonetically realized pronoun in comparison to age-matched typically developing children, adults, first class children and preschool children. Assuming that the computation of pronouns, and especially of overt pronouns, is expensive in terms of processing resources, the analysis of the performance shown by dyslexics can be useful for testing the hypothesis that dyslexia is associated with a working memory and processing deficit.

Since a control group composed of adults was also included in the protocol, specific attention was also devoted to the presence or absence of differences amongst adults' performance and children's performance.

4.1. Participants

The experimental task was performed on 96 subjects, divided in five distinct groups: 18 dyslexic children, 18 age-matched typically developing children, 18 control adults (30;2), and two groups of younger children, the former composed of 23 children attending to the first class of the primary school and the latter composed of 20 preschool children.

The group of Dyslexic children (DC) included 18 children (14 males), all native speakers of Italian. At the moment of testing, the group mean age was 9 years and 3 months (SD = 1;4). All children have been chosen from those who had independently received a diagnosis of dyslexia, specifically by the "Centro Audiofonetico" in Trento: in particular, dyslexic children were selected according to different factors: (i) absence of neurological diseases or genetic pathologies, (ii) absence of sensorial diseases, (iii) absence of psychopathological diseases, (iv) IQ > 80 (WISC – R) and (v) fluent and correct reading and writing abilities under 2 SD (Tressoldi et al. Battery, Prove MT).

The group of age-matched control children (AMCC) was composed by 18 primary school children (4 males), all native speakers of Italian. At the moment of testing, the group mean age was 9 years and 0 months (SD = 0;8). Children were selected from those who had no history of reading problems or language disorders.

The group of control adults (CA) was composed by 18 adults (7 males), all native speakers of Italian with no history of reading or language disorders. At the moment of testing, the group mean age was 30 years and 4 months (SD = 13;9).

The group of first-class children (FCC) was composed by 23 children attending to the first class of the primary school (11 males), all native speakers of Italian with no reports of language problems. At the moment of testing the group mean age was 7 years and 0 months (SD = 0;4). Finally, the last group of preschool children (PC) was composed by 19 children attending the kindergarten (10 males), all native speakers of Italian with no reports of language problems. At the moment of testing the group mean age was 4 years and 9 months (SD = 0;3).

The main features of the five groups are summarized in Table 7.1.

Table 7.1. Group data of the subjects who took part in Exp. 1.

Group	Number	Mean Age (SD)
DC	18	9;3 (1;4)
AMCC	18	9;0 (0;8)
CA	18	30;4 (13;9)
FCC	23	7;0 (0;4)
PC	20	4;9 (0;3)

4.2. Design and Procedure

The experimental protocol was designed to assess the subject's comprehension of anaphoric expressions, by means of a truth value judgment task. The subject was shown some pictures on a computer screen portraying a short story that always involved two characters performing some actions. The experimenter introduced the subject with a puppet, the Clumsy Detective, who had the task to explain what happened in the short story. The subject was told that the inspector was named "Clumsy" since he could not always describe correctly what happened in the story; thus, the participant's task was to decide whether the Clumsy Detective said the truth about what happened in the story or whether he lied. The task involved ten experimental items divided in four different conditions, two items each for Conditions A and C and three items each for Conditions B and D. An example of each condition and of the reasoning required for its interpretation is reported below:

(i) Condition A, Zero True (ZT): The Clumsy Detective described the story using a zero pronoun; if the zero pronoun was interpreted correctly as referring to the subject of the sentence, the utterance was true. An example is the sentence in (22), uttered by the Clumsy Detective in a context in which Piglet is indeed about to fly away. The sentence is true: the utterance, indeed, contains a zero pronoun selecting the subject as its correct referent, as established by the Rule for Reference Assignment to the Zero Pronoun.

(22) Pimpi è andato a fare una passeggiata con Winnie e sta per volare via!
'Piglet went for a walk with Winnie and Ø is about to fly away!'

(ii) Condition B, Zero False (ZF): The Clumsy Detective described the story using a zero pronoun; if the zero pronoun was interpreted correctly as referring to the subject of the sentence, the utterance was false. An example is the sentence in (23), uttered in a context in which Daisy Duck, instead of Minnie, prepared dinner. The sentence uttered by the Clumsy Detective is false. The utterance, in fact, contains a zero pronoun that selects the subject, i.e. Minnie, as a referent. At this point, the subject has to simulate the asserted state of affairs and to compare it with the picture. This operation has been described in Chapter 6, where we have observed that if she cannot resort to the picture to build the representation of the sentence, an additional step is required to create it. Finally, since the picture and the simulation of the asserted state of affairs are not mutually consistent, the subject should answer false. Given that the interpretation and verification of this kind of sentences requires a further step, imposing additional load on WM, greater difficulties are expected for those subjects whose processing resources are limited.

(23) Minnie ha ballato con Paperina e poi ha preparato la cena!
'Minnie danced with Daisy Duck and then Ø prepared dinner'

(iii) Condition C, Realized True (RT): The Clumsy Detective described the story using a phonetically realized pronoun; if the pronoun was interpreted correctly as not referring to the subject of the sentence, but to the object, the utterance was true. An example is the sentence in (24), uttered in a context in which Donald Duck did his homework. In this case, the utterance contains a phonetically realized pronoun, whose resolution involves the computation of an implicature. The subject has to reason that if the speaker had used the zero pronoun, the correct antecedent would have been the topic of the sentence, i.e. Goofy. However, since the Clumsy Detective preferred to use the overt pronoun, the interpretation cannot be that expressed by the alternative sentence with the zero pronoun. Therefore, the subject identifies Donald Duck as the correct antecedent of the phonetically realized pronoun. Finally, she has to compare the simulation of the asserted state of affairs with the picture. Given that they are mutually consistent, she should answer true. Note that in this case the interpretation of the sentence involves the computation of an implicature, increasing the amount of processing load required. Therefore, greater difficulties are expected in comparison to Condition A, where the zero was used and the computation of the implicature was not needed.

(24) Pippo è tornato a casa insieme a Paperino e poi lui ha fatto i compiti.
'Goofy came back home with Donald Duck and then he did his homework'

(iv) Condition D, Realized False: The Clumsy Detective described the story using a phonetically realized pronoun; if the pronoun is interpreted correctly as not referring to the subject of the sentence, but to the object, the utterance is false. An example is the sentence in (25), uttered in a context in which Winnie, and not Tigger, brought a cake. In this case the target sentence is false. As a matter of fact, it contains a phonetically realized pronoun, whose resolution involves the computation of an implicature. The subject has to reason that if the Clumsy Detective had used a zero pronoun, the correct referent would have been the topic of the sentence, i.e. Winnie. However, since he chose to use the overt pronoun, the appropriate antecedent must be the non-topic expression, i.e. Tigger.
Moreover, she has to make a further step in order to assign a truth value judgment to the sentence; more particularly, she must construct a simulation of the asserted state of affairs, since the picture cannot be used for it. Finally, since the picture and the simulation are not mutually consistent, the correct answer should be "false".
To summarize, Condition D is the most difficult one, since it requires both the computation of the implicature and the construction of a simulation of the expected state of affairs. Consequently, the highest error rates are expected.

(25) Winnie ha festeggiato insieme a Tigro e lui gli ha portato una torta.
'Winnie celebrated with Tigger and he brought him a cake'.

The experimental items were interspersed with 5 fillers and preceded by one warm-up item, presented at the beginning of the task to let the child get acquainted with the experimental procedure.

4.3. *Results*

All subjects included in the five groups gave the correct answer to the vast majority of the fillers; only one of the preschool children failed to give the correct answer to all fillers and therefore he was excluded from the sample.

Let us consider first the general performances reported by the five groups; descriptive statistics of the error rates are displayed in Table 7.2 and represented in Graph 7.1.

Table 7.2. Descriptive statistics of the error rates displayed by the five groups.

	Group	N	Mean	Std. Deviation
TOTAL ERROR RATES	DC	18	0.49	0.12
	AMCC	18	0.10	0.11
	CA	18	0.02	0.05
	FCC	23	0.35	0.13
	PC	19	0.51	0.13

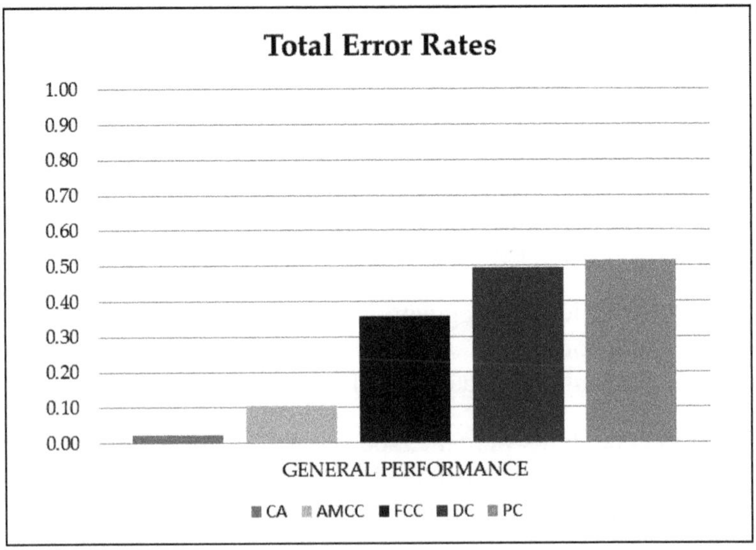

Graph. 7.1. Mean Error Rates of the five groups.

As the graph shows, it is possible to distinguish two different kinds of behavior amongst the five groups: DC display a very poor performance showing a high error rate that approaches chance performance. Their behavior resembles that of PC, whose error rate is only slightly higher.

Conversely, AMCC exhibit a substantially correct performance, with a low error rate, performing similarly to CA. FCC, instead, occupy a mid position between them, with an error rate significantly higher than that of AMCC and CA, but lower than that of DC and PC. Let us examine now the error rates reported in each condition; descriptive statistics are displayed in Table 7.3, whereas the error rates are represented in Graph 7.2.

Table 7.3. Descriptive statistics of the error rates displayed by the five groups in each condition.

	Group	N	Mean	Std. Deviation
COND. A – ZT	DC	18	0.02	0.11
	AMCC	18	0.00	0.00
	CA	18	0.00	0.00
	FCC	23	0.00	0.00
	PC	19	0.00	0.00
COND. B – ZF	DC	18	0.51	0.30
	AMCC	18	0.03	0.10
	CA	18	0.00	0.00
	FCC	23	0.34	0.27
	PC	19	0.70	0.36
COND. C – RT	DC	18	0.36	0.37
	AMCC	18	0.11	0.21
	CA	18	0.00	0.00
	FCC	23	0.23	0.33
	PC	19	0.18	0.29
COND. D – RF	DC	18	0.87	0.20
	AMCC	18	0.23	0.27
	CA	18	0.07	0.18
	FCC	23	0.68	0.36
	PC	19	0.89	0.19

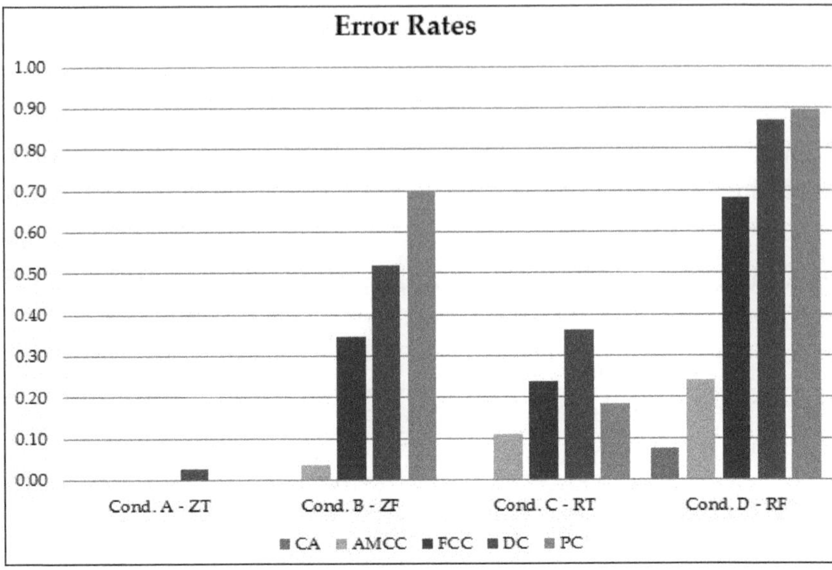

Graph. 7.2. Mean Error Rates of the five groups for each condition.

As the graph shows, the performance in each condition confirms the trend observed in the general performance, with DC behaving similarly to PC, AMCC showing an adultlike behavior and FCC occupying a mid position. With respect to Condition A ("Zero True"), the mean error rate obtained in the five groups is very low for DC, while it is absent for AMCC, CA, FCC and PC. Condition D ("Realized False") is the most difficult one for all groups, with DC performing much worse than AMCC and even than FCC, similarly to PC. The same trend is found also for Condition B ("Zero False"); in Condition C ("Realized True"), instead, DC underperformed in comparison to AMCC and FCC, whereas PC showed a lower error rate.

A statistical analysis was conducted on these data, to verify if there were statistically significant differences between the performances of the five groups of participant. A 2 x 2 x 2 repeated measure ANOVA was conducted. *Group* (DC; AMCC; CA; FCC; PC) was selected as the between-subject variable. *Type of pronoun* (zero; realized) was the first within subject variable, verifying if the type of pronoun used in the sentence affected performance (comparing Conditions "Zero True" and

"Zero False" with Conditions "Realized True" and "Realized False"). *Truth* was the second within subject variable, comparing true sentences with false sentences (Conditions "Zero True" and "Realized True" with Conditions "Zero False" and "Realized False").

The first interesting result showed that there is a highly significant *Group* effect, $F(4, 91)$ 65.089, $p < .001$, partial $\eta^2 = .741$, indicating that there are significant differences amongst the five groups. Post-hoc comparisons were then run to determine which group differed from the others. Levene's test for homogeneity of variances resulted significant for "Zero True" ($F(4, 91) = 4.910$, $p < .001$), for "Zero False" ($F(4, 91) = 15.849$, $p < .001$), for "Realized True" ($F(4, 91) = 16.669$, $p < .001$) and for "Realized False" ($F(4, 91) = 4.680$, $p < .01$). Therefore, subsequent post hoc comparison tests for equal variance not assumed (Dunnett's T3), with a α-level of 0.05 were administered. Results show that DC perform differently from AMCC ($p < .001$), from CA ($p < .001$) and even from FCC ($p < .001$), whereas there are not significant differences between DC and PC ($p = 1.000$). AMCC, instead, perform similarly to CA ($p = .061$), but differently from DC, FCC and PC ($p < .001$). Interestingly, FCC's performance is different from DC's performance ($p < .05$), CA's and AMCC's performance ($p < .001$) and even from PC's performance ($p < .01$).

Summarizing, the between-subject variable *Group* is highly significant, confirming that DC perform similarly to PC and differently from the other groups, whereas AMCC show a behavior similar to that of CA; FCC, instead, perform differently from all other groups.

Turning back to the statistical analysis, the within-subject variables were successively considered. The *Type of Pronoun* variable is highly significant, $F(1, 91) = 62.232$, $p < .001$, partial $\eta^2 = .406$, showing that the pronoun used (zero vs. phonetically realized) has a great influence on the performance; moreover, there is also a significant *Type of Pronoun – Group interaction*, $F(4, 91) = 4.191$, $p < .01$, partial $\eta^2 = .156$, showing that the form of the pronoun affects the performance of all the five groups. This result confirms that sentences containing a zero pronoun are easier to interpret than sentences containing a phonetically realized pronoun for all groups. The *Truth* variable is highly significant as well, $F(1, 91) = 157.408$, $p < .001$, partial $\eta^2 = .634$, showing that the truth value of the target sentences has an impact on the performance. In this case the significant *Truth – Group* interaction, $F(4, 91) = 20.666$, $p < .001$, partial $\eta^2 = .476$, indicates that this variable is not equally significant for all groups. Specifically, a separate analysis of the performances of the five groups reveals that truth does not affect significantly the performance of CA, and it affects only marginally the performance of AMCC. Conversely, false sentences are significantly more difficult than true sentences for DC, FCC and PC, arguably due to the additional step required to construct a mental simulation of the asserted state of affairs to be compared with the picture showed by the experimenter.

A Pearson correlation test was also performed, to verify if there was a significant correlation between the age of the participants and their performance. Results show that there is indeed a positive and highly significant correlation between age and the total error rates ($r = .541$, $p < .001$), as well as between age and Condition B, "Zero False" ($r = .419$, $p < .001$), Condition C, "Realized True" ($r = .236$, $p < .05$) and Condition D, "Realized False" ($r = .503$, $p < .001$). Conversely, there is no correlation between Condition A, "Zero True" and age ($r = .030$, $p= .772$), arguably due to the absence of errors in that condition (except for DC, whose error rate is however very low). These results confirm that there is a strong correlation between age and performance, demonstrating that growing up children can count on more efficient processing resources.

4.4. *Discussion*

As expected, dyslexic children are remarkably more impaired in the interpretation of pronouns in comparison to age-matched control children, who show an adultlike behavior, while, interestingly, their poor performance does not differ from the one shown by YC, more than four years younger than them. Even more significantly, DC show a poorer performance also in comparison to FCC, who, in spite of being younger, commit less errors.

As confirmed by the correlation analysis, strong support is provided for the hypothesis that children's WM develops with age, leading to performance enhancement. Indeed, AMCC already show an adult performance, even though they commit much more errors than CA in the most difficult condition, "Realized False", revealing that their behavior is not completely adult-like, presumably due to the fact that their WM development is not fully developed yet. PC, whose WM has just started to develop, show a very poor performance, whereas FCC, two years older, perform already significantly better, occupying a mid position between them and AMCC. In this scenario, the performance shown by DC is extremely interesting, since they do not simply perform worse than AMCC, but also significantly worse than FCC, two years younger than them. Interestingly, instead, their performance is not different from that of PC, more than four years younger than them. These data strongly confirm that they do perform differently from their peers in the interpretation of pronouns, a task that is arguably demanding in terms of processing costs and memory resources.

The results of this experimental protocol also confirm that it is more difficult to assign a referent to a phonetically realized pronoun in comparison to a zero pronoun; this is consistent with the hypothesis I proposed above, according to which the interpretation of an overt pronoun in a *pro-drop* language like Italian involves the computation of an implicature. This operation is complex and demanding in terms of WM resources, as argued by Reinhart (1999, 2006), who observed that the computation of an implicature requires the subject to construct and compare two alternative representations, an operation imposing high processing costs. Compatibly with this hypothesis, the statistical analysis conducted on the results of the experiment confirmed that the type of pronoun used in the target sentences affects sensibly the performance of the five groups tested. Moreover, results are also consistent with the prediction claiming that false sentences are more difficult to interpret than true sentences in a sentence-picture verification task like the one proposed in this protocol, at least for the three groups of subjects whose memory resources are lower (DC, FCC and PC). In the case of false sentences, the subject cannot resort to the picture to simulate the asserted state of affairs and therefore she has to construct a representation to be compared with the picture. In line with this prediction, the truth value of the target sentences has a significant impact on the performance for these groups, with Conditions B and D being generally more difficult than Conditions A and C. Arguably, the additional step required to check false sentences imposes an extra load on working memory and it can be held responsible for the lower performance shown in false sentences in comparison to true sentences.

Summarizing, then, PC are unable to cope with the task and show a very poor performance, while FCC, two years older, are more skilled and commit less errors in all four conditions; AMCC, finally, exhibit an adultlike performance, whereas CA do not display difficulties and provide, in the vast majority of the cases, correct answers. DC, instead, show a really different behavior: they are not only more impaired than AMCC, but they show a poorer performance also in comparison to children two years younger than them, whereas their performance does not differ significantly from that of preschool children.

To conclude, results point to the existence of a difficulty in the interpretation of pronouns in dyslexia. This difficulty is arguably triggered by the complexity of the task and it is due to the lower processing resources that dyslexics can rely on in comparison to age-matched typically developing children.

5. Summary and Conclusions

In this chapter, further evidence for the occurrence of a working memory deficit in developmental dyslexia has been reported. The experimental protocol, designed to investigate dyslexic children's reference assignment abilities, has taken into account, in particular, their interpretation of pronouns in the framework of Accessibility Theory. Dyslexic children's performance in the resolution of both zero pronouns and phonetically realized pronouns has been found remarkably poorer in comparison to that of age-matched typically developing children, who showed instead an adultlike behavior. Interestingly, dyslexics performed worse even in comparison to first-class children, more than two years younger than them, while their error rate did not differ significantly from the one shown by preschool children, more than four years younger than them. Furthermore, all groups of subjects committed more errors when required to interpret phonetically realized pronouns in comparison to zero pronouns, consistently with the proposal that the resolution of overt pronouns is more difficult, since it involves the computation of an implicature.

These results strongly confirm that developmental dyslexia should be considered as an impairment affecting different levels of linguistic representation, beyond the phonological domain. Moreover, since throughout the chapter it has been argued that the interpretation of pronominal expressions is highly demanding in terms of processing resources, the results obtained provide support in favor of the Phonological and Executive Working Memory Deficit Hypothesis.

Chapter 8

Concluding Remarks

1. Introduction

In this book I put forward an original proposal, the Phonological and Executive Working Memory Deficit Hypothesis, to account for the different disorders exhibited by individuals affected by developmental dyslexia, reported below for convenience.

> The Phonological and Executive Working Memory Deficit Hypothesis
>
> Dyslexic individuals suffer from a limitation affecting their Working Memory and hampering in particular their phonological memory and their executive functions. As a consequence, this impairment disrupts their phonological competence, as well as their performance in complex tasks that are particularly demanding in terms of Working Memory resources. On the contrary, dyslexics can rely on a spared visuo-spatial memory, to which they can resort for the accomplishment of compensatory strategies.

According to this hypothesis, dyslexic people suffer from an impairment affecting their phonological memory and their executive functions, which can be held responsible for their difficulties in those tasks that require a good phonological competence or that are particularly demanding in terms of processing resources.

Throughout the chapters of this book I have shown that the Phonological and Executive Working Memory Deficit Hypothesis is able to account for the whole range of deficits exhibited by dyslexic individuals and reviewed in Chapter 1. For its explicative power, this proposal differentiates from the other theories developed in the last decades and presented in Chapter 2. We have observed, for instance, that the Magnocellular Deficit Hypothesis, which resumes more precisely and elegantly the arguments put forward by the Visual and the Auditory Deficit

Hypotheses, cannot explain the occurrence of grammatical, vocabulary and attention deficits which are typically reported in dyslexia.

Nor can the Phonological Deficit Hypothesis, which provides a reliable account only for the poor phonological awareness shown by dyslexics, by proposing that their difficulties lie in the access to phonological representations.

A similar inadequacy is manifested by the Double Deficit Hypothesis, which, stemming from the Phonological Deficit Hypothesis, explains phonological and naming deficits but cannot account for grammatical and attention problems. The Phonological and Executive Working Memory Deficit Hypothesis tries to compensate for the incompleteness of these proposals, postulating the existence of an impairment affecting dyslexics' phonological memory and executive functions, which is able to account for the whole range of manifestations of dyslexia. Although further experimental studies and researches are needed to strengthen it, this proposal is already supported by extensive evidence confirming that the Phonological Loop and the Central Executive are disrupted in dyslexia. These findings are also consistent with the results of the experimental protocol presented in Chapter 3 and confirming the presence of phonological and executive impairments in dyslexic children, who underperformed on all Phonological Loop and Central Executive measures in comparison to age-matched typically developing children.

Assuming that developmental dyslexia is characterized by a limitation affecting phonological memory and executive functions, in Chapter 4 we have observed that the Phonological and Executive Working Memory Deficit Hypothesis can explain dyslexics' well-known reading and spelling difficulties, given that these tasks necessitate both of a good phonological awareness and of a considerable amount of cognitive resources, since they are indeed complex and costly activities. The phonological deficits found in the totality of the dyslexic population are also captured by the hypothesis that I am proposing: an impaired phonological memory can actually cause the difficulties exhibited by dyslexics in phonological awareness tasks.

The Phonological and Executive Working Memory Deficit Hypothesis is also able to explain dyslexics' naming deficits, which have proven to be even more specific to dyslexia than reading and spelling disorders.

Working Memory, and especially the Phonological Loop, has the fundamental task of retrieving items from Long-Term Memory; a disordered phonological memory hampers this retrieval process, causing the slower performance frequently reported in dyslexics asked to name as quick as possible pictures of objects, colors and alphanumeric characters. Similarly, this hypothesis can explain the vocabulary deficits manifested by dyslexic children: given that one of the functions accomplished by the Phonological Loop is that of supporting the learning of new words, its disruption can hinder this process. As a consequence, dyslexics' vocabulary appears to be poorer than that of their peers and characterized by both length and frequency effects.

Importantly, the Phonological and Executive Working Memory Deficit Hypothesis can offer a valid account also for the grammatical deficits exhibited by dyslexic individuals. Consistently with the Capacity Constrained Comprehension Theory developed by Just and Carpenter (1992, 2002), my proposal predicts that dyslexics' more limited WM capacity (where Working Memory is mainly intended as Central Executive functioning) is responsible for their difficulties in the comprehension of complex constructions, whose processing demands exceed their total amount of available resources. Adopting this perspective, we have shown that a deficient WM can be held responsible for dyslexic children's impaired comprehension of tough sentences, pronouns, relative clauses, passive sentences and grammatical aspect.

To further test my hypothesis and investigate dyslexics' linguistic competence, I developed three additional experimental protocols, presented respectively in Chapters 5, 6 and 7 and testing the computation of scalar implicatures, the interpretation of negative sentences and the reference assignment to phonetically realized and zero pronouns. As extensively discussed, all of these tasks are considerably complex and demanding in terms of memory resources. As expected, dyslexic children always performed worse than controls, manifesting a behavior that was more similar to that shown by younger children.

On the basis of the considerations and the results discussed throughout this book and of the formulation of the Phonological and Executive Working Memory Deficit Hypothesis, we can now propose a new definition of developmental dyslexia.

An original definition of Developmental Dyslexia

> Developmental Dyslexia is a specific learning disability that is genetically inheritable and neurologically determined. Dyslexic individuals suffer from an impairment affecting their phonological memory and their executive functions, which hinders their performance in those tasks which involve an accurate phonological awareness and which are particularly demanding in terms of processing resources. As a consequence, dyslexics are likely to exhibit difficulties in acquiring reading and spelling skills, attention problems and deficits affecting their phonological competence, their vocabulary development, their performance in rapid naming tasks and their comprehension and production of complex sentences and instructions.

In comparison to the existing definitions of developmental dyslexia, the one developed above does not identify dyslexia by exclusion, admitting thus that dyslexia can occur at any level of intelligence, exposure to instruction and socio-economical conditions. Moreover, the advantage of this definition is that it does not consider reading and spelling disorders as the only deficits characterizing dyslexia: as we have observed throughout this book, problems in reading and spelling acquisition cannot in fact be considered either the necessary or the sufficient symptom of dyslexia. A considerable amount of evidence has actually shown that dyslexics manifest a wider range of disorders: focusing only on reading and spelling deficits, therefore, can be risky, since children whose mother tongue has a transparent orthography are likely to show relatively spared literacy abilities, with the consequence that their real difficulties go unnoticed.

As the careful reader may have observed, the occurrence of motor disorders in dyslexic individuals has not been discussed in the Phonological and Executive Working Memory Deficit Hypothesis yet. The main reason is that, as observed in Chapter 1, the results of the studies suggesting the presence of motor deficits in dyslexia have often been considered controversial, while other studies have indeed not confirmed these findings.

Within the perspective of the Phonological and Executive Working Memory Deficit Hypothesis, one might tentatively argue that dyslexics' motor problems under dual-task conditions can be caused by the impairment affecting their Central Executive and hampering their ability to perform more than one task simultaneously or to properly comprehend the given instructions. This could be the case, for instance, of the experiment administered by Haslum (1989), showing that dyslexic children underperformed in a task in which they were asked to catch a ball, throw it in the air and clap a certain number of times before catching it again. In this case, the difficulty could depend on the complexity of the instructions, involving the rapid succession of a series of operations. The same explanation may be relevant for the deficits reported by Nicolson and Fawcett (1994) in dual-task balance and also to account for fine-motricity disorders, including, for instance, the problems reported in learning to tie shoelaces, which requires a complex procedure as well.

Similarly, handwriting and copying difficulties could be interpreted as a consequence of the general complexity of the task of writing, which is arguably demanding in terms of processing resources, involving the retrieval and application of a series of rules.

However, these speculations must be supported by further researches.

Before concluding this book, I will briefly present an alternative hypothesis, which considers motor deficits as the core feature of dyslexia. This hypothesis, known as the Cerebellar Deficit Hypothesis and developed in its refined version by Nicolson and Fawcett (1995), proposes an interesting account of dyslexia while presenting both similarities and differences with respect to the Phonological and Executive Working Memory Deficit Hypothesis.

2. The Cerebellar Deficit Hypothesis

The Cerebellar Deficit Hypothesis was proposed by Nicolson and Fawcett (1995, 1999) in order to offer an alternative account of developmental dyslexia, recognizing the importance of motor deficits. The main tenet of this hypothesis is that dyslexic individuals suffer from a cerebellar impairment affecting their ability to automatize skills. The presence of automatization deficits in dyslexic individuals was already reported by Nicolson and Fawcett in a previous theory, the Automatization Deficit Hypothesis, formulated in 1990 and maintaining that dyslexia is characterized by a failure to carry out tasks automatically. As explained by the authors, automatization constitutes the final stage in skills mastery: it is achieved through extensive practice and it decreases the general processing cost demanded by the task. In fact, when a skill is not automatic, it requires a controlled processing and high attentional and Working Memory resources; conversely, once the skill becomes automatic, it is stored in Long Term Memory and it operates unconsciously, decreasing thus the need of attention and memory resources.

In the first version of their hypothesis, Nicolson and Fawcett propose that dyslexic children show abnormal automatization difficulties, regardless of whether the skill they are trying to acquire is cognitive or motor. Since they are not able to automatize a skill as rapidly and efficiently as typically developing children, they make use of higher attentional and memory resources: as a consequence, their performance appears to be slower and more effortful. Nonetheless, a sort of compensation is also possible: dyslexics are generally able to compensate for their lack of automaticity by means of a process of "conscious compensation", that is, by concentrating and by controlling processes that otherwise would be automatic. Therefore, they can achieve an apparently normal behavior in easier tasks, whereas their performance becomes slower and effortful in more complex tasks or under dual-task conditions, in which they tend to get tired more quickly than normal.

To find support for their hypothesis, Nicolson and Fawcett (1990, 1994) analyzed dyslexics' and controls' performance in balance tasks, a non-phonological skill which should be fully automatic in children: as discussed in Chapter 1, dyslexic children were found more impaired in dual-task and blindfolded balance, whereas they performed as controls in single-task balance. The authors interpreted these results by arguing that dyslexics had not automatized balance, differently from their peers, but that they were able to consciously compensate for their deficit in the simplest, single-task, conditions. The authors extended this reasoning also to the impairments found in reading, arguing that this skill depends critically on automaticity: dyslexics' effortful and slow performance reveals that they have not automatized it yet.

In a later work, Nicolson and Fawcett (1995) refined their intuitive account, formulating the Cerebellar Deficit Hypothesis and proposing that the automatization deficit found in dyslexics is caused by a cerebellar abnormality. The idea that the cerebellum is involved in dyslexia can be traced back to the 1970s, with the studies conducted by Frank and Levinson (1973) and Denkla (1985), and it is supported by neurobiological data revealing the occurrence of cerebellar abnormalities in dyslexia. Importantly, the cerebellum is also involved in automatization processes, as well as in the learning of motor skills and in the acquisition of *language dexterity* (see Nicolson and Fawcett 2008). It has been shown, indeed, that the cerebellum is both linked to the frontal motor areas and to the frontal cortex, including Broca's area and that it is activated in reading and in verbal working memory tasks. The causal chain proposed for dyslexia by the Cerebellar Deficit Hypothesis, developed by Nicolson and colleagues (2001), is reported below.

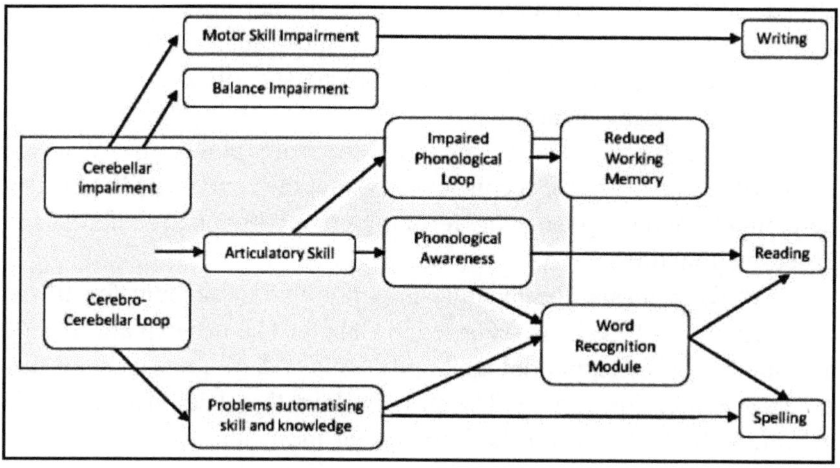

Figure 8.1. The Causal Chain of Dyslexia (Nicolson et al. 2001).

As the figure shows, Nicolson and colleagues argue that cerebellar abnormalities cause four different kinds of impairment in dyslexic individuals, such as (i) motor skills impairments (which are also responsible for writing disorders), (ii) balance impairments, (iii) articulatory impairments and (iv) problems in automatising skills and knowledge.

Articulatory deficits, in turn, are supposed to cause poor phonological awareness, affecting Working Memory, and to impair the functioning of the Phonological Loop, giving rise to problems for the word recognition module. Difficulties in automatising skill and knowledge, together with the impaired word recognition module, are finally responsible for reading and spelling deficits.

Even though the Cerebellar Deficit Hypothesis offers interesting insights to the research on dyslexia, some weaknesses can be individuated in the causal explanation put forward by Nicolson and colleagues. The first perplexity concerns the role of articulatory problems, which are considered the cause of poor phonological awareness and reduced Working Memory. Specifically, the authors argue that a less fluent articulation "leads to reduced effective working memory as reflected in the phonological loop" and that "this in turn leads to difficulties in language acquisition" (Nicolson et al. 2001: 510). However, some studies have already shown that articulatory disorders do not affect phonological awareness at all: as discussed in Chapter 2, individuals with articulatory problems, as people affected by anarthria, can actually show a normally functioning Phonological Loop.

A second perplexity concerns the role played by Working Memory in this model: it seems, namely, that the concept of WM refers here only to phonological short-term memory, without any reference to executive functions.

In these terms, the hypothesis is not able to account for all the manifestations of dyslexia reviewed in Chapter 1. It can explain reading and spelling deficits, phonological problems and, of course, motor disorders and attention deficits. The authors claim that it could also explain naming deficits, based on the impairment individuated at the level of the word recognition module. However, it is not clear why problems for this module, whose functioning is affected by poor phonological awareness and lack of automaticity skills, should cause naming deficits. Remember that it has been shown that a critical role in word retrieval is played by the Phonological Loop (see Chapter 2), which however does not affect the word recognition module in the causal chain reported in Figure 8.1.

More importantly, the Cerebellar Deficit Hypothesis is not able to account for the grammatical deficits identified in dyslexia. To offer a partial solution to this problem, Nicolson and Fawcett (2008) tried to link their account to a specific neurological framework, adopting the Declarative/Procedural Model developed by Ullman (2001, 2004), which will be briefly exposed in the following paragraph.

2.1. Ullman's Declarative/Procedural Model

According to the Declarative/Procedural Model, the distinction between lexicon and grammar characterizing human language is reflected by the distinction between two fundamental brain memory systems, that is, the Procedural Memory System and the Declarative Memory System (Ullman 2001, 2004).

The Procedural Memory System governs the learning of new procedures as well as the control of those skills and habits that have been already established. Specifically, it is involved in all aspects of rule-learning and in the acquisition of both cognitive and motor skills that are characterized by sequences of operations. In this system learning is gradual and it occurs through multiple presentations of stimuli and responses; once acquired, instead, skills are applied more quickly and automatically. Moreover, the Procedural Memory System is said to be implicit, since knowledge is generally not available to conscious access and retrieval, and informationally encapsulated, given that it operates rigidly, without being influenced by other mental systems. For what concerns the network of brain structures underlying this system, a fundamental role is carried out by the frontal/basal ganglia circuits, the parietal cortex, the superior temporal cortex and the cerebellum. Importantly, the basal ganglia are closely linked to the cortical regions and in particular to the frontal area, comprising Broca's area and the pre-motor cortex.

Conversely, the Declarative Memory System subserves the learning, representation and use of semantic knowledge (i.e. the information about facts), and episodic knowledge (i.e. the information about events). It is crucially involved in the acquisition of arbitrary relations between different pieces of information. Learning in this system is very rapid, since it can be based on a single stimulus presentation. Differently from the Procedural Memory System, the Declarative Memory System is defined as explicit, since knowledge can be, at least in part, consciously accessed, and is not informationally encapsulated, given that it can be accessible to other mental systems.

From a neurological point of view, declarative memory is served by the medial temporal lobe structures, comprising the hippocampus, the entorhinal cortex, the perirhinal cortex and the parahippocampal cortex.

Analyzing the peculiarities of these two memory systems, Ullman suggests that a similar subdivision can be extended to language, with mental grammar corresponding to the Procedural System and mental lexicon to the Declarative System. In this perspective, then, the learning and the use of the rules making part of grammar, including syntax, (regular) morphology and possibly non-lexical semantics, depend on procedural memory: knowledge is indeed implicit and, once acquired, it operates automatically.

The brain system that underlies declarative memory, instead, serves also the mental lexicon, which stores arbitrary word-specific knowledge, including both phonological and semantic information of words. Moreover, it is involved with the acquisition of idiosyncratic items, such as the irregular and unpredictable forms that a word may take (e.g. plurals, past tenses…). In Ullman's Declarative/Procedural Model, the two systems are supposed to be independent but to interact dynamically.

It is important to emphasize that the distinction between the two systems does not replace the concept of Working Memory, which instead plays a crucial and independent role, being concerned with retrieval processes in both declarative and procedural memory. Furthermore, Ullman and Pierpont (2005) observe that Working Memory is strongly linked to the Procedural System from a neurological point of view, since they depend on the same brain structures.

Adopting Ullman's perspective, Nicolson and Fawcett (2008) tentatively propose that dyslexia is caused by an impairment affecting the Procedural Memory System, which is responsible for automatization deficits as well as for the problems manifested by dyslexics in activities requiring the learning of sequences of procedures. Their

Declarative Memory System, instead, is supposed to be spared and available for "conscious compensation" strategies. Resorting to Ullman's Model, Nicolson and Fawcett (2008) implement the Cerebellar Deficit Hypothesis in order to account for language problems, beyond dyslexics' motor deficits (due to the involvement of the cerebellum in the Procedural Memory System), phonological disorders (which involve the learning of precise rules and procedures) and automatization difficulties.

Based on these considerations, they propose an outline definition of dyslexia, which is reported below.

> Developmental Dyslexia is one of the developmental disorders characterized by impaired functioning of the procedural learning system. The key diagnostic factor is impaired procedural learning in language areas, leading to specific difficulties in reading, writing and spelling. Early problems will emerge in terms of implicit awareness of phonological rules, but problems will also arise in learning other nonexplicit linguistic regularities, including orthography and morphology. Phonological difficulties, motor difficulties, automatization difficulties, and early speech difficulties frequently occur in dyslexia, but these are not defining characteristics of the disorder. Children with dyslexia will normally show a dissociation between aspects of their procedural learning and those of their declarative learning.
>
> (Nicolson and Fawcett 2008: 222)

As the reader may have noticed, this account involves an important prediction, as it assumes that dyslexics are impaired in all the abilities governed by the Procedural Memory System, whereas they are unimpaired in all the activities that depend on the Declarative Memory System. Crucially, if we consider language from this perspective, the mental grammar is expected to be impaired, while the mental lexicon is supposed to be spared.

In the following section, I will try to identify both commonalities and differences between the Phonological and Executive Working Memory Deficit Hypothesis and the Cerebellar Deficit Hypothesis as formulated by Nicolson and colleagues (1995, 1999, 2001) and subsequently implemented by Nicolson and Fawcett (2008) by resorting to Ullman's Declarative/Procedural Model.

3. The Phonological and Executive Working Memory Deficit Hypothesis and the Cerebellar Deficit Hypothesis: A comparison between the two hypotheses

As we observed in the previous sections, Nicolson and Fawcett proposed a new account for developmental dyslexia, the Cerebellar Deficit Hypothesis, according to which dyslexics suffer from a cerebellar impairment causing an automatization deficit responsible for their difficulties in performing complex tasks. More recently, they further implemented their theory, adopting the Declarative/Procedural Model developed by Ullman and identifying dyslexia as a disorder affecting procedural learning. According to this proposal, dyslexics' inability to automatize skills and procedures causes phonological and motor problems, as well as difficulties in reading, spelling and writing and, more generally, in all activities requiring sequences of operations.

The Phonological and Executive Working Memory Deficit Hypothesis and Nicolson and Fawcett (2008)'s account present an important similarity: both theories predict that dyslexics' difficulties will be more evident in complex tasks, imposing a high load in terms of processing resources. Moreover, both proposals argue that a sort of compensation is possible, through the individuation and employment of alternative strategies to bypass difficulties.

However, there is also a fundamental difference between the two hypotheses for what concerns the role of Working Memory in dyslexia. The Phonological and Executive Working Memory Deficit Hypothesis argues indeed that Working Memory, and in particular the Phonological Loop and the Central Executive, is disrupted in dyslexic individuals, and proposes that this impairment is responsible for the deficits experienced by affected individuals in phonological tasks and in those processes that are expensive in terms of memory resources. The Cerebellar Deficit Hypothesis, instead, proposes a different concept of Working Memory: as discussed above, the authors seem to conceive of Working Memory as simply associated with the Phonological Loop, without focusing on the role played by the Central Executive in language comprehension. Moreover, having adopted Ullman's model, Nicolson and Fawcett argue that dyslexics do not fail in the interpretation of complex structures because of a limited Working Memory capacity, but rather due to a procedural deficit preventing them from automatising skills and increasing the load imposed on their WM. In other words, dyslexics do not fail in complex tasks because their WM is impaired or less efficient, but rather because it is overloaded.

Nevertheless, as the reader may have observed, such a prediction is challenged by the results of a number of experimental protocols, as the one discussed in Chapter 3, showing that dyslexics' Central Executive is indeed severely impaired. Considering the nature of the tasks administered, namely the Listening Recall, the Counting Recall and the Backward Digit Recall, it cannot be argued that controls performed better because of their higher automaticity skills and without postulating a difference in the processing efficiency between the two groups.

Moreover, the grammatical deficits exhibited by dyslexics cannot be completely accounted for by Nicolson and Fawcett (2008)'s proposal. It is not plausible, in fact, that higher automaticity skills are responsible for controls' better performance in the computation of scalar implicatures, as well as in the resolution of zero pronouns and phonetically realized pronouns. As discussed in Chapter 5, in fact, the computation of implicatures is not at all automatic, but it is rather determined by the context.

Summarizing, although further studies are required to investigate more thoroughly the relationship between the two proposals at stake, it seems that the Phonological and Executive Working Memory Deficit Hypothesis is able to provide a better account for the whole range of deficits shown by dyslexic individuals. On the other hand, it would be very interesting to analyze the role of automaticity in dyslexia, and to verify if the two hypotheses can be, at least to some extent, combined together.

4. Summary and Conclusions

In this last chapter, I have summarized the arguments and considerations put forward in this volume. Specifically, I have argued that the main manifestations of dyslexia discussed in Chapter 1 cannot be successfully accounted for by the theories developed in the last decades.

For this reason, I have proposed a new hypothesis, the Phonological and Executive Working Memory Deficit Hypothesis, arguing that dyslexics' difficulties arise from an impairment affecting their phonological memory and their executive functions.

I have shown, in fact, that the Phonological and Executive Working Memory Deficit Hypothesis is able to account for:

(i) Reading deficits;
(ii) Spelling deficits;
(iii) Phonological deficits;
(iv) Vocabulary and naming speed deficits;
(v) Grammatical deficits;
(vi) Attention Deficits.

After explaining how this proposal is able to capture the whole range of deficits experienced by dyslexic individuals, I have proposed a new definition of developmental dyslexia, which focuses precisely on the central role played by Working Memory in this disorder.

Finally, I have compared my hypothesis with the Cerebellar Deficit Hypothesis proposed by Nicolson and colleagues (1995) and subsequently implemented by Nicolson and Fawcett (2008) by adopting Ullman's Declarative/Procedural Model. As observed above, this proposal claims that dyslexics suffer from an automatization deficit, preventing them from automatising skills and forcing them to resort to conscious compensations strategies in order to overcome their difficulties.

Although I have observed that the Phonological and Executive Working Memory Deficit Hypothesis and the Cerebellar Deficit Hypothesis present important commonalities, predicting that dyslexics' problems increase proportionally to the complexity of the tasks, I have noticed that they differ in some important respects. Specifically, the Cerebellar Deficit Hypothesis, as formulated at present, is not able to adequately explain the naming speed deficits and part of the grammatical problems shown by dyslexic individuals. However, further studies are required to better investigate the relationship between the two proposals and to analyze the role of automaticity in dyslexia.

To conclude, I would like to emphasize that the hypothesis put forward in this dissertation does not pretend to solve all the problems that have been discussed as to the nature of dyslexia, but rather it aspires to offer new perspectives and to show new directions for future research. I am, in fact, firmly convinced that further important steps can be made in the research on dyslexia, and that new findings and proposals will finally permit to develop more efficient tools for diagnosis and remediation programs, offering at the same time important contributions to research on other learning disabilities and, more generally, on language acquisition, production and comprehension.

> The doubter is a true man of science; he doubts only himself and his interpretations, but he believes in science.
>
> Claude Bernard

References

Adlard, A. / Hazan, V. 1997. Speech perception in children with specific reading difficulties (dyslexia). *Quarterly Journal of Experimental Psychology*, 51, 152–177.

Almor, A. / Kempler, D. / MacDonald M. C. / Andersen, E. S. / Tyler, L. K. 1999. Why do Alzheimer Patients have difficulty with pronouns? Working Memory, semantics, and reference in comprehension and production in Alzheimer's Disease. *Brain and Language*, 67, 202–227.

Aquinas, T., Saint 1496. *Expositio super libros Posteriorum et De Interpretatione Aristotelis*. Completed by Thomas Caietanus. Venice: Otinus de Cuna, for Alexander Calcedonius.

Araùjo, S. / Faìsca, L. / Bramao, I. / Petersson, K. M. / Reis, A. (2014). Lexical and Phonological Processes in Dyslexic Readers: Evidence from a Visual Lexical Decision Task. *Dyslexia*, 20, 18–53.

Ariel, M. 1990. *Accessing noun phrases antecedents*. London: Routledge.

Ariel, M. 1991. The function of accessibility in a theory of grammar. *Journal of Pragmatics*, 16, 443–463.

Ariel, M. 1994. Interpreting anaphoric expressions: a cognitive versus a pragmatic approach. *Journal of Linguistics*, 30, 3–42.

Ariel, M. 2001. Accessibility Theory: an overview. In T. Sanders, J. Schlipperoord / W. Spooren (eds.), *Text representation*. Amsterdam, Philadelphia: John Benjamins.

Aristotle 1961. *Works*. W. D. Ross, trans. London: Oxford University Press.

Asbjornsen, A. / Bryden, M. 1998. Auditory attentional shifts in reading-disabled students: quantification of attention effectiveness by the Attentional Shift Index. *Neuropsychologia*, 36, 143–148.

Atkinson, R. C. / Shiffrin, R. M. 1968. Human memory: A proposed system and its control processes. In K. W. Spence / J. T. Spence (eds.), *The psychology of learning and motivation*. New York: Academic Press.

Avrutin, S. / Wexler, K. 1992. Development of principle B in Russian: Coindexation at LF and coreference. *Language Acquisition*, 2, 259–306.

Baddeley, A. D. 1966. The influence of acoustic and semantic similarity on long-term memory for word sequences. *Quarterly Journal of Experimental Psychology*, 18, 302–309.

Baddeley, A. D. 1968. How does acoustic similarity influence short-term memory? *Quarterly Journal of Psychology,* 20, 249–264.

Baddeley, A. D. 1986. *Working memory*. Oxford: Oxford University Press.

Baddeley, A. D. 1992. Working memory. *Science*, 31, 556–559.

Baddeley, A. D. 1996. Exploring the central executive. *Quarterly Journal of Experimental Psychology*, 49, 5–28.

Baddeley, A. D. 1999. *Essentials of Human Memory*. Hove: Psychology Press.

Baddeley, A. D. 2000. The episodic buffer: a new component of working memory? *Trends in Cognitive Science*, 4, 417–423.

Baddeley A. D. 2002a. Is working memory still working? *European Psychologist*, 7, 85–97.

Baddeley, A. D. 2002b. The psychology of memory. In Baddeley, A. D. / Wilson, B. A. / Kopelma, M. (eds.), *Handbook of Memory Disorders*, 2nd Edition. Hove: Psychology Press.

Baddeley, A. D. 2003a. Working memory and language: An overview. *Journal of Communication Disorders*, 36, 189–208.

Baddeley, A. D. 2003b. Working Memory: Looking back and looking forward. *Nature Reviews Neuroscience*, 4, 829–839.

Baddeley, A. D. 2007. *Working memory, thought and action*. Oxford: Oxford University Press.

Baddeley, A. D. / Baddeley, H. / Wilcock, G. K. / Bucks, R. 2001. Attentional control in Alzheimer's disease. *Brain*, 124, 1492–1508.

Baddeley, A. D. / Bressi, S. / Della Sala, S. / Logie, R. / Spinnler, H. 1991. The decline of working memory in Alzheimer's disease: A longitudinal study. *Brain,* 114, 2521–2542.

Baddeley, A. D. / Gathercole, S. / Papagno, C. 1998. The phonological loop as a language learning device. *Psychological Review*, 105, 158–173.

Baddeley, A. D. / Hitch, G. J. 1974. Working memory. In Bower, G. A. (ed.), *The Psychology of Learning and Motivation*. New York: Academic Press.

Baddeley, A. D. / Jarrold, C. 2007. Working memory and Down Syndrome. *Journal of Intellectual Disability Research*, 51, 925–931.

Baddeley, A. D. / Lewis, V. J. / Vallar, G. 1984. Exploring the articulatory loop. *Quarterly Journal of Experimental Psychology*, 36, 233– 252.

Baddeley, A.D. / Logie, R. 1999. Working memory: The multiple component model. In Miyake, A. / Shah, P. (eds.), *Models of working memory*. New York: Cambridge University Press.

Baddeley, A. D. / Thomson, N. / Buchanan, M. 1975. Word length and the structure of short-term memory. *Journal of Verbal Learning and Verbal Behavior*, 14, 575–589.

Bar-Shalom, E. / Crain, S. / Shankweiler, D. 1993. Comparison of comprehension and production in good and poor readers. *Applied Psycholinguistics*, 14, 197–227.

Beaton, A. A. 2004. Dyslexia, reading and the brain: A sourcebook of psychological and biological research. New York: Psychology Press.

Beneventi, H. / Tonnessen, F. E. / Ersland, L. / Hugdahl, K. 2010. Executive working memory processes in dyslexia: Behavioral and fMRI evidence. *Scandinavian Journal of Psychology*, 51, 192–202.

Benton, A. L 1991. The prefrontal region: Its early history. In Levin, H. S. / Eisenberg, H. M. / Benton, A. L., *Frontal lobe function and dysfunction*. New York: Oxford University Press.

Bishop, D. V. M. 1991. Developmental reading disabilities: the role of phonological processing has been overemphasised. *Mind and Language*, 6, 97–101.

Bishop, D. V. M. / North, T. / Donlan, C. 1996. Nonword repetition as a phenotypic marker for inherited language impairment: Evidence from a twin study. *Journal of Child Psychology and Psychiatry*, 37, 391–342.

Bishop, D. V. M. / Robson, J. 1989. Unimpaired short-term memory and rhyme judgment in congenitally speechless individuals: Implications for the notion of "Articulatory Coding". *Quarterly Journal of Experimental Psychology*, 41, 123–140.

Blachman, B. A. 1994. Early literacy acquisition – the role of phonological awareness. In Wallach, G. / Butler, K. (eds.), *Language learning disabilities in schoolage children and adolescents: Some underlying principles and applications*. Columbus, OH: Merrill.

Blachman, B. A. 1997. *Foundations of reading acquisition and dyslexia*. Mahwah, NJ: Lawrence Erlbaum.

Blachman, B. A. 2000. Phonological awareness. In Kamil, M. L./ Mosenthal, P. B. / Pearson, P. D. / Barr, R. (eds.), *Handbook of reading research*. Mahwah, NJ: Lawrence Erlbaum.

Bott, L. / Noveck, I. A. 2004. Some utterances are underinformative: the onset and time course of scalar inferences. *Journal of Memory and Language*, 51, 437–457.

Bourassa, D. / Treiman, R. 2003. Spelling in Children With Dyslexia: Analyses From the Treiman–Bourassa Early Spelling Test. *Scientific Studies of Reading*, 4, 309–333.

Bowers, P. G. / Kennedy, A. 1993. Effects of naming speed differences on fluency of reading after practice. *Annals of the New York Academy of Sciences*, 682, 318–320.

Bowers, P. G. / Swanson, L. B. 1991. Naming speed deficits in reading disability: Multiple measures of a singular process. *Journal of Experimental Child Psychology,* 51, 195–219.

Bowey, J. A. 1994. Phonological sensitivity in novice readers and non-readers. *Journal of Experimental Child Psychology*, 58, 134–159.

Brady, S. A., Shankweiler, D. and Mann, V. 1983. Speech perception and memory coding in relation to reading ability. *Journal of Experimental Child Psychology*, 35, 345–367.

Braine, M. / Rumain, B. 1981. Children's comprehension of "or": evidence for a sequence of competencies. *Journal of Experimental Child Psychology*, 31, 46–70.

de Bree, E., 2007. Dyslexia and Phonology: A study of the phonological abilities of Dutch children at-risk of dyslexia. Doctoral dissertation. Utrecht Institute for Linguistics OTS. LOT Series.

Breheny R. / Katsos N. / Williams J. 2006. Are scalar implicatures generated by default? *Cognition*, 100, 434–463.

Broom, Y. V. / Doctor, E. A. 1995. Developmental phonological dyslexia: a case study of the efficacy of a remediation programme. *Cognitive Neuropsychology*, 12, 725–766.

Bruck, M. / Treiman R. 1990. Phonological awareness and spelling in normal children and dyslexics: the case of initial consonant cluster. *Journal of Experimental Psychology,* 50, 156–178.

Brunswick, N. / McCroy, E. / Price, C. J. / Frith, C. D. / Frith, U. 1999. Explicit and implicit processing of words and pseudowords by adult developmental dyslexics. *Brain*, 122, 1901–1917.

Bus, A. G. / van Ijzendoorn, M. H. 1999. Phonological awareness and early reading: a meta analysis of experimental training studies. *Journal of Educational Psychology*, 91, 403–414.

Byrne, B. (1981). Deficient syntactic control in poor readers: Is a weak phonetic memory code responsible? *Applied Psycholinguistics* 2, 201–212.

Caplan, D. / Waters, G. S. 1996. Syntactic processing in sentence comprehension under dual-task conditions in aphasic patients. *Language and Cognitive Processes*, 11, 525–551.

Caplan, D. / Waters, G. S. 1999. Verbal working memory and sentence comprehension. *Brain and Behavioral Sciences*, 22, 77–126.

Caravolas, M. / Hulme, C. / Snowling, M. J. 2001. The foundations of spelling ability: evidence from a 3-year longitudinal study. *Journal of Memory and Language*, 45, 751–774.

Cardinaletti, A. / Volpato, F. 2015. On the comprehension and production of passive and relative clauses by dyslexic University students. In Di Domenico, E. / Hamann, C. / Matteini, S. (a cura di), *Structures, Strategies and Beyond. Studies in Honour of Adriana Belletti*, Amsterdam/Philadelphia, Benjamins, 279–301.

Carpenter, P. A. / Just, M. A. 1975. Sentence comprehension: a psycholinguistic processing model of verification. *Psychological Review,* 82, 45–73.

Carston, R. 1998. Informativeness, relevance and scalar implicature. In R. Carson S. Uchida (eds.), *Relevance Theory: Applications and Implications*. Amsterdam: John Benjamins.

Casalini, C. / Brizzolara, D. / Chilosi, A. / Cipriani, P. / Marcolini, S. / Pecini, C. / Roncoli, S. / Burani, C. 2007. Non-Word Repetition in Children with Specific Language Impairment: A Deficit in Phonological Working Memory or in Long-Term Verbal Knowledge? *Cortex*, 43, 769–776.

Casco, C. / Ressoldi, P. / Dellantonio, A. 1998. Visual selective attention and reading efficiency are related in children. *Cortex*, 34, 531–546.

Chase, W. G. / Clark, H. H. 1972. Mental operations in the comparison of sentences and pictures. In Gregg, L. (ed.), *Cognition in Learning and Memory*. New York: Wiley.

Chien, Y. / Wexler, K. 1990. Children's Knowledge of Locality Conditions in Binding as Evidence for the Modularity of Syntax and Pragmatics, *Language Acquisition*, 1, 225–295.

Chierchia, G. / Crain, S. / Guasti, M. T. / Gualmini, A. / Meroni, L. 2001. The acquisition of disjunction: evidence for a grammatical view of scalar implicatures. *Proceedings of the 25th Boston University Conference on Language Development*, Somerville, MA: Cascadilla Press.

Chierchia, G. 2004. Scalar Implicatures, Polarity Phenomena and the Syntax/Pragmatics Interface. In Belletti, A. (ed.), *Structures and Beyond*. Oxford: Oxford University Press.

Chomsky, C. 1969. The acquisition of syntax in children from 5 to 10. Cambridge, MA: MIT Press.

Chomsky, N. 1980. On binding. *Linguistic Inquiry*, 11, 1–46.

Chomsky, N. 1981. *Lectures on Government and Binding*. Dordrecht: Foris.

Clark, H. H. / Chase, W. G. 1972. On the process of comparing sentences against pictures. *Cognitive Psychology*, 3, 472–517.

Colle, H. A. / Welsh, A. 1976. Acoustic masking in primary memory. *Journal of Verbal Learning and Verbal Behavior*, 15, 17–31.

Coltheart, M. 1985. Cognitive neuropsychology and the study of reading. In Posner M. I. and Marin O. S. M. (eds.), *Attention and Performance XI*. Hillsdale, NJ: Lawrence Erlbaum Associates Inc.

Coltheart, M. 1986. Graphemics and visual word recognition. In Augst, G. (ed.), *New Trends in Graphemics and Orthography*. Berlin: de Gruyter.

Coltheart, M. / Rastle K. / Perry C., Langdon R. / Ziegler J. 2001. DRC: A dual route cascaded model of visual word recognition and reading aloud. *Psychological Review*, 108, 204–256.

Conrad, R. / Hull, A. J. 1964. Information, acoustic confusion and memory span. *British Journal of Psychology*, 55, 429–432.

Cornish, E. R. / Wason, P. C. 1970. The recall of affirmative and negative sentences in an incidental learning task. *Quarterly Journal of Experimental Psychology,* 22, 109–114.
Cowan, N. / Kail, R. 1996. Covert processes and their development in short-term memory. In Gathercole, S. E. (ed.), *Models of short-term memory.* Hove, England: Psychology Press.
Cromer, R. F. 1970. Children are nice to understand: surface structures clues for the recovery of a deep structure. *British Journal of Psychology*, 61, 397–408.
Cubelli, R. / Nichelli, P. 1992. Inner speech in anarthria: neuropsychological evidence of differential effects of cerebral lesions on subvocal articulation. *Journal of Clinical and Experimental Neuropsychology,* 14, 499–517.
Daneman, M. / Carpenter, J. A. 1980. Individual differences in working memory and reading. *Journal of Verbal Learning and Verbal Behavior,* 19, 450–466.
Delfitto, D. 2002. *Genericity in language. Issues in Syntax, Logical Form and Interpretation*. Alessandria: Edizioni dell'Orso.
Delfitto, D. 2004. On the logical form of the imperfective aspect. In Géuron, J. and Lecarne, J. (eds.), *The syntax of tense*, 115–142, Cambridge, MA: MIT Press.
Della Sala, S. / Gray, C. / Baddeley, A.D. / Allamano, N. / Wilson, L. 1999. Pattern span: A tool for unwelding visuo-spatial memory. *Neuropsychologia*, 37, 1189–1199.
Denckla, M. B. 1972. Color-naming defects in dyslexic boys. *Cortex*, 8, 164–176.
Denckla, M. B. 1985. Motor coordination in dyslexic children: theoretical and clinical implications. In Duffy, F. H. / Geschwind, N. (eds.), *Dyslexia: a neuroscientific approach to clinical evaluation*. Boston, MA: Little, Brown, & Co.
Denckla, M. B. / Rudel, R. G. 1976a. Naming of objects by dyslexic and other learning-disabled children. *Brain and Language*, 3, 1–15.
Denckla, M. B. / Rudel, R. G. 1976b. Naming of object-drawings by dyslexic and other learning disabled children. *Brain and Language*, 3, 1–15.

Desmond, J. E. / Fiez, J. A. 1998. Neuroimaging studies of the cerebellum: Language, learning and memory. *Trends in Cognitive Sciences*, 2, 355–362.

Desroches, A. S. / Joanisse, M. F. / Robertson, E. K. 2006. Specific phonological impairments in dyslexia revealed by eyetracking. *Cognition*, 100, 32–42.

Dispaldro, M. / Leonard, L. B. / Deevy, P. 2011. Real-Word and Non-word Repetition in Italian-Speaking Children With Specific Language Impairment: A Study of Diagnostic Accuracy. *Journal of Speech, Language and Hearing Research*, 56, 323–336.

Ehri, L. C. 1991. The development of reading and spelling in children: An overview. In Snowling, M. J. and Thomson, M. (eds.), *Dyslexia: Integrating theory and practice*. London: Whurr.

Ehri, L. C. 1997. Learning to read and to spell are one and the same, almost. In Perfetti, C. A. / Rieben, L. / Fayol, M. (eds.), *Learning to Spell: Research, Theory and Practice across Languages*. Mahwah, NJ: Lawrence Erlbaum Associates Inc.

Elbro, C. 1996. Early linguistic abilities and reading development: a review and a hypothesis. *Reading and Writing: An Interdisciplinary Journal*, 8, 453–485.

Elbro, C. 1997. Early linguistic abilities and reading development: A review and a hypothesis about underlying differences in distinctiveness of phonological representations of lexical items. *Reading and Writing*, 8, 453–485.

Ellis, N. C. / Hennelley, R. A. 1980. A bilingual word-length effect: Implications for intelligence testing and the relative ease of mental calculation in Welsh and English. *British Journal of Psychology*, 50, 449–458.

Ellis, N. C. / Sinclair, S. G. 1996. Working memory in the acquisition of vocabulary and syntax: Putting language in a good order. *The Quarterly Journal of Experimental Psychology*, 49, 234–250.

Evans, B. J. W. / Drasdo, N. / Richards, I. L. 1994. An investigation of some sensory and refractive visual factors in dyslexia. *Vision Research*, 34, 1913–1926.

Everatt, J. / Turner, J. / Miles, T. R. 1997. The incidence of Stroop Interference in Dyslexia. *Dyslexia*, 3, 222–228.

Facoetti, A. / Paganoni, P. / Lorusso, M. L. 2000. The spatial distribution of visual attention in developmental dyslexia. *Experimental Brain Research*, 132, 531–538.

Fawcett, A. J. / Nicolson, R. I. 1992. Automatization Deficits in Balance for Dyslexic Children. *Perceptual and Motor Skills*, 75, 507–529.

Fawcett, A. J. / Nicolson, R. I. 1994. Naming speed in children with dyslexia. *Journal of Learning Disabilities*, 27, 641–646.

Fawcett, A. J. / Nicolson, R. I. 1995. Persistent deficits in motor skill for children with dyslexia. *Journal of Motor Behavior*, 27, 235–241.

Fedorenko, E. / Gibson, E. / Rohde, D. 2006. The nature of working memory capacity in sentence comprehension: Evidence against domain-specific resources. *Journal of Memory and Language*, 54, 541–553.

Fedorenko, E. / Gibson, E. / Rohde, D. 2007. The nature of working memory in linguistic, arithmetic and spatial integration processes. *Journal of Memory and Language*, 56, 246–269.

Felton, R. H. / Naylor, C. E. / Wood, F. B. 1990. Neuropsychological profile of adult dyslexics. *Brain and Language*, 39, 485–497.

Ferreira, E. / Clifton, C. 1986. The independence of syntactic processing. *Journal of Memory and Language*, 25, 348–368.

Fiorin, G. / Vender, M. 2009. The interpretation of pronominal expressions in developmental dyslexia. *Proceedings of the 1st Patras International Conference of Graduate Students in Linguistics,* University of Patras, Patras, 64–74.

Fiorin, G. 2009. The interpretation of imperfective aspect in developmental dyslexia. *Proceedings of the 2nd International Clinical Linguistics Conference*, Universidad Autónoma de Madrid, Universidad Nacional de Educación a Distancia and Euphonia Ediciones.

Fiorin, G. 2010. *Meaning and dyslexia: a study on pronouns, aspect and quantification*. Doctoral dissertation. Utrecht Institute for Linguistics OTS. LOT Series.

Fowler, A. E. 1991. How early phonological development might set the stage for phoneme awareness. In Brady, S. A. / Shankweiler, D. P. (eds.), *Phonological processes in literacy: a tribute to Isabelle Y. Liberman*. Hillsdale, NJ: Lawrence Erlbaum Associates Inc.

Frank, J. / Levinson, H. N. 1973. Dysmetric dyslexia and dyspraxia: Hypothesis and study. *Journal of American Academy of Child Psychiatry*, 12, 690–701.

Frege, G. 1892. Über Sinn und Bedeutung. *Zeitschrift für Philosophie und philosophische Kritik*, 100, 25–50.

Frith, U. 1986. A developmental framework for developmental dyslexia. *Annals of Dyslexia,* 36, 69–81.

Frith, U. 1999. Paradoxes in the definition of dyslexia. *Dyslexia*, 5, 192–214.

Fry, A. F. / Hale, S. 1996. Processing speed, working memory, and fluid intelligence: evidence for a developmental cascade. *Psychological Science*, 7, 237–241.

Fry, A. F. / Hale, S. 2000. Relationship among processing speed, working memory, and fluid intelligence in children. *Biological Psychology*, 54, 1–34.

Fry, M. A. / Johnson, C. S. / Muehl, S. 1970. Oral language production in relation to reading achievement among select second graders. In Bakker, D. J. / Satz, P. (eds.), *Specific reading disability: advances in theory and method.* Rotterdam: Rotterdam University Press.

Fulbright, R. K. / Jenner, A. R. / Mencl, W. E. / Pugh, K. R. / Shaywitz, B. A. / Shaywitz, S. E. 1999. The cerebellum's role in reading: A functional MR imaging study. *American Journal of Neuroradiology*, 20, 1925–1930.

Gahni, K. A. / Gathercole, S. E. 2013. Working memory and study skills: a comparison between dyslexic and non-dyslexic adult learners. *Procedia – Social and Behavioral Sciences*, 97, 271–277.

Galaburda, A. M. / Kemper, T. L. 1979. Cytoarchitectonic abnormalities in developmental dyslexia: a case study. *Annals of Neurology*, 6, 94–100.

Galaburda, A. M. / Sherman, G. F. / Rosen, G. D. / Aboitiz, F. / Geschwind, N. 1985. Developmental dyslexia: four consecutive patients with cortical anomalies. *Annals of Neurology*, 18, 222–233.

Gathercole, S. E. 1995. Is nonword repetition a test of phonological memory or long-term knowledge? It all depends on the nonwords. *Memory & Cognition*, 23, 83–94.

Gathercole, S. E. 1999. Cognitive approaches to the development of short-term memory. *Trends in Cognitive Science*, 3, 410–418.

Gathercole, S. E. / Adams, A. M. 1993. Phonological working memory in very young children. *Developmental Psychology*, 29, 770–778.

Gathercole, S. E. / Alloway T. P. 2006. Practitioner Review: Short-term and working memory impairments in neurodevelopmental disorders: diagnosis and remedial support. *Journal of Child Psychology and Psychiatry*, 47, 1, 4–15.

Gathercole, S. E. / Alloway, T. P. / Willis, C. / Adams, A. M. 2006. Working memory in children with reading disabilities. *Journal of Experimental Child Psychology*, 93, 265–281.

Gathercole, S. E. / Alloway, T. P. / Kirkwood, H. J. / Elliott, J. G. / Holmes, J. / Hilton, K. A. 2008. Attentional and executive function behaviours of children with poor working memory. *Learning and Individual Differences*, 18, 214–223.

Gathercole, S. E. / Alloway, T. P. / Willis, C. / Adams A. M. 2006. Working memory in children with reading disabilities. *Journal of Experimental Child Psychology*, 93, 265–281.

Gathercole, S. E. / Baddeley, A. D. 1993. *Working Memory and Language*. Hillsdale, New Jersey: Lawrence Erlbaum Associates Inc.

Gathercole, S. E. / Baddeley, A. D. 1990. Phonological memory deficits in language disordered children: Is there a causal connection? *Journal of Memory and Language*, 29, 336–360.

Gathercole, S. E. / Hitch, G. 1993. Developmental Changes in Short-Term Memory: A Revised Working Memory Perspective. In Collins, A. F. / Gathercole, S. E. / Conway, M. A. / Morris, P. E. (eds.), *Theories of Memory*. Hillsdale, New Jersey: Lawrence Erlbaum Associates Inc.

Gathercole, S. E. / Pickering, S. J. / Ambridge, B. / Wearing, H. 2004. The structure of working memory from 4 to 15 years of age. *Developmental Psychology*, 40, 177–190.

Gathercole, S. E. / Willis, C. / Emslie, H. / Baddeley, A. D. 1992. Phonological memory and vocabulary development during the early school years: A longitudinal study. *Developmental Psychology*, 28, 887–898.

Gayan, J. / Olson, R. K. 1999. Reading disability: Evidence for a genetic etiology. *European Child & Adolescent Psychiatry*, 8, 52–55.

Gazdar, G. 1979. Pragmatics: Implicature, presupposition, and logical form. New York: Academic Press.

Geary, D. C. / Hoard, M. K. / Byrd-Craven, J. / De Soto, M. C. 2004. Strategy choices in simple and complex addition: Contributions of working memory and counting knowledge for children with mathematical disability. *Journal of Experimental Child Psychology*, 88, 121–151.

de Gelder, B. / Vrooman, J. 1991. Phonological deficits: Beneath the surface of reading acquisition. *Psychological Review,* 53, 88–97.

Gibson, E. 1991. A computational Theory of Human Linguistic Processing: Memory Limitations and Processing Breakdown. Doctoral Dissertation. Carnegie Mellon University, Pittsburgh, P. A.

Gibson, E. 1998. Linguistic complexity: Locality of syntactic dependencies. *Cognition*, 68, 1–76.

Givón, T. 1978. Negation in language: pragmatics, function, ontology. In Cole P. (ed.), *Syntax and Semantics 9: Pragmatics*. New York: Academic Press.

Glenberg, A. M. / Robertson, D. A. / Jansen, J. L. / Johnson-Glenberg, M. C. 1999. Not propositions. *Journal of Cognitive System Research*, 1, 19–33.

Gordon, P. C. / Hendrick, R. / Levine, W. H. 2002. Memory load interference in syntactic processing. *Psychological Science*, 13, 425–430.

Gough, P. B. 1965. Grammatical transformations and speed of understanding. *Journal of Verbal Learning and Verbal Behavior*, 5, 107–111.

Gough, P. B. 1966. The verification of sentences: the effects of delay of evidence and sentence length. *Journal of Verbal Learning and Verbal Behavior*, 5, 492–496.

Greenberg, J. 1966. Language universals, with special reference to feature hierarchies. The Hague: Mouton.

Grice, H. P. 1975. Logic and conversation. In Cole P. and Morgan J. (eds.), *Syntax and semantics 3: Speech acts*. Academic Press: New York.

Grodzinsky, Y. / Reinhart, T. 1993. The innateness of binding and coreference. *Linguistic Inquiry*, 24, 69–101.

Gross-Glenn, K. / Jallad, B. / Novoa, L. / Helgren-Lempesis, V. / Lubs, H. A. 1990. Nonsense passage reading as a diagnostic aid in the study of familial dyslexia. *Reading and Writing*, 2, 161–174.

Gualmini, A. / Crain, S. / Meroni, L. / Chierchia, G. / Guasti, M. T. 2001. At the semantics/pragmatics interface in child language, *Proceedings of Semantics and Linguistic Theory,* 11, 231–247, Cornell University, Ithaca, NY.

Guasti, M. T. / Branchini, Ch. / Vernice, M. / Barbieri, L. / Arosio, F. 2015, *Language disorders in children with Developmental Dyslexia*, Specific Language Impairment. Current trends in research, Amsterdam, John Benjamins Publishing Company, 35–55.

Hall, J. W. / Wilson, K. P. / Humphreys, M. S. / Tinzmann, M. B. / Bowyer, P. M. 1983. Phonemic-similarity effects in good vs. poor readers. *Memory and Cognition*, 11, 520–527.

Hari, R. / Valta, M. / Uutela, K. 1999. Prolonged attentional dwell time in dyslexics adults. *Neuroscience Letters*, 271, 202–204.

Haslum, M. N. 1989. Predictors of dyslexia? *Irish Journal of Psychology*, 10, 622–630.

Hasson, U. / Glucksberg, S. 2006. Does understanding negation entail affirmation? *Journal of Pragmatics*, 38, 1015–1032.

Heiervang, E. / Stevenson, J. / Lund, A. / Hugdahl, K. 2001. Behaviour problems in children with dyslexia. *Nordic Journal of Psychiatry*, 55, 251–256.

Helland, T. / Asbjornsen, A. 2004. Digit span in dyslexia: Variations according to language comprehension and mathematics skills. *Journal of Clinical and Experimental Neuropsychology*, 26, 31–42.

Hinshelwood, J. 1895. Word-blindness and visual memory. *The Lancet*, 2, 1564–1570.

Hollebrandse, B. / Van Hout, A. 2001. On the acquisition of the aspects in Italian. In Kim, J. Y. / Werle, A. (eds.), *The Proceedings of SULA: the Semantics of Underrepresented Languages in the Americas.* Amherst: GLSA.

Horn, L. R. 1989. *A natural history of negation*. Chicago: University of Chicago Press.

Horn, L. R. 1996. Presupposition and implicature. In Lappin, S. (ed.), *The Handbook of Contemporary Semantic Theory*. Oxford: Blackwell Publishers.

Houghton G. / Zorzi M. 2003. Normal and impaired spelling in a connectionist dual-route architecture. *Cognitive Neuropsychology*, 20, 115–162.

Hulme, C. 1988. The implausibility of low-level visual deficits as a cause of children's reading difficulties. *Cognitive Neuropsychology, 5*, 369–374.
Hulme, C. / Roodenrys, S. 1995. Practitioner review: verbal working memory development and its disorders. *Journal of Child Psychology and Psychiatry*, 36, 373–398.
Hulme, C. / Thomson, N. / Muir C. / Lawrence A. 1984. Speech rate and the development of short term memory span. *Journal of Experimental Child Psychology*, 43, 35–52.
Hulme, C. / Tordoff V. 1989. Working memory development: The effects of speech rate, word length, and acoustic similarity on serial recall. *Journal of Experimental Child Psychology*, 47, 72–87.
Humphreys, P. / Kaufmann, W. E. / Galaburda, A. M. 1990. Developmental dyslexia in women: Neuropathological findings in three patients. *Annals of Neurology*, 28, 727–738.
Jarrold, C. / Baddeley, A. D. 1997. Short-term memory for verbal and visuo-spatial information in Down's Syndrome. *Cognitive Neuropsychiatry*, 2, 102–122.
Jeffries, S. A. / Everatt J. E. 2003. Differences between dyspraxics and dyslexics in sequence learning and working memory. *Dyspraxia Foundation Professional Journal* 2, 12–21.
Jeffries, S. / Everatt J. E. 2004. Working memory: Its role in dyslexia and other specific learning difficulties. *Dyslexia*, 10, 196–214.
Jiménez, J. E. / Garcìa, E. / Estévez, A. / Dìaz, A. / Guzman R. / Hernandez-Valle, I. / Rosario M. / Rodrigo, M. / Hernandéz, S. 2004. An evaluation of syntactic-semantic processing in developmental dyslexia. *Electronic Journal of Research in Educational Psychology*, 2, 127–142.
Joanisse, M. F. / Manis, F. / Keating, P. / Seidenberg, M. S. 2000. Language deficits in dyslexic children: speech perception, phonology and morphology. *Journal of Experimental Child Psychology*, 77, 30–60.
Johnston, R. S. / Anderson, M. / Holligan, C. 1996. Knowledge of the alphabet and explicit awareness of phonemes in prereaders: the nature of the relationship. *Reading and Writing,* 8, 217–234.

Johnston, R. S. / Rugg, M. / Scott, T. 1987. Phonological similarity effects, memory span and developmental reading disorders: The nature of the relationship. *British Journal of Psychology*, 78, 205–211.

De Jong, P. / Leij, A. van der 1999. Specific contributions of phonological abilities to early reading acquisition: results from a Dutch latent variable longitudinal study. *Journal of Educational Psychology*, 91, 450–475.

Just, M. A. / Carpenter, P. A. 1971. Comprehension of negation with quantification. *Journal of Verbal Learning and Verbal Behavior*, 12, 21–31.

Just, M. A. / Carpenter, P. A. 1992. A capacity theory of comprehension: individual differences in working memory. *Psychological Review*, 99, 122–149.

Just, M. A. / Carpenter, P. A. 2002. A capacity theory of comprehension: individual differences in working memory. In Polk, T. A. / Seifert C.M., *Cognitive Modeling*. Cambridge, MA: MIT Press.

Kane, M. J. / Bleckley, M. K. / Conway, A. R. / Engle, R. W. 2001. A controlled-attention view of working-memory capacity. *Journal of Experimental Psychology: General*, 130, 169–183.

Karttunen, L. 1974. Presupposition and linguistic context. *Theoretical Linguistics,* 1, 181–194.

Katsos, N. / Breheny, R. / Williams, J. 2005. The interaction of structural and contextual constraints during the on-line generation of scalar inferences. In Bara, B. / Barsalou, L. / Bucciarelli (eds.), *Proceedings of the 27th Annual Conference of the Cognitive Science Society*. Mahwah, NJ: Erlbaum.

Kaup, B. 1997. The processing of negatives during discourse comprehension. In Shafto, M. G. / Langley, P. (eds.), *Proceedings of the nineteenth conference of the cognitive science society*, Mahwah, NJ: Erlbaum.

Kaup, B. 2001. Negation and its impact on the accessibility of text information. *Memory and Cognition*, 20, 960–967.

Kaup, B. / Lüdtke, J. / Zwaan, R. A. 2006. Processing negated sentences with contradictory predicates: Is a door that is not open mentally closed? *Journal of Pragmatics*, 38, 1033–1050.

Kaup, B. / Yaxley, R. H. / Madden, C. J. / Zwaan, R. A. / Lüdtke, J. 2007. Experiential simulations of negated text information. *Quarterly Journal of Experimental Psychology*, 60, 976–990.

Kaup, B. / Zwaan, R. A. / Lüdtke, J. 2007. The experiential view of language comprehension: How is negated text information represented? In Schmalhofer, F. / Perfetti, C.A. (eds.), *Higher level language processes in the brain: Inference and comprehension processes*. Mahwah, NJ: Erlbaum.

King, J. / Just, M. A. 1991. Individual differences in syntactic processing: The role of working memory. *Journal of Memory and Language*, 30, 580–602.

Kyllonen, P. C. / Christal, R. E. 1990. Reasoning ability is (little more than) working-memory capacity? *Intelligence*, 14, 389–433.

Ladusaw, W. A. 1996. Negation and polarity items. In Lappin, S. (ed.), *The Handbook of Contemporary Semantic Theory*. Oxford: Blackwell Publishers.

Leech, G. 1981. Pragmatics and conversational rhetoric. In Parrett, H. Sbisà, M. / Verschueren, J. (eds.), *Possibilities and limitations of pragmatics*. Amsterdam: Benjamins.

Leiner, H. C. / Leiner, A. L. / Dow, R. S. 1989. Reappraising the cerebellum: What does the hindbrain contribute to the forebrain. *Behavioural Neuroscience*, 103, 998–1008.

Leiner, H. C. / Leiner, A. L. / Dow, R. S. 1991. The human cerebro-cerebellar system: Its computing, cognitive and language skills. *Behavioral Brain Research*, 44, 113–128.

Leonard, L. 1998. *Children with specific language impairment*. Cambridge, MA: MIT Press.

Levinson 2000. *Presumptive meaning*. Cambridge, MA: MIT Press.

Lewis, D. 1979. Scorekeeping in a language game. *Journal of Philosophical Logic*, 8, 339–359.

Logie, R. H. 1995. *Visuo-spatial working memory.* Hove, England: Erlbaum.

Lovegrove, W. J. / Martin, F. / Slaghuis, W. L. 1986. A theoretical and experimental case for a visual deficit in specific reading disability. *Cognitive Neuropsychology*, 3, 225–227.

Lovett, M.W. / Lacerenza, L. / Borden, S. L. / Frijters, J. C. / Steinbach, K. A. / De Palma, M. 2000. Components of effective remediation for developmental reading disabilities: combining phonological and strategy based instruction to improve outcomes. *Journal of Educational Psychology*, 92, 263–283.

Lüdtke, J. / Kaup, B. 2006. Context effects when reading negative and affirmative sentences. In Sun, R. (ed.), *Proceedings of the 28th Annual Conference of the Cognitive Science Society*. Mahwah, NJ: Lawrence Erlbaum.

Lukasiewicz, J. 1930. Philosophical remarks on many-valued systems of propositional logic. Reprinted in: *Selected Works: Studies in Logic and the Foundations of Mathematics* (1970). North-Holland, Amsterdam: Borkowski.

Lukasiewicz, J. 1957. Aristotle's Syllogistic from the Standpoint of Modern Formal Logic. Oxford: Oxford University Press.

MacDonald, M. C. / Just, M. A. 1989. Changes in activation level with negation. *Journal of Experimental Psychology: Learning, Memory and Cognition*, 15, 633–642.

Manis, F. R. / Szeszuiski, P. A. / Hoit, I. K. / Graves, K. 1988. A developmental perspective on dyslexic subtypes. *Annals of Dyslexia*, 38, 139–153.

Manis, F. R. / Custodio, R. / Szeszulski, P. A. 1993. Development of phonological and orthographic skill: a 2-year longitudinal study of dyslexic children. *Journal of Experimental Child Psychology*, 56, 64–86.

Manis, F. R. / McBride-Chang, C. / Seidenberg, M. S. / Keating, P. / Doi, L. M. / Munson, B. / Petersen, A. 1997. Are speech perception deficits associated with developmental dyslexia? *Journal of Experimental Child Psychology*, 66,m 211–235.

Mann, V. A. / Shankweiler, D. / Smith, S. T. 1984. The association between comprehension of spoken sentences and early reading ability: the role of phonetic representation. *Journal of Child Language*, 11, 627–643.

Martin, F. / Lovegrove, W. 1987. Flicker contrast sensitivity in normal and specifically disabled readers. *Perception*, 16, 215–221.

Maughan B. / Pickles A. / Hagell A. / Rutter M. / Yule W. 1996. Reading problems and antisocial behaviour: developmental trends in comorbidity. *Journal of Child Psychology and Psychiatry*, 37, 405–18.

McLoughlin D. / Fitzgibbon G. / Young V. 1994. *Adult Dyslexia: Assessment, Counselling and Training*. London: Whurr.
McLoughlin, D. / Leather, C. / Stringer, P. 2002. *The adult dyslexic: interventions and outcomes*. London: Whurr.
Miles, T. R. 1993. *Dyslexia: the pattern of difficulties*. London: Whurr.
Miller, G. A. / Galanter, E. / Pribram, K. H. 1960. *Plans and the Structure of Behavior*. New York: Holt, Rinehart & Winston.
Moores, E. / Nicolson, R. I. / Fawcett, A. J. 2003. Attention deficits in dyslexia: evidence for an automatization deficit? *European Journal of Cognitive Psychology,* 15, 231–348.
Mundy I. R. / J. M. Carroll 2012. Speech prosody and developmental dyslexia: reduced phonological awareness in the context of intact phonological representations. *Journal of Cognitive Psychology*, 24, 560–81.
Murray, D. J. 1967. The role of speech responses in short-term memory. *Canadian Journal of Psychology*, 21, 263–276.
Murray, D. J. 1968. Articulation and acoustic confusability in short term memory. *Journal of Experimental Psychology*, 78, 679–684.
Muter, V. / Snowling, M. 1998. Concurrent and longitudinal predictors of reading: the role of metalinguistic and short-term memory skills. *Reading Research Quarterly*, 33, 320–337.
Nelson, H. E. / Warrington, E. K. 1980. An investigation of memory functions in dyslexic children. *British Journal of Psychology,* 71, 487–503.
Nicolson, R. I. / Fawcett, A. J. 1990. Automaticity: a new framework for dyslexia research? *Cognition*, 35, 159–182.
Nicolson, R. I. / Fawcett, A. J. 1994. Comparison of deficits in cognitive and motor skills among children with dyslexia. *Annals of Dyslexia*, 44, 147–163.
Nicolson, R. I. / Fawcett, A. J. 1995. Dyslexia is more than a phonological disability. *Dyslexia: An international journal of research and practice*, 1, 19–37.
Nicolson, R. I. / Fawcett, A. J. 1999. Developmental dyslexia: the role of the cerebellum. *Dyslexia: International Journal of Research and Practice*, 5, 155–177.
Nicolson, R. I. / Fawcett, A. J. 2008. *Dyslexia, learning and the Brain.* Cambridge, MA: The MIT Press.

Nicolson, R. I. / Fawcett, A. J. / Berry, E. L. / Jenkins, I. H. / Dean, P. / Brooks, D. J. 1999. Association of abnormal cerebellar activation with motor learning difficulties in dyslexic adults. *Lancet*, 353, 1662–1667.

Nicolson, R. I. / Fawcett, A. J. / Dean, P. 2001. Developmental dyslexia: The cerebellar deficit hypothesis. *Trends in Neurosciences*, 24, 508–511.

Noveck, I. A. 2001. When children are more logical than adults: experimental investigations of scalar implicature. *Cognition*, 78, 165–188.

Noveck, I. A. / Posada, A. 2003. Characterizing the time course of an implicature: an evoked potentials study. *Brain and Language*, 85, 203–210.

Olson, R. K. 2002. Dyslexia: nature and nurture. *Dyslexia*, 8, 143–159.

Orton, S. T. 1925. Word-blindness in school children. *Archives of Neurology and Psychiatry*, 14, 582–615.

Papagno, C. / Valentine, T. / Baddeley, A. D. 1991. Phonological short-term memory and foreign-language vocabulary learning. *Journal of Memory and Language*, 30, 331–347.

Papagno, C. / Vallar, G. 1995. Verbal short-term memory and vocabulary learning in polyglots. *Quarterly Journal of Experimental Psychology*, 38, 98–107.

Partee, B. H. 1970. Negation, conjunction and quantifiers: Syntax vs. semantics. *Foundations of Language,* 6, 153–165.

Paulesu, E. / Démonet, J. F. / Fazio, F. / McCrory, E. / Chanoine, V. / Brunswick, N. / Cappa, S. F. / Cossu, G. / Habib, M. / Frith, C.D. / Frith, U. 2001. Dyslexia: cultural diversity and biological unity. *Science*, 291, 2165–2167.

Paulesu, E. / Frith, U. / Snowling, M. / Gallagher, A. / Morton, J. / Frackowiak, R. S. J. / Frith, C. D. 1996. Is developmental dyslexia a disconnection syndrome? Evidence from PET scanning. *Brain*, 119, 143–157.

Pennington, B. F. / Filipek, P. A. / Lefly, D. / Churchwell, J. / Kennedy, D. N. / Simon, J. H. / Filley, C. M. / Galaburda, A. / Alarcon, M. / de Fries, J. C. 1999. Brain morphometry in reading disabled twins. *Neurology*, 53, 723–729.

Philip, W. / Coopmans, P. 1996. The double Dutch delay of Principle B effect. In Stringfellow, A. / Cahana-Amitay, D. / Hughes, E. / Zukowski, A. (eds.), *Proceedings of the Annual Boston University Conference on Language Development,* 20. Somerville, MA: Cascadilla Press.

Phillips, C. E. / Jarrold, C. / Baddeley, A. / Grant, J. / Karmiloff-Smith, A. 2004. Comprehension of spatial language terms in Williams syndrome: Evidence for an interaction between domains of strength and weakness. *Cortex*, 40, 85–10.

Pickering, S. J. / Gathercole, S. E. 2001. *Working Memory Test Battery for Children*. London: Pearson Assessment.

Pickering S. J. / Gathercole, S. E. / Hall, M. / Lloyd, S. A. 2001. Development of memory for pattern and path: Further evidence for the fractionation of visuo-spatial memory. *The Quarterly Journal of Experimental Psychology*, 54, 397–420.

Pivi M. / Del Puppo G. 2014. L'acquisizione delle frasi relative restrittive in bambini italiani con sviluppo tipico e con dislessia evolutiva. *Atti del XIV Congresso AItLa*, Verona.

Plato 1937. *The Sophist*. Jowett, B., trans., New York: Random House.

Plisson, A. / D. Daigle / Montésinon-Gelet, I. 2013. The Spelling Skills of French-Speaking Dyslexic Children. *Dyslexia,* 19, 79–91.

Pugh, K. R. / Mencl, W. E. / Jenner, A. R. / Katz, L. / Frost, S. J. / Lee, J. R. / Shaywitz, S. E. / Shaywitz, B. A. 2000. Functional neuroimaging studies of reading and reading disability (developmental dyslexia). *Mental Retardation and Developmental Disabilities Research Review*, 6, 207–213.

Pulvermüller, F. A. 2002. Brain perspective on language mechanisms: From discrete neuronal ensembles to serial order. *Progress in Neurobiology*, 67, 85–111.

Rack, J. P. / Snowling, M. J. / Olson, R. K. 1992. The nonword reading deficit in developmental dyslexia: a review. *Reading Research Quarterly*, 27, 29–53.

Rae, C. / Harasty, J. A. / Dzendrowskyj, T. E. / Talcott, J. B. / Simpson, J. M. / Blamire, A. M. 2002. Cerebellar morphology in developmental dyslexia. *Neuropsychologia*, 40, 1285–1292.

Rae, C. / Lee, M. A. / Dixon, R. M. / Blamire, A. M. / Thompson, C. H. / Styles, P. 1998. Metabolic abnormalities in developmental dyslexia detected by H-1 magnetic resonance spectroscopy. *Lancet*, 351, 1849–1852.

Ramus, F. 2003. Developmental dyslexia: specific phonological deficit or sensorimotor dysfunction? *Current Opinion in Neurobiology*, 13, 212–218.

Ramus, F. / Rosen, S. / Dakin, S. C. / Day, B. L. / Castellote, J. M. / White, S. / Frith, U. 2003. Theories of developmental dyslexia: insight from a multiple case study of dyslexic adults. *Brain*, 126, 841–865.

Ramus, F. / Szenkovits, G. 2008. What phonological deficit? *The Quarterly Journal of Experimental Psychology*, 61, 129–141.

Ramus F. M. / Ahissar M. 2012. Developmental dyslexia: the difficulties of interpreting poor performance, and the importance of normal performance. *Cognitive Neuropsychology*, 29, 104–22.

Ramus, F. / Marshall, C. R. / Rosen, S. / Van der Lely, H. K. J. 2013. Phonological deficits in specific language impairment and developmental dyslexia: towards a multidimensional model. *Brain*, 136, 630–645.

Recanati, F. 2003. *Literal meaning*. Cambridge: Cambridge University Press.

Reggiani, D. 2010. Dyslexia and the acquisition of syntax: passive and control. Doctoral Dissertation. University of Verona, Verona.

Reinhart, T. 1983a. *Anaphora and Semantic Interpretation*. London: Croom Helm.

Reinhart, T. 1983b. Coreference and Bound Anaphora: A Restatement of the Anaphora Questions. *Linguistics and Philosophy*, 6, 47–88.

Reinhart, T. 1999. The Processing Cost of Reference-Set Computation: Guess Patterns in Acquisition. UiL OTS Working Papers in Linguistics.

Reinhart, T. 2000. Strategies of anaphora resolution. In Bennis, H. / Everaert, M. (eds.), *Interface Strategies*. North-Holland, Amsterdam.

Reinhart, T. 2006. *Interface Strategies*. Cambridge, MA: MIT Press.

Rice, M. L. 2004. Growth models of developmental language disorders. In M. L. Rice, M. L. / S. Warren 2004. *Developmental language disorders: From phenotypes to etiologies*. Mahwah, NJ: Erlbaum.
Rispens, J. E. 2004. *Syntactic and phonological processing in developmental dyslexia.* Doctoral dissertation. University of Groningen, Groningen.
Rudel, R. G. 1985. The definition of dyslexia: language and motor deficits. In Duffy, F. H. / Geschwind, N. (eds.), *Dyslexia: a neuroscientific approach to clinical evaluation.* Boston, MA: Little, Brown, & Co.
Rumsey J. M. / Horwitz, B. / Donohue, K. 1997. Phonological and orthographic components of word recognition a PET-rCBF study. *Brain*, 120, 739–759.
Russell, B. 1905. On denoting. *Mind,* 14, 479–493.
Scarborough, H. S. 1989. Prediction of reading disability from familial and individual differences. *Journal of Educational Psychology*, 81, 101–108.
Scarborough, H. S. 1990. Very early language deficits in dyslexic children. *Child Development*, 61, 1728–1743.
Scarborough, H. S. 1991a. Early syntactic development of dyslexic children. *Annals of Dyslexia*, 41, 207–220.
Scarborough, H. S. 1991b. Antecedents to reading disability: Preschool language development and literacy experiences of children from dyslexic families. *Reading and Writing: An Interdisciplinary Journal*, 3, 219–233.
Schwartz, M. F. / Saffran, E. M. / Marin, O. S. M. 1980. Fractionating the reading process in dementia. In Coltheart, M. / Patterson, K. E. / Marshall J. C. (eds.), *Deep dyslexia*. London: Routledge & Kegan Paul.
Seymour, P. H. K. / Aro, M. / Erskine, J. M. 2003. Foundation literacy acquisition in European orthographies. *British Journal of Psychology*, 94, 143–174.
Seymour, P. H. K. / Elder, L. 1986. Beginning reading without phonology. *Cognitive Neuropsychology*, 3, 1–36.
Shaywitz, S. E. / Shaywitz, B. A. / Pugh, K. R. 1998. Functional disruption in the organization of the brain for reading in dyslexia. *Proceedings of the Natural Academy of Science*, 95, 2636–2641.

Sheldon, A. 1974. The role of parallel function in the acquisition of relative clauses in English. *Journal of Verbal Learning and Verbal Behavior*, 13, 272–281.
Schlösser, R. G. M. / Wagner, G. / Sauer, H. 2006. Assessing the working memory network: studies with functional magnetic resonance imagining and structural equation modeling. *Neuroscience*, 139, 91–103.
Skottun, B. C. 2000. The magnocellular deficit theory of dyslexia: the evidence from contrast sensitivity. *Vision Research*, 40, 111–127.
Simos, P. G. / Breier, J. I. / Fletcher, J. M. / Foorman, B. R. / Bergman, E. / Fishbeck, E. K. / Papanicolau, A. C. 2000. Brain activation profiles in dyslexic children during nonword reading: A magnetic source imaging study. *Neuroscience Reports*, 290, 61–65.
Smith, C. L. 1980. Quantifiers and question answering in young children. *Journal of Experimental Child Psychology*, 30, 191–205.
Smith, E. E. / Jonides, J. 1996. Working memory in humans: Neuropsychological evidence. In Gazzaniga, M. (ed.), *The cognitive neurosciences*. Cambridge, MA: MIT Press.
Smith, E. S. / Geva, A. 2000. Verbal working memory and its connection to language processing. In Grodzinsky, Y., Shapiro, L. P. and Swinney, D. (eds.), *Language and the Brain: Representation and Processing*. San Diego: Academic Press.
Smith, S. T. / Macaruso, P. / Shankweiler, D. / Crain, S. (1989). Syntactic comprehension in young poor readers. *Applied psycholinguistics*, 10, 429–454.
Snowling, M. J. 1995. Phonological processing and developmental dyslexia. *Journal of Research in Reading,* 18, 132–138.
Snowling, M. J. 2001. From language to reading and dyslexia. *Dyslexia*, 7, 37–46.
Snowling, M. J. / Gallagher, A. / Frith, U. 2003. Family risk of dyslexia is continuous: Individual differences in the precursors of reading skill. *Child Development*, 74, 358–373.
Snowling, M. / Goulandris, N. / Defty, N. 1996. A longitudinal study of reading development in dyslexic children. *Journal of Educational Psychology,* 88, 653–669.

Snowling, M. J. / Hulme, C. 1989. A longitudinal study of developmental phonological dyslexia. *Cognitive Neuropsychology*, 6, 379–401.

Snowling, M. J. / Hulme, C. 1994. The development of phonological skills. *Philosophical Transactions of the Royal Society of London*, 346, 21–27.

Snowling, M. / Nation, K. / Moxham, P. / Gallagher, A. / Frith, U. 1997. Phonological processing skills of dyslexic students in higher education: a preliminary report. *Journal of Research in Reading*, 20, 31–41.

Sperber, D. / Wilson, D. 1986. *Relevance: Communication and Cognition*. Cambridge MA: Blackwell, Oxford and Harvard University Press.

Sperber, D. / Wilson, D. 1995. *Relevance: Communication and Cognition*. Oxford: Blackwell.

Stalnaker, R. 1974. Pragmatic presuppositions. In Munitz, M. K. / Unger, P.K. (eds.), *Semantics and Philosophy*. New York: New York University Press.

Stein, C. L. / Cairns, H. S. / Zurif, E. B. 1984, Sentence comprehension limitations related to syntactic deficits in reading-disabled children. *Applied Psycholinguistics*, 5, 305–322.

Stein, J. F. 2001. The magnocellular theory of developmental dyslexia. *Dyslexia*, 7, 12–36.

Stein, J. F. / Walsh, V. 1997. To see but not to read; the magnocellular theory of dyslexia. *Trends in Neuroscience*, 20, 147–152.

Stalnaker, R. 1978. Assertion. *Syntax and Semantics*, 9, 315–332.

Strawson, P. F. 1950. On referring. *Mind,* 59, 320–344.

Strawson, P. F. 1964. Identifying reference and truth values. *Theoria*, 30, 96–118.

Stroop, J. R. 1935. Studies of interference in serial verbal reactions. *Journal of Experimental Psychology*, 18, 643–662.

Swan, D. / Goswami, U. 1997a. Phonological awareness deficits in developmental dyslexia and the phonological representations hypothesis. *Journal of Experimental Child Psychology*, 66, 18–41.

Swan, D., / Goswami, U. 1997b. Picture naming deficits in developmental dyslexia: the phonological representations hypothesis. *Brain and Language*, 56, 334–353.

Swanson, H. L. / Beebe-Frankenberger, M. 2004. The relationship between working memory and mathematical problem solving in children at risk and not at risk for math disabilities. *Journal of Education Psychology*, 96, 471–491.

De Swart, H. 2009. *Expression and interpretation of negation*. Dordrecht: Springer.

Tallal, P. 1980. Auditory temporal perception, phonics and reading disabilities in children. *Brain and Language*, 9, 182–198.

Tallal, P. 1984. Temporal or phonetic processing deficit in dyslexia? That is the question. *Applied Psycholinguistics*, 5, 167–169.

Tomatis, A. 1969. *Dyslexia*. Ottawa, Ontario, Canada: University of Ottawa Press.

Torgesen, J. K. / Alexander, A. W. / Wagner, R. K. / Rashotte, C. A. / Voeller, K. K. S. / Conway, T. 2001. Intensive remedial instruction for children with severe reading disabilities: Immediate and long-term outcomes from two instructional approaches. *Journal of Learning Disabilities*, 34, 33–58.

Torgesen, J. K. / Rose, E. / Lindamood, P. / Conway, T. / Garvan C. 1999. Preventing reading failure in young children with phonological processing disabilities: Group and individual responses to instruction. *Journal of Educational Psychology*, 91, 579–594.

Towse, J. N. / Hitch, G. / Hutton, U. 1998. A reevaluation of working memory capacity in children. *Journal of Memory and Language* 39, 195–217.

Trojano, L. / Grossi, D. 1995. Phonological and lexical coding in verbal short-term memory and learning. *Brain and Cognition*, 21, 336–354.

Ulatowska, H. K. / Allard, L. / Donnell, A. 1988. Discourse performance in subjects with dementia of the Alzheimer's type. In Whitaker, H. (ed.), *Neuropsychological studies in nonfocal brain damage*. New York: Springer-Verlag.

Ulatowska, H. K. / Chapman, S. B. 1995. Discourse studies. In Lubinski, R. (ed.), *Dementia and communication*. San Diego: Singular.

Ullman, M. T. 2001. The declarative/procedural model of lexicon and grammar. *Journal of Psycholinguistic Research*, 30, 37–69.

Ullman, M. T. 2004. Contributions of memory circuits to language: The declarative/procedural model. *Cognition*, 92, 231–270.

Ullman, M. T. / Pierpont, E. 2005. Specific Language Impairment is not Specific to Language: The Procedural Deficit Hypothesis. *Cortex*, 41, 399–433.
Vallar, G. / Papagno, C. 2002. Neuropsychological impairments of verbal short-term memory. In Baddeley, A. / Wilson, B. / Kopelman, M. (eds.), *Handbook of memory disorders*. Chichester, England: Wiley.
Vellutino, F. R. 1979. *Dyslexia: Theory and Research*. Cambridge, MA: MIT Press.
Vellutino, F. R. / Fletcher, J. M. / Snowling, M. J. / Scanlon, D. M. 2004. Specific reading disability (dyslexia): what have we learned in the past four decades? *Journal of Child Psychology and Psychiatry*, 45, 2–40.
Vender, M. 2009. Scalar implicatures and developmental dyslexia. *Proceedings of the 2nd International Clinical Linguistics Conference*, Universidad Autónoma de Madrid, Universidad Nacional de Educación a Distancia, and Euphonia Ediciones, Victoria Marrero / Idaira Pineda (Eds.), 239–246.
De Villiers, J. G. / Flusberg, H. B. T. 1975. Some facts one simply cannot deny. *Journal of Child Language*, 2, 279–286.
Waltzman, D. / Cairns, H. 2000. Grammatical knowledge of third grade good and poor readers. *Applied Psycholinguistics*, 21, 263–284.
Wang, S. / Gathercole, S. E. 2013. Working memory deficits in children with reading difficulties: Memory span and dual task coordination. *Journal of Experimental Child Psychology*, 115, 188–197.
Wason, P. C. 1959. The processing of positive and negative information. *Quarterly Journal of Experimental Psychology*, 11, 92–107.
Wason, P. C. 1961. Response to affirmative and negative binary statements. *British Journal of Psychology*, 52, 133–142.
Wason, P. C. 1965. The context of plausible denial. *Journal of Verbal Learning and Verbal Behaviour*, 4, 7–11.
White, S. / Frith, U. / Milne, E. / Rosen, S. / Swettenham, J. / Ramus, F. 2006. A double dissociation between sensorimotor impairments and reading disability: a comparison of autistic and dyslexic children. *Cognitive Neuropsychology*, 23, 748–761.

Wilsenach, C. 2006. Syntactic processing in Developmental Dyslexia and in Specific Language Impairment: A study on the acquisition of the past participle construction in Dutch. Doctoral dissertation. Utrecht Institute for Linguistics OTS. LOT Series.

Wilsenach, C. / Wijnen, F. 2004. Perceptual sensitivity to morphosyntactic agreement in language learners. Evidence from Dutch children at risk for developing dyslexia. *Proceedings of BUCLD 28*, Somerville, MA: Cascadilla Press.

Wimmer, H. 1993. Characteristics of developmental dyslexia in a regular writing system. *Applied Psycholinguistics*, 14, 1–33.

Wimmer, H. / Goswami, U. 1994. The influence of orthographic consistency on reading development-word recognition in English and German children. *Cognition*, 51, 91–103.

Wimmer, H. / Schruz, M. 2010. Dyslexia in regular orthographies: Manifestations and causation. *Dyslexia*, 16, 283–299.

Wolf, M. / Bally, H. / Morris, R. 1986. Automaticity, retrieval processes, and reading: A longitudinal study in average and impaired readers. *Child Development*, 57, 988–1000.

Wolf, M. / Bowers, P. G. 1999. The double-deficit hypothesis for the developmental dyslexias. *Journal of Educational Psychology, 91,* 415–438.

Wolf, M. / Bowers, P. G. / Biddle, K. 2000. Naming speed processes, timing, and reading: a conceptual review. *Journal of Learning Disabilities*, 33, 387–407.

Wolf, M. / Obregón, M. 1992. Early naming deficits, developmental dyslexia, and a specific deficit hypothesis. *Brain and Language*, 42, 219–247.

Wolff, P. H. / Michel, G. F. / Ovrut, M. / Drake, C. 1990. Rate and timing precision of motor coordination in developmental dyslexia. *Developmental Psychology,* 26, 349–359.

Wolff, P. H. / Melngailis, I. 1994. Family patterns of developmental dyslexia: clinical findings. *American Journal of Medical Genetics*, 54, 122–131.

Zempleni, M. Z. / Renken, R. / Hoeks, J. C. J. / Hoogduin, J. M. / Stowe, L. A. 2006. Semantic ambiguity processing in sentence context: Evidence from event-related fMRI. *NeuroImage*, 34, 1270–1279.

Ziegler, J. C. / Perry, C. / Ma-Wyatt, A. / Ladner, D. / Schulte-Körne, G. 2003. Developmental dyslexia in different languages: Language-specific or universal? *Journal of Experimental Child Psychology*, 86, 169–193.

Zwaan, R. A. / Radvansky, G. A. 1998. Situation models in language comprehension and memory. *Psychological Bulletin*, 123, 162–185.

Linguistic Insights

Studies in Language and Communication

This series aims to promote specialist language studies in the fields of linguistic theory and applied linguistics, by publishing volumes that focus on specific aspects of language use in one or several languages and provide valuable insights into language and communication research. A cross-disciplinary approach is favoured and most European languages are accepted.

The series includes two types of books:

- **Monographs** – featuring in-depth studies on special aspects of language theory, language analysis or language teaching.
- **Collected papers** – assembling papers from workshops, conferences or symposia.

Each volume of the series is subjected to a double peer-reviewing process.

Vol. 1 Maurizio Gotti & Marina Dossena (eds)
Modality in Specialized Texts. Selected Papers of the 1st CERLIS Conference.
421 pages. 2001. ISBN 3-906767-10-8 · US-ISBN 0-8204-5340-4

Vol. 2 Giuseppina Cortese & Philip Riley (eds)
Domain-specific English. Textual Practices across Communities and Classrooms.
420 pages. 2002. ISBN 3-906768-98-8 · US-ISBN 0-8204-5884-8

Vol. 3 Maurizio Gotti, Dorothee Heller & Marina Dossena (eds)
Conflict and Negotiation in Specialized Texts. Selected Papers of the 2nd CERLIS Conference.
470 pages. 2002. ISBN 3-906769-12-7 · US-ISBN 0-8204-5887-2

Vol. 4 Maurizio Gotti, Marina Dossena, Richard Dury, Roberta Facchinetti & Maria Lima
Variation in Central Modals. A Repertoire of Forms and Types of Usage in Middle English and Early Modern English.
364 pages. 2002. ISBN 3-906769-84-4 · US-ISBN 0-8204-5898-8

Editorial address:

Prof. Maurizio Gotti Università di Bergamo, Dipartimento di Lingue, Letterature Straniere e Comunicazione, Piazza Rosate 2, 24129 Bergamo, Italy
Fax: +39 035 2052789, E-Mail: m.gotti@unibg.it

Vol. 5 Stefania Nuccorini (ed.)
Phrases and Phraseology. Data and Descriptions.
187 pages. 2002. ISBN 3-906770-08-7 · US-ISBN 0-8204-5933-X

Vol. 6 Vijay Bhatia, Christopher N. Candlin & Maurizio Gotti (eds)
Legal Discourse in Multilingual and Multicultural Contexts.
Arbitration Texts in Europe.
385 pages. 2003. ISBN 3-906770-85-0 · US-ISBN 0-8204-6254-3

Vol. 7 Marina Dossena & Charles Jones (eds)
Insights into Late Modern English. 2nd edition.
378 pages. 2003, 2007.
ISBN 978-3-03911-257-9 · US-ISBN 978-0-8204-8927-8

Vol. 8 Maurizio Gotti
Specialized Discourse. Linguistic Features and Changing Conventions.
351 pages. 2003, 2005.
ISBN 3-03910-606-6 · US-ISBN 0-8204-7000-7

Vol. 9 Alan Partington, John Morley & Louann Haarman (eds)
Corpora and Discourse.
420 pages. 2004. ISBN 3-03910-026-2 · US-ISBN 0-8204-6262-4

Vol. 10 Martina Möllering
The Acquisition of German Modal Particles. A Corpus-Based Approach.
290 pages. 2004. ISBN 3-03910-043-2 · US-ISBN 0-8204-6273-X

Vol. 11 David Hart (ed.)
English Modality in Context. Diachronic Perspectives.
261 pages. 2003. ISBN 3-03910-046-7 · US-ISBN 0-8204-6852-5

Vol. 12 Wendy Swanson
Modes of Co-reference as an Indicator of Genre.
430 pages. 2003. ISBN 3-03910-052-1 · US-ISBN 0-8204-6855-X

Vol. 13 Gina Poncini
Discursive Strategies in Multicultural Business Meetings.
2nd edition. 338 pages. 2004, 2007.
ISBN 978-3-03911-296-8 · US-ISBN 978-0-8204-8937-7

Vol. 14 Christopher N. Candlin & Maurizio Gotti (eds)
Intercultural Aspects of Specialized Communication.
2nd edition. 369 pages. 2004, 2007.
ISBN 978-3-03911-258-6 · US-ISBN 978-0-8204-8926-1

Vol. 15 Gabriella Del Lungo Camiciotti & Elena Tognini Bonelli (eds)
Academic Discourse. New Insights into Evaluation.
234 pages. 2004. ISBN 3-03910-353-9 · US-ISBN 0-8204-7016-3

Vol. 16 Marina Dossena & Roger Lass (eds)
Methods and Data in English Historical Dialectology.
405 pages. 2004. ISBN 3-03910-362-8 · US-ISBN 0-8204-7018-X

Vol. 17 Judy Noguchi
The Science Review Article. An Opportune Genre in
the Construction of Science.
274 pages. 2006. ISBN 3-03910-426-8 · US-ISBN 0-8204-7034-1

Vol. 18 Giuseppina Cortese & Anna Duszak (eds)
Identity, Community, Discourse. English in Intercultural Settings.
495 pages. 2005. ISBN 3-03910-632-5 · US-ISBN 0-8204-7163-1

Vol. 19 Anna Trosborg & Poul Erik Flyvholm Jørgensen (eds)
Business Discourse. Texts and Contexts.
250 pages. 2005. ISBN 3-03910-606-6 · US-ISBN 0-8204-7000-7

Vol. 20 Christopher Williams
Tradition and Change in Legal English. Verbal Constructions in Prescriptive Texts.
2nd revised edition. 216 pages. 2005, 2007. ISBN 978-3-03911-444-3.

Vol. 21 Katarzyna Dziubalska-Kolaczyk & Joanna Przedlacka (eds)
English Pronunciation Models: A Changing Scene.
2nd edition. 476 pages. 2005, 2008. ISBN 978-3-03911-682-9.

Vol. 22 Christián Abello-Contesse, Rubén Chacón-Beltrán, M. Dolores López-Jiménez & M. Mar Torreblanca-López (eds)
Age in L2 Acquisition and Teaching.
214 pages. 2006. ISBN 3-03910-668-6 · US-ISBN 0-8204-7174-7

Vol. 23 Vijay K. Bhatia, Maurizio Gotti, Jan Engberg & Dorothee Heller (eds)
Vagueness in Normative Texts.
474 pages. 2005. ISBN 3-03910-653-8 · US-ISBN 0-8204-7169-0

Vol. 24 Paul Gillaerts & Maurizio Gotti (eds)
Genre Variation in Business Letters. 2nd printing.
407 pages. 2008. ISBN 978-3-03911-681-2.

Vol. 25 Ana María Hornero, María José Luzón & Silvia Murillo (eds)
Corpus Linguistics. Applications for the Study of English.
2nd printing. 526 pages. 2006, 2008. ISBN 978-3-03911-726-0

Vol. 26 J. Lachlan Mackenzie & María de los Ángeles Gómez-González (eds)
Studies in Functional Discourse Grammar.
259 pages. 2005. ISBN 3-03910-696-1 · US-ISBN 0-8204-7558-0

Vol. 27 Debbie G. E. Ho
Classroom Talk. Exploring the Sociocultural Structure of Formal ESL Learning.
2nd edition. 254 pages. 2006, 2007. ISBN 978-3-03911-434-4

Vol. 28 Javier Pérez-Guerra, Dolores González-Álvarez, Jorge L. Bueno-Alonso & Esperanza Rama-Martínez (eds)
'Of Varying Language and Opposing Creed'. New Insights into Late Modern English.
455 pages. 2007. ISBN 978-3-03910-788-9

Vol. 29 Francesca Bargiela-Chiappini & Maurizio Gotti (eds)
Asian Business Discourse(s).
350 pages. 2005. ISBN 3-03910-804-2 · US-ISBN 0-8204-7574-2

Vol. 30 Nicholas Brownlees (ed.)
News Discourse in Early Modern Britain. Selected Papers of CHINED 2004.
300 pages. 2006. ISBN 3-03910-805-0 · US-ISBN 0-8204-8025-8

Vol. 31 Roberta Facchinetti & Matti Rissanen (eds)
Corpus-based Studies of Diachronic English.
300 pages. 2006. ISBN 3-03910-851-4 · US-ISBN 0-8204-8040-1

Vol. 32 Marina Dossena & Susan M. Fitzmaurice (eds)
Business and Official Correspondence. Historical Investigations.
209 pages. 2006. ISBN 3-03910-880-8 · US-ISBN 0-8204-8352-4

Vol. 33 Giuliana Garzone & Srikant Sarangi (eds)
Discourse, Ideology and Specialized Communication.
494 pages. 2007. ISBN 978-3-03910-888-6

Vol. 34 Giuliana Garzone & Cornelia Ilie (eds)
The Use of English in Institutional and Business Settings.
An Intercultural Perspective.
372 pages. 2007. ISBN 978-3-03910-889-3

Vol. 35 Vijay K. Bhatia & Maurizio Gotti (eds)
Explorations in Specialized Genres.
316 pages. 2006. ISBN 3-03910-995-2 · US-ISBN 0-8204-8372-9

Vol. 36 Heribert Picht (ed.)
Modern Approaches to Terminological Theories and Applications.
432 pages. 2006. ISBN 3-03911-156-6 · US-ISBN 0-8204-8380-X

Vol. 37 Anne Wagner & Sophie Cacciaguidi-Fahy (eds)
Legal Language and the Search for Clarity / Le langage juridique et la quête de clarté.
Practice and Tools / Pratiques et instruments.
487 pages. 2006. ISBN 3-03911-169-8 · US-ISBN 0-8204-8388-5

Vol. 38 Juan Carlos Palmer-Silveira, Miguel F. Ruiz-Garrido &
Inmaculada Fortanet-Gómez (eds)
Intercultural and International Business Communication.
Theory, Research and Teaching.
2nd edition. 343 pages. 2006, 2008. ISBN 978-3-03911-680-5

Vol. 39 Christiane Dalton-Puffer, Dieter Kastovsky, Nikolaus Ritt &
Herbert Schendl (eds)
Syntax, Style and Grammatical Norms. English from 1500–2000.
250 pages. 2006. ISBN 3-03911-181-7 · US-ISBN 0-8204-8394-X

Vol. 40 Marina Dossena & Irma Taavitsainen (eds)
Diachronic Perspectives on Domain-Specific English.
280 pages. 2006. ISBN 3-03910-176-0 · US-ISBN 0-8204-8391-5

Vol. 41 John Flowerdew & Maurizio Gotti (eds)
Studies in Specialized Discourse.
293 pages. 2006. ISBN 3-03911-178-7

Vol. 42 Ken Hyland & Marina Bondi (eds)
Academic Discourse Across Disciplines.
320 pages. 2006. ISBN 3-03911-183-3 · US-ISBN 0-8204-8396-6

Vol. 43 Paul Gillaerts & Philip Shaw (eds)
The Map and the Landscape. Norms and Practices in Genre.
256 pages. 2006. ISBN 3-03911-182-5 · US-ISBN 0-8204-8395-4

Vol. 44 Maurizio Gotti & Davide Giannoni (eds)
New Trends in Specialized Discourse Analysis.
301 pages. 2006. ISBN 3-03911-184-1 · US-ISBN 0-8204-8381-8

Vol. 45 Maurizio Gotti & Françoise Salager-Meyer (eds)
Advances in Medical Discourse Analysis. Oral and Written Contexts.
492 pages. 2006. ISBN 3-03911-185-X · US-ISBN 0-8204-8382-6

Vol. 46 Maurizio Gotti & Susan Šarcević (eds)
Insights into Specialized Translation.
396 pages. 2006. ISBN 3-03911-186-8 · US-ISBN 0-8204-8383-4

Vol. 47 Khurshid Ahmad & Margaret Rogers (eds)
Evidence-based LSP. Translation, Text and Terminology.
584 pages. 2007. ISBN 978-3-03911-187-9

Vol. 48 Hao Sun & Dániel Z. Kádár (eds)
It's the Dragon's Turn. Chinese Institutional Discourses.
262 pages. 2008. ISBN 978-3-03911-175-6

Vol. 49 Cristina Suárez-Gómez
Relativization in Early English (950-1250). the Position of Relative Clauses.
149 pages. 2006. ISBN 3-03911-203-1 · US-ISBN 0-8204-8904-2

Vol. 50 Maria Vittoria Calvi & Luisa Chierichetti (eds)
Nuevas tendencias en el discurso de especialidad.
319 pages. 2006. ISBN 978-3-03911-261-6

Vol. 51 Mari Carmen Campoy & María José Luzón (eds)
Spoken Corpora in Applied Linguistics.
274 pages. 2008. ISBN 978-3-03911-275-3

Vol. 52 Konrad Ehlich & Dorothee Heller (Hrsg.)
Die Wissenschaft und ihre Sprachen.
323 pages. 2006. ISBN 978-3-03911-272-2

Vol. 53 Jingyu Zhang
The Semantic Salience Hierarchy Model. The L2 Acquisition of Psych Predicates
273 pages. 2007. ISBN 978-3-03911-300-2

Vol. 54 Norman Fairclough, Giuseppina Cortese & Patrizia Ardizzone (eds)
Discourse and Contemporary Social Change.
555 pages. 2007. ISBN 978-3-03911-276-0

Vol. 55 Jan Engberg, Marianne Grove Ditlevsen, Peter Kastberg & Martin Stegu (eds)
New Directions in LSP Teaching.
331 pages. 2007. ISBN 978-3-03911-433-7

Vol. 56 Dorothee Heller & Konrad Ehlich (Hrsg.)
Studien zur Rechtskommunikation.
322 pages. 2007. ISBN 978-3-03911-436-8

Vol. 57 Teruhiro Ishiguro & Kang-kwong Luke (eds)
Grammar in Cross-Linguistic Perspective.
The Syntax, Semantics, and Pragmatics of Japanese and Chinese.
304 pages. 2012. ISBN 978-3-03911-445-0

Vol. 58 Carmen Frehner
Email – SMS – MMS
294 pages. 2008. ISBN 978-3-03911-451-1

Vol. 59 Isabel Balteiro
The Directionality of Conversion in English. A Dia-Synchronic Study.
276 pages. 2007. ISBN 978-3-03911-241-8

Vol. 60 Maria Milagros Del Saz Rubio
English Discourse Markers of Reformulation.
237 pages. 2007. ISBN 978-3-03911-196-1

Vol. 61 Sally Burgess & Pedro Martín-Martín (eds)
English as an Additional Language in Research Publication and Communication.
259 pages. 2008. ISBN 978-3-03911-462-7

Vol. 62 Sandrine Onillon
Pratiques et représentations de l'écrit.
458 pages. 2008. ISBN 978-3-03911-464-1

Vol. 63 Hugo Bowles & Paul Seedhouse (eds)
Conversation Analysis and Language for Specific Purposes.
2nd edition. 337 pages. 2007, 2009. ISBN 978-3-0343-0045-2

Vol. 64 Vijay K. Bhatia, Christopher N. Candlin & Paola Evangelisti Allori (eds)
Language, Culture and the Law.
The Formulation of Legal Concepts across Systems and Cultures.
342 pages. 2008. ISBN 978-3-03911-470-2

Vol. 65 Jonathan Culpeper & Dániel Z. Kádár (eds)
Historical (Im)politeness.
300 pages. 2010. ISBN 978-3-03911-496-2

Vol. 66 Linda Lombardo (ed.)
Using Corpora to Learn about Language and Discourse.
237 pages. 2009. ISBN 978-3-03911-522-8

Vol. 67 Natsumi Wakamoto
Extroversion/Introversion in Foreign Language Learning.
Interactions with Learner Strategy Use.
159 pages. 2009. ISBN 978-3-03911-596-9

Vol. 68 Eva Alcón-Soler (ed.)
Learning How to Request in an Instructed Language Learning Context.
260 pages. 2008. ISBN 978-3-03911-601-0

Vol. 69 Domenico Pezzini
The Translation of Religious Texts in the Middle Ages.
428 pages. 2008. ISBN 978-3-03911-600-3

Vol. 70 Tomoko Tode
Effects of Frequency in Classroom Second Language Learning.
Quasi-experiment and stimulated-recall analysis.
195 pages. 2008. ISBN 978-3-03911-602-7

Vol. 71 Egor Tsedryk
Fusion symétrique et alternances ditransitives.
211 pages. 2009. ISBN 978-3-03911-609-6

Vol. 72 Cynthia J. Kellett Bidoli & Elana Ochse (eds)
English in International Deaf Communication.
444 pages. 2008. ISBN 978-3-03911-610-2

Vol. 73 Joan C. Beal, Carmela Nocera & Massimo Sturiale (eds)
Perspectives on Prescriptivism.
269 pages. 2008. ISBN 978-3-03911-632-4

Vol. 74 Carol Taylor Torsello, Katherine Ackerley & Erik Castello (eds)
Corpora for University Language Teachers.
308 pages. 2008. ISBN 978-3-03911-639-3

Vol. 75 María Luisa Pérez Cañado (ed.)
English Language Teaching in the European Credit Transfer System. Facing the Challenge.
251 pages. 2009. ISBN 978-3-03911-654-6

Vol. 76 Marina Dossena & Ingrid Tieken-Boon van Ostade (eds)
Studies in Late Modern English Correspondence. Methodology and Data.
291 pages. 2008. ISBN 978-3-03911-658-4

Vol. 77 Ingrid Tieken-Boon van Ostade & Wim van der Wurff (eds)
Current Issues in Late Modern English.
436 pages. 2009. ISBN 978-3-03911-660-7

Vol. 78 Marta Navarro Coy (ed.)
Practical Approaches to Foreign Language Teaching and Learning.
297 pages. 2009. ISBN 978-3-03911-661-4

Vol. 79 Qing Ma
Second Language Vocabulary Acquisition.
333 pages. 2009. ISBN 978-3-03911-666-9

Vol. 80 Martin Solly, Michelangelo Conoscenti & Sandra Campagna (eds)
Verbal/Visual Narrative Texts in Higher Education.
384 pages. 2008. ISBN 978-3-03911-672-0

Vol. 81 Meiko Matsumoto
From Simple Verbs to Periphrastic Expressions: The Historical Development of Composite Predicates, Phrasal Verbs, and Related Constructions in English.
235 pages. 2008. ISBN 978-3-03911-675-1

Vol. 82 Melinda Dooly
Doing Diversity. Teachers' Construction of Their Classroom Reality.
180 pages. 2009. ISBN 978-3-03911-687-4

Vol. 83 Victoria Guillén-Nieto, Carmen Marimón-Llorca & Chelo Vargas-Sierra (eds)
Intercultural Business Communication and Simulation and Gaming Methodology.
392 pages. 2009. ISBN 978-3-03911-688-1

Vol. 84 Maria Grazia Guido
English as a Lingua Franca in Cross-cultural Immigration Domains.
285 pages. 2008. ISBN 978-3-03911-689-8

Vol. 85 Erik Castello
Text Complexity and Reading Comprehension Tests.
352 pages. 2008. ISBN 978-3-03911-717-8

Vol. 86 Maria-Lluisa Gea-Valor, Isabel García-Izquierdo & Maria-José Esteve (eds)
Linguistic and Translation Studies in Scientific Communication.
317 pages. 2010. ISBN 978-3-0343-0069-8

Vol. 87 Carmen Navarro, Rosa Mª Rodríguez Abella, Francesca Dalle Pezze & Renzo Miotti (eds)
La comunicación especializada.
355 pages. 2008. ISBN 978-3-03911-733-8

Vol. 88 Kiriko Sato
The Development from Case-Forms to Prepositional Constructions in Old English Prose.
231 pages. 2009. ISBN 978-3-03911-763-5

Vol. 89 Dorothee Heller (Hrsg.)
Formulierungsmuster in deutscher und italienischer Fachkommunikation. Intra- und interlinguale Perspektiven.
315 pages. 2008. ISBN 978-3-03911-778-9

Vol. 90 Henning Bergenholtz, Sandro Nielsen & Sven Tarp (eds)
Lexicography at a Crossroads. Dictionaries and Encyclopedias Today, Lexicographical Tools Tomorrow.
372 pages. 2009. ISBN 978-3-03911-799-4

Vol. 91 Manouchehr Moshtagh Khorasani
The Development of Controversies. From the Early Modern Period to Online Discussion Forums.
317 pages. 2009. ISBN 978-3-3911-711-6

Vol. 92 María Luisa Carrió-Pastor (ed.)
Content and Language Integrated Learning. Cultural Diversity.
178 pages. 2009. ISBN 978-3-3911-818-2

Vol. 93 Roger Berry
Terminology in English Language Teaching. Nature and Use.
262 pages. 2010. ISBN 978-3-0343-0013-1

Vol. 94 Roberto Cagliero & Jennifer Jenkins (eds)
Discourses, Communities, and Global Englishes
240 pages. 2010. ISBN 978-3-0343-0012-4

Vol. 95 Facchinetti Roberta, Crystal David, Seidlhofer Barbara (eds)
From International to Local English – And Back Again.
268 pages. 2010. ISBN 978-3-0343-0011-7

Vol. 96 Cesare Gagliardi & Alan Maley (eds)
EIL, ELF, Global English. Teaching and Learning Issues
376 pages. 2010. ISBN 978-3-0343-0010-0

Vol. 97 Sylvie Hancil (ed.)
The Role of Prosody in Affective Speech.
403 pages. 2009. ISBN 978-3-03911-696-6

Vol. 98 Marina Dossena & Roger Lass (eds)
Studies in English and European Historical Dialectology.
257 pages. 2009. ISBN 978-3-0343-0024-7

Vol. 99 Christine Béal
Les interactions quotidiennes en français et en anglais. De l'approche comparative à l'analyse des situations interculturelles.
424 pages. 2010. ISBN 978-3-0343-0027-8

Vol. 100 Maurizio Gotti (ed.)
Commonality and Individuality in Academic Discourse.
398 pages. 2009. ISBN 978-3-0343-0023-0

Vol. 101 Javier E. Díaz Vera & Rosario Caballero (eds)
Textual Healing. Studies in Medieval English Medical, Scientific and Technical Texts.
213 pages. 2009. ISBN 978-3-03911-822-9

Vol. 102 Nuria Edo Marzá
The Specialised Lexicographical Approach. A Step further in Dictionary-making.
316 pages. 2009. ISBN 978-3-0343-0043-8

Vol. 103 Carlos Prado-Alonso, Lidia Gómez-García, Iria Pastor-Gómez &
David Tizón-Couto (eds)
New Trends and Methodologies in Applied English Language Research.
Diachronic, Diatopic and Contrastive Studies.
348 pages. 2009. ISBN 978-3-0343-0046-9

Vol. 104 Françoise Salager-Meyer & Beverly A. Lewin
Crossed Words. Criticism in Scholarly Writing?
371 pages. 2011. ISBN 978-3-0343-0049-0.

Vol. 105 Javier Ruano-García
Early Modern Northern English Lexis. A Literary Corpus-Based Study.
611 pages. 2010. ISBN 978-3-0343-0058-2

Vol. 106 Rafael Monroy-Casas
Systems for the Phonetic Transcription of English. Theory and Texts.
280 pages. 2011. ISBN 978-3-0343-0059-9

Vol. 107 Nicola T. Owtram
The Pragmatics of Academic Writing.
A Relevance Approach to the Analysis of Research Article Introductions.
311 pages. 2009. ISBN 978-3-0343-0060-5

Vol. 108 Yolanda Ruiz de Zarobe, Juan Manuel Sierra &
Francisco Gallardo del Puerto (eds)
Content and Foreign Language Integrated Learning.
Contributions to Multilingualism in European Contexts
343 pages. 2011. ISBN 978-3-0343-0074-2

Vol. 109 Ángeles Linde López & Rosalía Crespo Jiménez (eds)
Professional English in the European context. The EHEA challenge.
374 pages. 2010. ISBN 978-3-0343-0088-9

Vol. 110 Rosalía Rodríguez-Vázquez
The Rhythm of Speech, Verse and Vocal Music. A New Theory.
394 pages. 2010. ISBN 978-3-0343-0309-5

Vol. 111 Anastasios Tsangalidis & Roberta Facchinetti (eds)
Studies on English Modality. In Honour of Frank Palmer.
392 pages. 2009. ISBN 978-3-0343-0310-1

Vol. 112 Jing Huang
Autonomy, Agency and Identity in Foreign Language Learning and Teaching.
400 pages. 2013. ISBN 978-3-0343-0370-5

Vol. 113 Mihhail Lotman & Maria-Kristiina Lotman (eds)
Frontiers in Comparative Prosody. In memoriam: Mikhail Gasparov.
426 pages. 2011. ISBN 978-3-0343-0373-6

Vol. 114 Merja Kytö, John Scahill & Harumi Tanabe (eds)
Language Change and Variation from Old English to Late Modern English.
A Festschrift for Minoji Akimoto
422 pages. 2010. ISBN 978-3-0343-0372-9

Vol. 115 Giuliana Garzone & Paola Catenaccio (eds)
Identities across Media and Modes. Discursive Perspectives.
379 pages. 2009. ISBN 978-3-0343-0386-6

Vol. 116 Elena Landone
Los marcadores del discurso y cortesía verbal en español.
390 pages. 2010. ISBN 978-3-0343-0413-9

Vol. 117 Maurizio Gotti & Christopher Williams (eds)
Legal Discourse across Languages and Cultures.
339 pages. 2010. ISBN 978-3-0343-0425-2

Vol. 118 David Hirsh
Academic Vocabulary in Context.
217 pages. 2010. ISBN 978-3-0343-0426-9

Vol. 119 Yvonne Dröschel
Lingua Franca English. The Role of Simplification and Transfer.
358 pages. 2011. ISBN 978-3-0343-0432-0

Vol. 120 Tengku Sepora Tengku Mahadi, Helia Vaezian & Mahmoud Akbari
Corpora in Translation. A Practical Guide.
135 pages. 2010. ISBN 978-3-0343-0434-4

Vol. 121 Davide Simone Giannoni & Celina Frade (eds)
Researching Language and the Law. Textual Features and Translation Issues.
278 pages. 2010. ISBN 978-3-0343-0443-6

Vol. 122 Daniel Madrid & Stephen Hughes (eds)
Studies in Bilingual Education.
472 pages. 2011. ISBN 978-3-0343-0474-0

Vol. 123 Vijay K. Bhatia, Christopher N. Candlin & Maurizio Gotti (eds)
The Discourses of Dispute Resolution.
290 pages. 2010. ISBN 978-3-0343-0476-4

Vol. 124 Davide Simone Giannoni
Mapping Academic Values in the Disciplines. A Corpus-Based Approach.
288 pages. 2010. ISBN 978-3-0343-0488-7

Vol. 125 Giuliana Garzone & James Archibald (eds)
Discourse, Identities and Roles in Specialized Communication.
419 pages. 2010. ISBN 978-3-0343-0494-8

Vol. 126 Iria Pastor-Gómez
The Status and Development of N+N Sequences in
Contemporary English Noun Phrases.
216 pages. 2011. ISBN 978-3-0343-0534-1

Vol. 127 Carlos Prado-Alonso
Full-verb Inversion in Written and Spoken English.
261 pages. 2011. ISBN 978-3-0343-0535-8

Vol. 128 Tony Harris & María Moreno Jaén (eds)
Corpus Linguistics in Language Teaching.
214 pages. 2010. ISBN 978-3-0343-0524-2

Vol. 129 Tetsuji Oda & Hiroyuki Eto (eds)
Multiple Perspectives on English Philology and History of Linguistics.
A Festschrift for Shoichi Watanabe on his 80th Birthday.
378 pages. 2010. ISBN 978-3-0343-0480-1

Vol. 130 Luisa Chierichetti & Giovanni Garofalo (eds)
Lengua y Derecho. líneas de investigación interdisciplinaria.
283 pages. 2010. 978-3-0343-0463-4

Vol. 131 Paola Evangelisti Allori & Giuliana Garzone (eds)
Discourse, Identities and Genres in Corporate Communication.
Sponsorship, Advertising and Organizational Communication.
324 pages. 2011. 978-3-0343-0591-4

Vol. 132 Leyre Ruiz de Zarobe & Yolanda Ruiz de Zarobe (eds)
Speech Acts and Politeness across Languages and Cultures.
402 pages. 2012. 978-3-0343-0611-9

Vol. 133 Thomas Christiansen
Cohesion. A Discourse Perspective.
387 pages. 2011. 978-3-0343-0619-5

Vol. 134 Giuliana Garzone & Maurizio Gotti
Discourse, Communication and the Enterprise. Genres and Trends.
451 pages. 2011. ISBN 978-3-0343-0620-1

Vol. 135 Zsuzsa Hoffmann
Ways of the World's Words.
Language Contact in the Age of Globalization.
334 pages 2011. ISBN 978-3-0343-0673-7

Vol. 136 Cecilia Varcasia (ed.)
Becoming Multilingual.
Language Learning and Language Policy between Attitudes and Identities.
213 pages. 2011. ISBN 978-3-0343-0687-5

Vol. 137 Susy Macqueen
The Emergence of Patterns in Second Language Writing.
A Sociocognitive Exploration of Lexical Trails.
325 pages. 2012. ISBN 978-3-0343-1010-9

Vol. 138 Maria Vittoria Calvi & Giovanna Mapelli (eds)
La lengua del turismo. Géneros discursivos y terminología.
365 pages. 2011. ISBN 978-3-0343-1011-6

Vol. 139 Ken Lau
Learning to Become a Professional in a Textually-Mediated World.
A Text-Oriented Study of Placement Practices.
261 pages. 2012. ISBN 978-3-0343-1016-1

Vol. 140 Sandra Campagna, Giuliana Garzone, Cornelia Ilie & Elizabeth Rowley-Jolivet (eds)
Evolving Genres in Web-mediated Communication.
337 pages. 2012. ISBN 978-3-0343-1013-0

Vol. 141 Edith Esch & Martin Solly (eds)
The Sociolinguistics of Language Education in International Contexts.
263 pages. 2012. ISBN 978-3-0343-1009-3

Vol. 142 Forthcoming.

Vol. 143 David Tizón-Couto
Left Dislocation in English. A Functional-Discoursal Approach.
416 pages. 2012. ISBN 978-3-0343-1037-6

Vol. 144 Margrethe Petersen & Jan Engberg (eds)
Current Trends in LSP Research. Aims and Methods.
323 pages. 2011. ISBN 978-3-0343-1054-3

Vol. 145 David Tizón-Couto, Beatriz Tizón-Couto, Iria Pastor-Gómez & Paula Rodríguez-Puente (eds)
New Trends and Methodologies in Applied English Language Research II.
Studies in Language Variation, Meaning and Learning.
283 pages. 2012. ISBN 978-3-0343-1061-1

Vol. 146 Rita Salvi & Hiromasa Tanaka (eds)
Intercultural Interactions in Business and Management.
306 pages. 2011. ISBN 978-3-0343-1039-0

Vol. 147 Francesco Straniero Sergio & Caterina Falbo (eds)
Breaking Ground in Corpus-based Interpreting Studies.
254 pages. 2012. ISBN 978-3-0343-1071-0

Vol. 148 Forthcoming.

Vol. 149 Vijay K. Bhatia & Paola Evangelisti Allori (eds)
Discourse and Identity in the Professions. Legal, Corporate and Institutional Citizenship.
352 pages. 2011. ISBN 978-3-0343-1079-6

Vol. 150 Maurizio Gotti (ed.)
Academic Identity Traits. A Corpus-Based Investigation.
363 pages. 2012. ISBN 978-3-0343-1141-0

Vol. 151 Priscilla Heynderickx, Sylvain Dieltjens, Geert Jacobs, Paul Gillaerts & Elizabeth de Groot (eds)
The Language Factor in International Business.
New Perspectives on Research, Teaching and Practice.
320 pages. 2012. ISBN 978-3-0343-1090-1

Vol. 152 Paul Gillaerts, Elizabeth de Groot, Sylvain Dieltjens, Priscilla Heynderickx & Geert Jacobs (eds)
Researching Discourse in Business Genres. Cases and Corpora.
215 pages. 2012. ISBN 978-3-0343-1092-5

Vol. 153 Yongyan Zheng
Dynamic Vocabulary Development in a Foreign Language.
262 pages. 2012. ISBN 978-3-0343-1106-9

Vol. 154 Carmen Argondizzo (ed.)
Creativity and Innovation in Language Education.
357 pages. 2012. ISBN 978-3-0343-1080-2

Vol. 155 David Hirsh (ed.)
Current Perspectives in Second Language Vocabulary Research.
180 pages. 2012. ISBN 978-3-0343-1108-3

Vol. 156 Seiji Shinkawa
Unhistorical Gender Assignment in Laȝamon's *Brut*. A Case Study of a Late Stage in the Development of Grammatical Gender toward its Ultimate Loss.
186 pages. 2012. ISBN 978-3-0343-1124-3

Vol. 157 Yeonkwon Jung
Basics of Organizational Writing: A Critical Reading Approach.
151 pages. 2014. ISBN 978-3-0343-1137-3.

Vol. 158 Bárbara Eizaga Rebollar (ed.)
Studies in Linguistics and Cognition.
301 pages. 2012. ISBN 978-3-0343-1138-0

Vol. 159 Giuliana Garzone, Paola Catenaccio, Chiara Degano (eds)
Genre Change in the Contemporary World. Short-term Diachronic Perspectives.
329 pages. 2012. ISBN 978-3-0343-1214-1

Vol. 160 Carol Berkenkotter, Vijay K. Bhatia & Maurizio Gotti (eds)
Insights into Academic Genres.
468 pages. 2012. ISBN 978-3-0343-1211-0

Vol. 161 Beatriz Tizón-Couto
Clausal Complements in Native and Learner Spoken English. A corpus-based study with Lindsei and Vicolse. 357 pages. 2013. ISBN 978-3-0343-1184-7

Vol. 162 Patrizia Anesa
Jury Trials and the Popularization of Legal Language. A Discourse Analytical Approach.
247 pages. 2012. ISBN 978-3-0343-1231-8

Vol. 163 David Hirsh
Endangered Languages, Knowledge Systems and Belief Systems.
153 pages. 2013. ISBN 978-3-0343-1232-5

Vol. 164 Eugenia Sainz (ed.)
De la estructura de la frase al tejido del discurso. Estudios contrastivos español/italiano.
305 pages. 2014. ISBN 978-3-0343-1253-0

Vol. 165 Julia Bamford, Franca Poppi & Davide Mazzi (eds)
Space, Place and the Discursive Construction of Identity.
367 pages. 2014. ISBN 978-3-0343-1249-3

Vol. 166 Rita Salvi & Janet Bowker (eds)
Space, Time and the Construction of Identity.
Discursive Indexicality in Cultural, Institutional and Professional Fields.
324 pages. 2013. ISBN 978-3-0343-1254-7

Vol. 167 Shunji Yamazaki & Robert Sigley (eds)
Approaching Language Variation through Corpora. A Festschrift in Honour of Toshio Saito.
421 pages. 2013. ISBN 978-3-0343-1264-6

Vol. 168 Franca Poppi
Global Interactions in English as a Lingua Franca. How written communication is changing under the influence of electronic media and new contexts of use.
249 pages. 2012. ISBN 978-3-0343-1276-9

Vol. 169 Miguel A. Aijón Oliva & María José Serrano
Style in syntax. Investigating variation in Spanish pronoun subjects.
239 pages. 2013. ISBN 978-3-0343-1244-8

Vol. 170 Inés Olza, Óscar Loureda & Manuel Casado-Velarde (eds)
Language Use in the Public Sphere. Methodological Perspectives and Empirical Applications
564 pages. 2014. ISBN 978-3-0343-1286-8

Vol. 171 Aleksandra Matulewska
Legilinguistic Translatology. A Parametric Approach to Legal Translation.
279 pages. 2013. ISBN 978-3-0343-1287-5

Vol. 172 Maurizio Gotti & Carmen Sancho Guinda (eds)
Narratives in Academic and Professional Genres.
513 pages. 2013. ISBN 978-3-0343-1371-1

Vol. 173 Madalina Chitez
Learner corpus profiles. The case of Romanian Learner English.
244 pages. 2014. ISBN 978-3-0343-1410-7

Vol. 174 Chihiro Inoue
Task Equivalence in Speaking Tests.
251 pages. 2013. ISBN 978-3-0343-1417-6

Vol. 175 Gabriel Quiroz & Pedro Patiño (eds.)
LSP in Colombia: advances and challenges.
339 pages. 2014. ISBN 978-3-0343-1434-3

Vol. 176 Catherine Resche
Economic Terms and Beyond: Capitalising on the Wealth of Notions.
How Researchers in Specialised Varieties of English Can Benefit from Focusing on Terms.
332 pages. 2013. ISBN 978-3-0343-1435-0

Vol. 177 Forthcoming.

Vol. 178 Cécile Desoutter & Caroline Mellet (dir.)
Le discours rapporté: approches linguistiques et perspectives didactiques.
270 pages. 2013. ISBN 978-3-0343-1292-9

Vol. 179 Ana Díaz-Negrillo & Francisco Javier Díaz-Pérez (eds)
Specialisation and Variation in Language Corpora.
341 pages. 2014. ISBN 978-3-0343-1316-2

Vol. 180 Pilar Alonso
A Multi-dimensional Approach to Discourse Coherence. From Standardness to Creativity.
247 pages. 2014. ISBN 978-3-0343-1325-4

Vol. 181 Alejandro Alcaraz-Sintes & Salvador Valera-Hernández (eds)
Diachrony and Synchrony in English Corpus Linguistics.
393 pages. 2014. ISBN 978-3-0343-1326-1

Vol. 182 Runhan Zhang
Investigating Linguistic Knowledge of a Second Language.
207 pages. 2015. ISBN 978-3-0343-1330-8

Vol. 183 Hajar Abdul Rahim & Shakila Abdul Manan (eds.)
English in Malaysia. Postcolonial and Beyond.
267 pages. 2014. ISBN 978-3-0343-1341-4

Vol. 184 Virginie Fasel Lauzon
Comprendre et apprendre dans l'interaction. Les séquences d'explication en classe de français langue seconde.
292 pages. 2014. ISBN 978-3-0343-1451-0

Vol. 185 Forthcoming.

Vol. 186 Wei Ren
L2 Pragmatic Development in Study Abroad Contexts
256 pages. 2015. ISBN 978-3-0343-1358-2

Vol. 187 Marina Bondi & Rosa Lorés Sanz (eds)
Abstracts in Academic Discourse. Variation and Change.
361 pages. 2014. ISBN 978-3-0343-1483-1

Vol. 188 Forthcoming.

Vol. 189 Paola Evangelisti Allori (ed.)
Identities in and across Cultures.
315 pages. 2014. ISBN 978-3-0343-1458-9

Vol. 190 Erik Castello, Katherine Ackerley & Francesca Coccetta (eds).
Studies in Learner Corpus Linguistics. Research and Applications for Foreign Language Teaching and Assessment.
358 pages. 2015. ISBN 978-3-0343-1506-7

Vol. 191 Ruth Breeze, Maurizio Gotti & Carmen Sancho Guinda (eds)
Interpersonality in Legal Genres.
389 pages. 2014. ISBN 978-3-0343-1524-1

Vol. 192 Paola Evangelisti Allori, John Bateman & Vijay K. Bhatia (eds)
Evolution in Genre. Emergence, Variation, Multimodality.
364 pages. 2014. ISBN 978-3-0343-1533-3

Vol. 193 Jiyeon Kook
Agency in Arzt-Patient-Gesprächen. Zur interaktionistischen Konzeptualisierung von Agency
271 pages. 2015. ISBN 978-3-0343-1666-8

Vol. 194 Susana Nicolás Román & Juan José Torres Núñez (eds)
Drama and CLIL. A new challenge for the teaching approaches in bilingual education.
170 pages. 2015. ISBN 978-3-0343-1629-3

Vol. 195 Alessandra Molino & Serenella Zanotti (eds)
Observing Norm, Observing Usage. Lexis in Dictionaries and in the Media.
430 pages. 2015. ISBN 978-3-0343-1584-5

Vol. 196 Begoña Soneira
A Lexical Description of English for Architecture. A Corpus-based Approach.
267 pages. 2015. ISBN 978-3-0343-1602-6

Vol. 197 M Luisa Roca-Varela
False Friends in Learner Corpora. A corpus-based study of English false friends in the written and spoken production of Spanish learners.
348 pages. 2015. ISBN 978-3-0343-1620-0

Vol. 198 Rahma Al-Mahrooqi & Christopher Denman
Bridging the Gap between Education and Employment. English Language Instruction in EFL Contexts.
416 pages. 2015. ISBN 978-3-0343-1681-1

Vol. 199 Rita Salvi & Janet Bowker (eds)
The Dissemination of Contemporary Knowledge in English. Genres, discourse strategies and professional practices.
171 pages. 2015. ISBN 978-3-0343-1679-8

Vol. 200 Maurizio Gotti & Davide S. Giannoni (eds)
Corpus Analysis for Descriptive and Pedagogical Purposes. ESP Perspectives.
432 pages. 2014. ISBN 978-3-0343-1516-6

Vol. 201 Ida Ruffolo
The Perception of Nature in Travel Promotion Texts. A Corpus-based Discourse Analysis.
148 pages. 2015. ISBN 978-3-0343-1521-0

Vol. 202 Ives Trevian
English suffixes. Stress-assignment properties, productivity, selection and combinatorial processes.
471 pages. 2015. ISBN 978-3-0343-1576-0

Vol. 203 Maurizio Gotti, Stefania Maci & Michele Sala (eds)
Insights into Medical Communication.
422 pages. 2015. ISBN 978-3-0343-1694-1

Vol. 204 Carmen Argondizzo (ed.)
European Projects in University Language Centres. Creativity, Dynamics, Best Practice.
371 pages. 2015. ISBN 978-3-0343-1696-5

Vol. 205 Aura Luz Duffé Montalván (ed.)
Estudios sobre el léxico. Puntos y contrapuntos.
502 pages. 2016. ISBN 978-3-0343-2011-5

Vol. 206 Maria Pavesi, Maicol Formentelli & Elisa Ghia (eds)
The Languages of Dubbing. Mainstream Audiovisual Translation in Italy.
275 pages. 2014. ISBN 978-3-0343-1646-0

Vol. 207 Ruth Breeze & Inés Olza (eds)
Evaluation in media discourse. European perspectives.
268 pages. 2017. ISBN 978-3-0343-2014-6

Vol. 208 Vijay K. Bhatia & Maurizio Gotti (eds)
Arbitration Discourse in Asia.
331 pages. 2015. ISBN 978-3-0343-2032-0

Vol. 209 Sofía Bemposta-Rivas, Carla Bouzada-Jabois, Yolanda Fernández-Pena, Tamara Bouso, Yolanda J. Calvo-Benzies, Iván Tamaredo (eds)
New trends and methodologies in applied English language research III. Synchronic and diachronic studies on discourse, lexis and grammar processing.
280 pages. 2017. ISBN 978-3-0343-2039-9

Vol. 210 Francisco Alonso Almeida, Laura Cruz García & Víctor González Ruiz (eds)
Corpus-based studies on language varieties.
285 pages. 2016. ISBN 978-3-0343-2044-3

Vol. 211 Juan Pedro Rica Peromingo
Aspectos lingüísticos y técnicos de la traducción audiovisual (TAV).
177 pages. 2016. ISBN 978-3-0343-2055-9

Vol. 212 Maria Vender
Disentangling Dyslexia. VenderPhonological and Processing Deficit in Developmental Dyslexia.
338 pages. 2017. ISBN 978-3-0343-2064-1

Vol. 213 Zhilong Xie
Bilingual Advantages. Contributions of Different Bilingual Experiences to Cognitive Control Differences Among Young-adult Bilinguals.
221 pages. 2016. ISBN 978-3-0343-2081-8

Vol. 214 Larissa D'Angelo
Academic posters. A textual and visual metadiscourse analysis.
367 pages. 2016. ISBN 978-3-0343-2083-2

Vol. 215 Evelyne Berger
Prendre la parole en L2. Regard sur la compétence d'interaction en classe de langue.
246 pages. 2016. ISBN 978-3-0343-2084-9

Vol. 216 David Lasagabaster and Aintzane Doiz (eds)
CLIL experiences in secondary and tertiary education: In search of good practices.
262 pages. 2016. ISBN 978-3-0343-2104-4

Vol. 217 Elena Kkese
Identifying Plosives in L2 English: The Case of L1 Cypriot Greek Speakers.
317 pages. 2016. ISBN 978-3-0343-2060-3

Vol. 218 Sandra Campagna, Elana Ochse, Virginia Pulcini & Martin Solly (eds)
Languaging in and across Communities: New Voices, New Identities. Studies in Honour of Giuseppina Cortese.
507 pages. 2016. ISBN 978-3-0343-2073-3

Vol. 219 Adriana Orlandi & Laura Giacomini (ed.)
Defining collocation for lexicographic purposes. From linguistic theory to lexicographic practice.
328 pages. 2016. ISBN 978-3-0343-2054-2

Vol. 220 Pietro Luigi Iaia
Analysing English as a Lingua Franca in Video Games. Linguistic Features, Experiential and Functional Dimensions of Online and Scripted Interactions.
139 pages. 2016. ISBN 978-3-0343-2138-9

Vol. 221 Forthcoming.

Vol. 222 Katherine Ackerley, Marta Guarda & Francesca Helm (eds)
Sharing Perspectives on English-Medium Instruction.
308 pages. 2017. ISBN 978-3-0343-2537-0

Vol. 223 Juana I. Marín-Arrese, Julia Lavid-López, Marta Carretero, Elena Domínguez Romero, Mª Victoria Martín de la Rosa & María Pérez Blanco (eds)
Evidentiality and Modality in European Languages. Discourse-pragmatic perspectives.
427 pages. 2017. ISBN 978-3-0343-2437-3

Vol. 224 Forthcoming.

Vol. 225 Forthcoming.

Vol. 226 Xu Zhang
English Quasi-Numeral Classifiers. A Corpus-Based Cognitive-Typological Study.
360 pages. 2017. ISBN 978-3-0343-2818-0

Vol. 227 María Ángeles Orts, Ruth Breeze & Maurizio Gotti (eds)
Power, Persuasion and Manipulation in Specialised Genres. Providing Keys to the Rhetoric of Professional Communities.
368 pages. 2017. ISBN 978-3-0343-3010-7

Vol. 228 Maurizio Gotti, Stefania Maci & Michele Sala (eds)
Ways of Seeing, Ways of Being: Representing the Voices of Tourism.
453 pages. 2017. ISBN 978-3-0343-3031-2

Vol. 229 Forthcoming.

Vol. 230 Forthcoming.

Vol. 231 Xiaodong Zhang
Understanding Chinese EFL Teachers' Beliefs and Practices in the Textbook-Based Classroom.
189 pages. 2017. ISBN 978-3-0343-3053-4

www.ingramcontent.com/pod-product-compliance
Ingram Content Group UK Ltd.
Pitfield, Milton Keynes, MK11 3LW, UK
UKHW020720041026
15590UKWH00002B/785